# 60 Hikes Within 60 Miles: San Antonio and Austin

| | | | |
|---|---|---|---|
| Featured trail | Alternate trail | Stairs | Boardwalk |
| Freeway | Highway with bridge | | Minor road |
| Unpaved road | Power line | | Railroad |
| Park/forest | Water body | | River/creek/ intermittent stream |

- 🔺 Amphitheater
- 🧍 Baseball field
- ⛱ Beach access
- ⌐ Bench
- 🚣 Boat launch
- ⛺ Campground
- 🛶 Canoe access
- / Dam
- 🚰 Drinking water
- $ Fee station
- 🎣 Fishing access
- ✕ Footbridge
- ✳ Garden
- •—• Gate
- ● General point of interest

- 🏌 Golf course
- ⛺ Group campground
- ⓘ Information kiosk
- 🔭 Lookout/fire tower
- 〰 Marsh
- ⚒ Mine/quarry
- ✝ Mission
- ⚐ Monument
- 🏠 Park office
- P Parking
- ▲ Peak/hill
- 🎋 Picnic area
- 🏕 Picnic shelter
- 🚻 Pit toilet
- 🛝 Playground

- ⚠ Primitive campsite
- 〰 Rapids
- 🚻 Restrooms
- 🚐 RV campground
- 🔭 Scenic view
- ⊂ Shelter
- 🚿 Shower access
- ⚽ Soccer field
- ○ Spring
- 🏊 Swimming access
- 🎾 Tennis court
- 🚶 Trailhead
- 🏗 Viewing platform
- ⚽ Volleyball court
- 〰 Waterfall/cascades

# Overview Map Key

## Other cities in the 60 Hikes Within 60 Miles series:

Albuquerque

Atlanta

Baltimore

Boston

Chicago

Cincinnati

Cleveland

Dallas and Fort Worth

Denver and Boulder

Harrisburg

Houston

Los Angeles

Madison

Minneapolis and St. Paul

Nashville

New York City

Philadelphia

Phoenix

Pittsburgh

Richmond

Sacramento

Salt Lake City

San Diego

San Francisco

Seattle

St. Louis

Washington, D.C.

# 60 HIKES WITHIN 60 MILES

## SAN ANTONIO AND AUSTIN

INCLUDING
The Hill Country

Fourth Edition

# Charlie Llewellin and Johnny Molloy

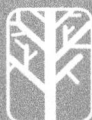

**MENASHA RIDGE PRESS**
Birmingham, Alabama

## 60 Hikes Within 60 Miles: San Antonio and Austin

Published by Menasha Ridge Press

Fourth edition, first printing

Cover design by Scott McGrew
Text design by Annie Long
Cover photo © INTERFOTO/Alamy
All other photos by Charlie Llewellin except where noted.
Maps by Scott McGrew and Thomas Hertzel

Library of Congress Cataloging-in-Publication Data
    Names: Llewellin, Charlie, 1959- author. | Molloy, Johnny, 1961- author.
    Title: 60 hikes within 60 miles : San Antonio and Austin including the hill
    country / by Charlie Llewellin and Johnny Molloy.
    Other titles: Sixty hikes within sixty miles
    Description: 4th Edition. | Birmingham, AL : Menasha Ridge Press, [2016] |
    Previous edition: 2010.
    Identifiers: LCCN 2016027902| ISBN 9781634040402 (paperback) |
    ISBN 9781634040419 (ebook); ISBN 9781634041737 (hardcover)
    Subjects: LCSH: Hiking—Texas—San Antonio Region—Guidebooks. |
    Hiking—Texas—Austin Region—Guidebooks. | Trails—Texas—San Antonio Region—Guidebooks. |
    Trails—Texas—Austin Region—Guidebooks. | San Antonio Region (Tex.) —Guidebooks. |
    Austin Region (Tex.) —Guidebooks.
    Classification: LCC GV199.42.T492 S366 2016 | DDC 796.5109764/3—dc23
                LC record available at https://lccn.loc.gov/2016027902

**MENASHA RIDGE PRESS**
An imprint of AdventureKEEN
2204 First Ave. S, Ste. 102
Birmingham, AL 35233
menasharidge.com

Visit menasharidge.com for a complete listing of our books and for ordering information. Contact us at our website, at facebook.com/menasharidge, or at twitter.com/menasharidge with questions or comments. To find out more about who we are and what we're doing, visit our blog, blog.menasharidge.com.

## DISCLAIMER

This book is meant only as a guide to select trails in the San Antonio and Austin area and does not guarantee hiker safety in any way—you hike at your own risk. Neither Menasha Ridge Press, Charlie Llewellin nor Johnny Molloy is liable for property loss or damage, personal injury, or death that result in any way from accessing or hiking the trails described in the following pages. Please be aware that hikers have been injured in the San Antonio and Austin area. Be especially cautious when walking on or near boulders, steep inclines, and drop-offs, and do not attempt to explore terrain that may be beyond your abilities. To help ensure an uneventful hike, please read carefully the introduction to this book, and perhaps get further safety information and guidance from other sources. Familiarize yourself thoroughly with the areas you intend to visit before venturing out. Ask questions, and prepare for the unforeseen. Familiarize yourself with current weather reports, maps of the area you intend to visit, and any relevant park regulations.

# Table of Contents

# Acknowledgments

THIS BOOK WOULD NOT BE POSSIBLE without the ceaseless efforts of volunteers and employees from Texas Parks & Wildlife, San Antonio Parks & Recreation, Austin Parks & Recreation, the San Marcos Parks and Recreation Department, the Lower Colorado River Authority, The Trail Foundation, and other city and county departments of parks and recreation who make the Texas Hill Country one of the finest hiking destinations in the USA.

I would also like to thank the entire staff at Menasha Ridge Press, who presented me with the opportunity to share my enthusiasm and guided the work to completion.

—*Charlie Llewellin*

# Foreword

WELCOME TO MENASHA RIDGE PRESS'S 60 Hikes Within 60 Miles, a series designed to provide hikers with the information they need to find and hike the very best trails surrounding metropolitan areas.

Our strategy was simple: First, find a hiker who knows the area and loves to hike. Second, ask that person to spend a year researching the most popular and very best trails around. And third, have that person describe each trail in terms of difficulty, scenery, condition, elevation change, and all other categories of information that are important to hikers. "Pretend you've just completed a hike and met up with other hikers at the trailhead," we told each author. "Imagine their questions; be clear in your answers."

Authors Charlie Llewellin and Johnny Molloy selected 60 of the best hikes in and around the San Antonio and Austin metropolitan areas. They provide hikers (and walkers) with a great variety of hikes—and all within roughly 60 miles of San Antonio or Austin.

You'll get more out of this book if you take a moment to read the Introduction, which explains how to read the trail listings. The "Topo Maps" section will help you understand how useful topos are on a hike and will also tell you where to get them. And though this is a where-to, not a how-to, guide, readers who have not hiked extensively will find the Introduction of particular value.

As much for the opportunity to free the spirit as to free the body, let these hikes elevate you above the urban hurry.

*All the best,*
*The Editors at Menasha Ridge Press*

# Preface

EVEN THOUGH I'M NOT ONE who walks for the sake of walking, I'll tramp for miles to see something that's out of the ordinary or extremely beautiful. I hike to get away from it all. I think the walks in this book reflect this. My hope is that you'll enjoy them and find them just as interesting as I did.

There are many scenic sights on these trails, from crystalline springs to historic homesteads to waves of Texas Hill Country expanding to the horizon. Sometimes, just the opportunity to see something interesting is enough. The San Antonio Botanical Garden is not even really a hike, but it's crammed so full of interesting exhibits and plants that it is probably the first hike from this book that you should complete. The information found there will greatly enhance your Texas hiking if you are the slightest bit interested in the native flora.

Following the Twin Peaks hike to its apex will give you the best chance in this part of the country of seeing a mountain lion. They are out there, but you'll have to sit still to catch one in the distance. This won't be a problem, though, because by the time you reach the peak, you'll be ready to rest. Just keep your eyes open.

All of the trails, even ones in the middle of San Antonio or Austin, contain a wide variety of wildlife. McAllister Park, one of the busiest, has one of the largest deer populations of any of the hikes in this book. It's also where I saw the most snakes. If you look hard enough, and are quiet enough, you could see deer at every park and preserve in this book.

You'll also find abundant and diverse species of birds, of which Texas hosts more than 600. Being located in the South Central part of the state, near the woods and the coast, allows you to see a lot of them right here. Rare painted buntings are at McKinney Falls on the Homestead Trail; a large variety of sparrows and finches are everywhere; and cardinals, jays, titmice, and more can be seen on these trails. I've spotted a pileated woodpecker in Buescher State Park—very rare for these parts. To enrich your bird-watching, pick up a bird guide before you go hiking. I never leave home without my binoculars and bird guide.

Keep your eyes on the ground and you could see everything from coral snakes to the rare Houston toad. Big tarantulas (especially in Buescher) live deeper in the woods too. One of the most fascinating trails for local wildlife is in Lockhart State Park. Huge garden spiders build webs more than 10 feet wide across the trails. You can't miss them, so don't walk into them. Although toads and spiders are creepy to some, these kinds of encounters are worth the drive for me.

Over time, some trails change. Some parks close and others open. For example, Commons Ford Ranch was sold and is now in private hands. Yet other places have begun to welcome visitors. Government Canyon State Natural Area, just west of San Antonio, offers 8,000 acres to explore via 20-plus miles of hiking trails. Medina River Natural Area has opened. Hikers can travel the river bottoms and see giant ancient cypress and cottonwoods. Other places, such as Palmetto State Park, have revamped their trail systems, bringing about new experiences at old destinations. Guadalupe River State Park expanded its trail network. With this book in hand, you can enjoy the new hikes that include the above areas.

Many hikers in the region make regular use of our extensive range of trails and tend to take good care of them too. Some of the most beautiful trails, and some that would seem more out of the way, see a lot of traffic on weekends. For a better chance at solitude, any of your trips would benefit from going during the week rather than the weekend.

However, at some parks, crowding doesn't seem to be related to the time of day or year. McAllister Park is always busy—all day, every day, all year long. The Hill Country State Natural Area sees an awful lot of traffic for its remote location as well. If you're looking for a rugged hike, it's your place, but if you're looking for solitude, it might not be for you. This leads me to my favorite hike of all those in the book, Friedrich Wilderness Park. This trail is located close to San Antonio and is unique among most trails in our area. It offers a lot of elevation change and seems to have more in common with the mountain states than with Texas. It is very secluded and sees little use. After you've hiked—and climbed—to the stone fence halfway through and realize that you haven't seen anyone else, it'll sink in. Just sit on the fence and listen to the silence. It's a great trail, my personal favorite.

All of the parks and trails, however, are worth visiting and, more so, worth preserving. If you get a chance to contribute to a donation box for maintenance, please do so, especially if you enjoyed the trail. Every trail in this book is worth a few dollars to visit.

*—Charlie Llewellin*

# 60 Hikes by Category

## Hike Categories

- Mileage
- Difficulty*
- Kid-Friendly
- Urban
- Lake
- Scenic

\* Difficulty: **E** = easy, **M** = moderate, **D** = difficult, **S** = strenuous

| REGION<br>Hike Name | page# | Mileage | Difficulty | Kid-friendly | Urban | Lake | Scenic |
|---|---|---|---|---|---|---|---|
| **AUSTIN** | | | | | | | |
| Barton Creek Greenbelt (East) | 12 | 11.2 | M | | ✓ | | ✓ |
| Homestead Trail at McKinney Falls State Park | 17 | 4.8 | M | | ✓ | | ✓ |
| Inga VanNynatten Memorial Trail at Lower Bull Creek Greenbelt | 23 | 3.4 | E | ✓ | ✓ | | ✓ |
| Lady Bird Lake: Boardwalk Loop | 27 | 3.9 | E | ✓ | ✓ | ✓ | ✓ |
| Lady Bird Lake: West Loop | 31 | 6.9 | E | ✓ | ✓ | ✓ | ✓ |
| Mayfield Park and Preserve | 35 | 1 | E | ✓ | ✓ | ✓ | |
| McKinney Roughs Nature Park: Bluffs and Bottoms | 40 | 4.5 | M–D | | | | ✓ |
| Onion Creek Trail at McKinney Falls State Park | 44 | 2.7 | E | ✓ | ✓ | | |
| Pace Bend Park | 47 | 6.1 | M | | | ✓ | |
| Pine Ridge Loop at McKinney Roughs Nature Park | 51 | 3.7 | M | | | | ✓ |
| River Place Nature Trail | 55 | 5.4 | D | | | | ✓ |
| Shoal Creek Greenbelt | 59 | 6.4 | M | | ✓ | | |
| Spicewood Valley Trail | 63 | 2.6 | E | | ✓ | | |
| Three Falls Hike at Barton Creek Greenbelt | 67 | 6.8 | M | | ✓ | | ✓ |
| Turkey Creek Trail at Emma Long Metropolitan Park | 71 | 2.7 | M | | ✓ | | ✓ |
| Wild Basin Wilderness Preserve | 75 | 1.8 | M | | ✓ | | |
| **NORTH OF AUSTIN** | | | | | | | |
| Bluffs of the North Fork San Gabriel River | 82 | 3.6 | E | | | ✓ | ✓ |
| Brushy Creek Regional Trail | 86 | 13* | E | | ✓ | ✓ | |
| Comanche Bluff Trail | 91 | 7.8* | M | | | ✓ | ✓ |
| Crockett Gardens and Falls at Cedar Breaks Park | 95 | 5 | M | | | ✓ | ✓ |

\* with options for shorter hikes

| REGION<br>Hike Name | page# | Mileage | Difficulty | Kid-friendly | Urban | Lake | Scenic |
|---|---|---|---|---|---|---|---|
| **NORTH OF AUSTIN** (continued) | | | | | | | |
| Dana Peak Park at Stillhouse Hollow Lake | 99 | 4 | M–D | | | ✓ | |
| Overlook Trail at Lake Georgetown | 103 | 7.2 | M | | | ✓ | |
| Randy Morrow Trail | 107 | 11.2 | M | | ✓ | ✓ | |
| Rimrock, Shin Oak, and Creek Trails at Doeskin Ranch | 111 | 2.3 | M | | | | ✓ |
| **SOUTHEAST OF AUSTIN** | | | | | | | |
| Bastrop State Park Loop | 118 | 3.2 | M | | | | ✓ |
| Bastrop State Park: Purple Trail | 121 | 4.3 | M | | | | |
| Lockhart State Park Loop | 125 | 4.9 | E–M | | | | ✓ |
| Monument Hill History and Nature Walk | 129 | 1 | E–M | ✓ | ✓ | | ✓ |
| Palmetto State Park Loop | 133 | 2.8 | E | ✓ | | | ✓ |
| **WEST OF AUSTIN** | | | | | | | |
| 5.5-Mile Loop at Pedernales Falls State Park | 140 | 5.8 | E–M | | | | |
| Hamilton Pool Preserve Trail | 144 | 2 | E | ✓ | ✓ | | ✓ |
| Inks Lake State Park | 149 | 4.6 | M–D | | | ✓ | ✓ |
| Loop and Summit Trails at Enchanted Rock State Natural Area | 154 | 4 | D | | | | ✓ |
| Turkey Pass Loop at Enchanted Rock State Natural Area | 159 | 2.6 | M–D | | | | ✓ |
| Wolf Mountain Trail at Pedernales Falls State Park | 163 | 7.4 | M | | | | ✓ |
| **SAN ANTONIO** | | | | | | | |
| Bluff Spurs Overlooks | 170 | 4.1 | M–D | | | | ✓ |
| Chula Vista Loop | 174 | 6.6 | D | | | | ✓ |
| Comanche Lookout Loop | 179 | 1.7 | M | ✓ | ✓ | | ✓ |
| Crownridge Canyon Natural Area Loop | 182 | 1.9 | E | ✓ | ✓ | | ✓ |
| Friedrich Wilderness Park Loop | 186 | 5.2 | D | ✓ | ✓ | | ✓ |
| Government Canyon Loop | 191 | 6.2 | M | | | | ✓ |
| Hillview Natural Trail | 196 | 2.8 | M | | ✓ | | |
| Leon Creek Greenway | 200 | 4.2 | E | ✓ | ✓ | | |
| McAllister Park Loop | 203 | 4.2 | E | | ✓ | | |
| Medina River Natural Area Loop | 207 | 2.3 or 4.5 | E | | | | ✓ |

| REGION<br>Hike Name | page# | Mileage | Difficulty | Kid-friendly | Urban | Lake | Scenic |
|---|---|---|---|---|---|---|---|
| **SAN ANTONIO** *(continued)* | | | | | | | |
| San Antonio Botanical Garden Trail | 211 | 1.4 | E | ✓ | ✓ | | |
| San Antonio Mission Trail | 216 | 6 | E | ✓ | ✓ | | ✓ |
| **NORTH OF SAN ANTONIO** | | | | | | | |
| Bamberger Trail | 222 | 4.8 | E | | | | |
| Cibolo Nature Center Hike | 226 | 2 | E | ✓ | ✓ | | |
| Dry Comal Nature Trail | 231 | 1.6 | E | ✓ | ✓ | | |
| Guadalupe River State Park Loop | 235 | 2.7 | E | ✓ | | | |
| Guadalupe River Trail | 239 | 2 | M | | | | |
| Hightower Trail | 243 | 4.5 | M | | | | ✓ |
| Hill Country Cougar Canyon Trek | 247 | 10.5 | D | | | | ✓ |
| Kerrville-Schreiner Park Loop | 252 | 5.8 | M | | | | |
| Panther Canyon Nature Trail | 256 | 1.6 | M | | ✓ | | ✓ |
| Purgatory Creek Natural Area: Dante's and Beatrice Trails | 260 | 6.9 | M | | ✓ | | |
| Spring Lake Natural Area | 265 | 4.3 | M | | ✓ | | |
| Twin Peaks Trek | 269 | 2.3 | M | | | | ✓ |
| Wilderness Trail at Hill Country State Natural Area | 273 | 5.1 | M–D | | | | ✓ |

## Hike Categories *(continued)*

- Historical
- Wildlife
- Wildflowers
- Bicyclists
- Runners
- Less Busy
- Heavily Traveled

| REGION<br>Hike Name | page# | Historical | Wildlife | Wildflowers | Bicyclists | Runners | Less Busy | Heavily Traveled |
|---|---|---|---|---|---|---|---|---|
| **AUSTIN** | | | | | | | | |
| Barton Creek Greenbelt (East) | 12 | | | | ✓ | ✓ | | ✓ |
| Homestead Trail at McKinney Falls State Park | 17 | ✓ | ✓ | ✓ | ✓ | | | ✓ |
| Inga VanNynatten Memorial Trail at Lower Bull Creek Greenbelt | 23 | | | | | | | ✓ |
| Lady Bird Lake: Boardwalk Loop | 27 | | | | ✓ | ✓ | | ✓ |
| Lady Bird Lake: West Loop | 31 | ✓ | | | ✓ | ✓ | | ✓ |
| Mayfield Park and Preserve | 35 | ✓ | | | | | ✓ | |
| McKinney Roughs Nature Park: Bluffs and Bottoms | 40 | ✓ | ✓ | | | | | |
| Onion Creek Trail at McKinney Falls State Park | 44 | ✓ | ✓ | | ✓ | | | ✓ |
| Pace Bend Park | 47 | | ✓ | ✓ | ✓ | | ✓ | |
| Pine Ridge Loop at McKinney Roughs Nature Park | 51 | ✓ | | | | | | |
| River Place Nature Trail | 55 | | | | | | | ✓ |
| Shoal Creek Greenbelt | 59 | ✓ | | | ✓ | ✓ | | ✓ |
| Spicewood Valley Trail | 63 | ✓ | | | | | | |
| Three Falls Hike at Barton Creek Greenbelt | 67 | | | | | | | ✓ |
| Turkey Creek Trail at Emma Long Metropolitan Park | 71 | | | | | | | ✓ |
| Wild Basin Wilderness Preserve | 75 | | | | | | | |
| **NORTH OF AUSTIN** | | | | | | | | |
| Bluffs of the North Fork San Gabriel River | 82 | | ✓ | ✓ | | | ✓ | |
| Brushy Creek Regional Trail | 86 | | | | ✓ | ✓ | | ✓ |
| Comanche Bluff Trail | 91 | | ✓ | ✓ | | | ✓ | |
| Crockett Garden and Falls at Cedar Breaks Park | 95 | ✓ | | | | | | |
| Dana Peak Park at Stillhouse Hollow Lake | 99 | | | | | | ✓ | |
| Overlook Trail at Lake Georgetown | 103 | ✓ | | ✓ | | | | |

| REGION<br>Hike Name | page# | Historical | Wildlife | Wildflowers | Bicyclists | Runners | Less Busy | Heavily Traveled |
|---|---|---|---|---|---|---|---|---|
| **NORTH OF AUSTIN** *(continued)* | | | | | | | | |
| Randy Morrow Trail | 107 | ✓ | | | ✓ | ✓ | | |
| Rimrock, Shin Oak, and Creek Trails at Doeskin Ranch | 111 | | ✓ | | | | ✓ | |
| **SOUTHEAST OF AUSTIN** | | | | | | | | |
| Bastrop State Park Loop | 118 | ✓ | | | | | | |
| Bastrop State Park: Purple Trail | 121 | | | | | | | |
| Lockhart State Park Loop | 125 | | ✓ | ✓ | | | ✓ | |
| Monument Hill History and Nature Walk | 129 | ✓ | | | | | | |
| Palmetto State Park Loop | 133 | | | | | | ✓ | |
| **WEST OF AUSTIN** | | | | | | | | |
| 5.5-Mile Loop at Pedernales Falls State Park | 140 | | ✓ | | ✓ | | | |
| Hamilton Pool Preserve Trail | 144 | | ✓ | | | | | ✓ |
| Inks Lake State Park | 149 | | ✓ | ✓ | | | ✓ | |
| Loop and Summit Trails at Enchanted Rock State Natural Area | 154 | | ✓ | | | | | ✓ |
| Turkey Pass Loop at Enchanted Rock State Natural Area | 159 | | | | | | ✓ | |
| Wolf Mountain Trail at Pedernales Falls State Park | 163 | | ✓ | | ✓ | | | ✓ |
| **SAN ANTONIO** | | | | | | | | |
| Bluff Spurs Overlooks | 170 | | | | | | | |
| Chula Vista Loop | 174 | | ✓ | ✓ | | | ✓ | |
| Comanche Lookout Loop | 179 | ✓ | | | | | | |
| Crownridge Canyon Natural Area Loop | 182 | | | | | | | |
| Friedrich Wilderness Park Loop | 186 | | | | | | | ✓ |
| Government Canyon Loop | 191 | ✓ | | | | | | ✓ |
| Hillview Natural Trail | 196 | | | | ✓ | ✓ | | |
| Leon Creek Greenway | 200 | | | | ✓ | ✓ | | ✓ |
| McAllister Park Loop | 203 | | ✓ | | ✓ | ✓ | | |
| Medina River Natural Area Loop | 207 | ✓ | | | ✓ | | ✓ | |
| San Antonio Botanical Garden Trail | 211 | ✓ | | ✓ | | | | ✓ |
| San Antonio Mission Trail | | | | | | | | |

| REGION<br>Hike Name | page# | Historical | Wildlife | Wildflowers | Bicyclists | Runners | Less Busy | Heavily Traveled |
|---|---|---|---|---|---|---|---|---|
| **NORTH OF SAN ANTONIO** | | | | | | | | |
| Bamberger Trail | 222 | | ✓ | ✓ | | | ✓ | |
| Cibolo Nature Center Hike | 226 | | ✓ | | | | | |
| Dry Comal Nature Trail | 231 | | | | | | | |
| Guadalupe River State Park Loop | 235 | | ✓ | | | | | |
| Guadalupe River Trail | 239 | | ✓ | | | | ✓ | |
| Hightower Trail | 243 | ✓ | ✓ | ✓ | | | ✓ | |
| Hill Country Cougar Canyon Trek | 247 | | | | | | ✓ | |
| Kerrville-Schreiner Park Loop | 252 | | | | | | ✓ | |
| Panther Canyon Nature Trail | 256 | | | | | | | |
| Purgatory Creek Natural Area: Dante's and Beatrice Trails | 260 | | | | ✓ | ✓ | | ✓ |
| Spring Lake Natural Area | 265 | | | | | | | |
| Twin Peaks Trek | 269 | | | | | | | |
| Wilderness Trail at Hill Country State Natural Area | 273 | | ✓ | ✓ | | | ✓ | |

# Introduction

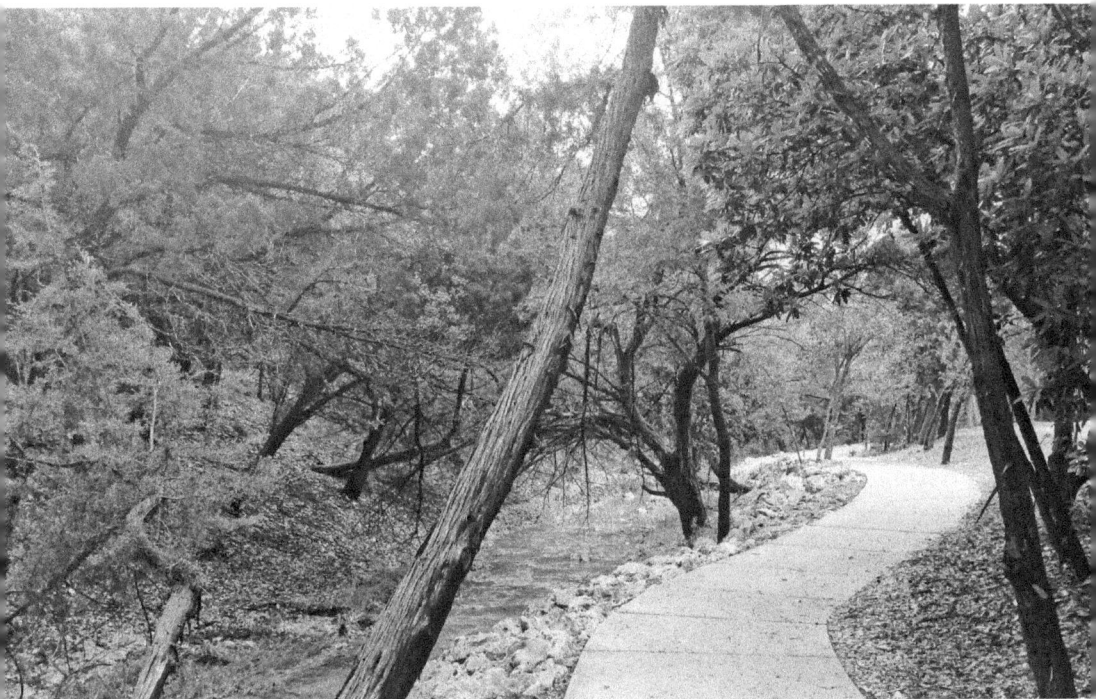

*Brushy Creek Regional Trail in Cedar Park (see page 86)*

WELCOME TO THE FOURTH EDITION OF *60 Hikes Within 60 Miles: San Antonio and Austin*. Whether you are new to hiking or a seasoned trailsmith, take a few minutes to read the following introduction. We explain how this book is organized and how to use it.

## Hike Descriptions

Each hike contains six key items: a brief description of the trail, a key at-a-glance information box, directions to the trail, a trail map, an elevation profile (if the change in elevation is 100 feet or more), and a more detailed trail description, and many hikes also include information about nearby activities. Combined, the maps and information provide a clear method to assess each trail from the comfort of your favorite reading chair.

### IN BRIEF

A taste of the trail. Think of this section as a snapshot focused on the historical landmarks, beautiful vistas, and other sights that you may encounter on the trail.

## KEY AT-A-GLANCE INFORMATION

The At-a-Glance boxes give you a quick idea of the specifics of each hike. Fourteen basic elements are covered:

**LENGTH**    The length of the trail from start to finish. There may be options to shorten or extend the hikes, but the mileage corresponds to the described hike. Consult the hike description to help decide how to customize the hike for your ability or time constraints.

**CONFIGURATION**    A description of what the trail might look like from overhead. Trails can be loops, out-and-backs (trails on which one enters and leaves along the same path), figure eights, or balloons (trails on which one enters and leaves on the same path with a loop in between). The descriptions might surprise you.

**DIFFICULTY**    The degree of effort an "average" hiker should expect on a given hike. For simplicity, difficulty is described as "easy," "moderate," or "difficult."

**SCENERY**    A rating of the overall environs of the hike and what to expect in terms of plant life, wildlife, streams, and historic buildings.

**EXPOSURE**    A quick check of how much sun you can expect during the hike. Descriptors used include terms such as "shady," "exposed," and "sunny."

**TRAFFIC**    Indicates how busy the trail might be on an average day, and if you might be able to find solitude. Trail traffic, of course, varies from day to day and season to season.

**TRAIL SURFACE**    A description of the trail surface, be it paved, rocky, dirt, or a mixture of elements.

**HIKING TIME**    The length of time it takes to hike the trail. A slow but steady hiker will average 2–3 miles an hour, depending on the terrain. Most of the estimates in this book reflect a speed of about 2 miles per hour. Take the miles of the hike and divide by 2, and this will give a rough estimate of hiking time. For example, an 8-mile hike should take the average hiker 4 hours.

**DRIVING DISTANCE**    This is how far to drive from a given point—in this case, from the state capitol in Austin or the Alamo in San Antonio.

**ACCESS**    A notation of fees or permits needed to access the trail (if any) and whether the trail has specific hours.

**WHEELCHAIR ACCESSIBILITY**    Notes whether the trail is wheelchair compatible.

**MAPS**    Which map is the best for this hike and where to get it.

**FACILITIES**    What to expect in terms of restrooms, water, and other amenities at the trailhead or nearby.

**CONTACT INFORMATION**    Phone number and website, if you need more information.

## DIRECTIONS TO THE TRAIL

The detailed directions will lead you to each trailhead. If you use GPS technology, latitude and longitude coordinates are provided to allow you to navigate directly to the trailhead.

## TRAIL DESCRIPTIONS

The heart of each hike. Here, the author provides a summary of the trail's essence and highlights any special traits that the hike offers. Ultimately, the hike description will help you choose which hikes are best for you.

## NEARBY ACTIVITIES

Look here for information on nearby dining opportunities or other activities to fill out your day.

# Maps

The maps in this book have been produced with great care and, used with the hiking directions, will help you stay on course. But as any experienced hiker knows, things can get tricky off the beaten path.

The maps in this book, when used with the route directions presented in each chapter, are sufficient to direct you to the trail and guide you on it. However, you will find superior detail and valuable information in the United States Geological Survey's 7.5-minute series topographic maps. Topo maps are available online in many locations, including from the U.S. Geological Survey at store.usgs.gov. The downside to topos is that most are outdated, having been created 20–30 years ago. But they still provide excellent topographic detail.

If you're new to hiking, you might be wondering, "What's a topographic map?" In short, a topo indicates not only linear distance but elevation as well, using contour lines. Wavy contour lines spread across topo maps, each line representing a particular elevation. At the base of each topo, a contour's interval designation is given. If the contour interval is 200 feet, then the distance between each contour line is 200 feet. Follow five contour lines up on a map and the elevation has increased by 1,000 feet.

Let's assume that the 7.5-minute series topo reads "contour interval 40 feet," that the short trail we'll be hiking is 2 inches long on the map, and that it crosses five contour lines from beginning to end. What do we know? Well, because the linear scale of this series is 2,000 feet to the inch, we know our trail is 4,000 feet, or approximately 0.8 mile, long (1 mile is 5,280 feet). But we also know that we'll be climbing or descending 200 vertical feet (one contour line is 40 feet) over that distance. And the elevation designations written on occasional contour lines will tell us if we're heading up or down.

In addition to outdoors shops and bike shops, you'll find topos at major universities and some public libraries, where you might try photocopying the ones you need to avoid the cost of buying them. I also recommend topozone.com and others mentioned in the appendix as resources for topographic maps and software.

## THE OVERVIEW MAP AND KEY

Use the overview map on the inside front cover to find the exact location of each hike's primary trailhead. Each hike's number appears on the overview map, on the hike list facing the overview map, and in the table of contents. As you flip through the book, you'll see that a hike's full profile is easy to locate by watching for the hike number at the top of each page. The book is organized by region, as indicated in the table of contents. A map legend that details the symbols found on trail maps appears on the inside back cover.

## REGIONAL MAPS

The book is divided into regions, and prefacing each regional section is an overview map of that region. The regional map provides more detail than the overview map does, bringing you closer to the hike.

## TRAIL MAPS

Each hike contains a detailed map that shows the trailhead, route, significant features, facilities, and topographic landmarks such as creeks, overlooks, and peaks. The author gathered map data by carrying Garmin eTrex or Garmin 60CS GPS units while hiking. This data was downloaded into the digital mapping program Topo USA and processed by expert cartographers to produce the highly accurate maps found in this book. Each trailhead's GPS coordinates are included with each profile (see below).

## ELEVATION PROFILES

For trails with significant changes in elevation, the hike description will contain a detailed elevation profile that corresponds directly to the trail map. The elevation profile provides a quick look at the trail from the side, enabling you to visualize how it rises and falls. Note the number of feet between each tick mark on the vertical axis (the height scale). To avoid making flat hikes look steep and steep hikes appear flat, height scales are used throughout the book to provide an accurate assessment of each hike's climbing difficulty.

## GPS TRAILHEAD COORDINATES

In addition to highly specific trail outlines, this book also includes the latitude/longitude coordinates for each trailhead. The latitude and longitude grid system is likely quite familiar to you, but here is a refresher.

Imaginary lines of latitude—called parallels and approximately 69 miles apart— run horizontally around the globe. Each parallel is indicated by degrees from the equator (established to be 0°): up to 90°N at the North Pole and down to 90°S at the South Pole.

Imaginary lines of longitude—called meridians—run perpendicular to latitude lines. Longitude lines are likewise indicated by degrees: Starting from 0° at the Prime Meridian, in Greenwich, England, they continue to the east and west until they meet 180° later at the International Date Line in the Pacific Ocean. At the equator, longitude lines also are approximately 69 miles apart, but that distance narrows as the meridians converge toward the North and South Poles.

Each degree can be divided into 60 minutes and each minute into 60 seconds. This system provides a precise location based on the coordinates of the latitude and longitude lines.

For more on GPS technology, the USGS offers a good deal of information regarding UTM (Universal Transverse Mercator) coordinates at its website, usgs.gov.

## Weather

With the exception of July, August, and September, the weather for hiking in the Hill Country can be great. Even the summer months have cool mornings. The best times are October–November and March–May. Depending on the severity of winter, December can be just as pleasant as early fall. The main things to watch out for are the heat, which can be brutal in the summer, and the rain. With all the rivers in the area, flash floods can be a real problem for unwary hikers. The Guadalupe River, for example, has flooded to the point of washing homes away twice in less than 10 years, and it doesn't take long for the waters to reach dangerous levels. What might seem like a pleasant light rain could turn into a disaster. With the heat, hydration is key. Carry lots of water, and get off the trails before morning is gone.

| AVERAGE DAILY TEMPERATURES BY MONTH | | | | | | |
|---|---|---|---|---|---|---|
|  | JAN | FEB | MAR | APR | MAY | JUN |
| HIGH | 62°F | 65°F | 72°F | 80°F | 87°F | 92°F |
| LOW | 42°F | 45°F | 51°F | 59°F | 67°F | 72°F |
|  | JUL | AUG | SEP | OCT | NOV | DEC |
| HIGH | 96°F | 97°F | 91°F | 82°F | 71°F | 63°F |
| LOW | 74°F | 75°F | 69°F | 61°F | 51°F | 42°F |

Source: usclimatedata.com/climate/austin/texas/united-states/ustx2742

## Trail Etiquette

Whether you're on a city, county, state, or national park trail, always remember that great care and resources (from nature as well as from your tax dollars) have gone into creating these trails. Treat the trail, wildlife, and fellow hikers with respect.

➢ Hike on open trails only. Respect trail and road closures (ask if not sure), avoid trespassing on private land, and obtain permits and authorization as required. Leave gates as you found them or as marked.

➢ Leave only footprints. Be sensitive to the ground beneath you. This also means staying on the trail and not creating any new ones. Be sure to pack out what you pack in. No one likes to see the trash someone else has left behind.

➢ Never spook animals. An unannounced approach, a sudden movement, or a loud noise startles all animals. This can be dangerous for you, for others, and for the animals. Give animals extra room and time to adjust to you.

➢ Plan ahead. Know your equipment, your ability, and the area in which you are hiking—and prepare accordingly. Be self-sufficient at all times; carry necessary supplies for changes in weather or other conditions. A well-executed trip is a satisfaction to you and to others.

➢ Make sure the park or trail allows pets before bringing your dog.

➢ Be courteous to other hikers, bikers, or equestrians you meet on the trails.

## Water

"How much is enough? One bottle? Two? Three? But think of all that extra weight!" Well, one simple physiological fact should convince you to err on the side of excess: A hiker working hard in 90° heat needs approximately 10 quarts of fluid every day. That's 2.5 gallons—12 large water bottles or 16 small ones. In other words, pack along one or two bottles even for short hikes.

Serious backpackers hit the trail prepared to purify water found along the route. Purifiers with ceramic filters are the safest but are also the most expensive. Many hikers pack along the slightly distasteful tetraglycine hydroperiodide tablets (sold under the names Potable Aqua, Coughlan's, and others). If you're tempted to drink "found" water, do so only if you understand the risks involved. Probably the most common waterborne "bug" is giardia, which may not hit until one to four weeks after ingestion. It will have you passing noxious rotten-egg gas, vomiting, shivering with chills, and living in the bathroom. But there are other parasites to worry about, including *E. coli* and cryptosporidium (that are harder to kill than giardia).

For day hikes, however, you can avoid these risks altogether. Simply hydrate prior to your hike, carry (and drink) 6 ounces of water for every mile you plan to hike, and hydrate after the hike. For most people, the pleasures of hiking make carrying water a relatively minor price to pay to remain healthy.

## First Aid Kit

A typical kit may contain more items than you might think necessary. But these are just the basics. Pack the items in a waterproof bag, such as a plastic zip-top bag.

- ➤ Ace bandages or Spenco joint wraps
- ➤ Adhesive bandages
- ➤ Antibiotic ointment (Neosporin or the generic equivalent)
- ➤ Aspirin, ibuprofen, or acetaminophen
- ➤ Benadryl or the generic equivalent, diphenhydramine (in case of allergic reactions)
- ➤ Butterfly-closure bandages
- ➤ Epinephrine in a prefilled syringe (for people known to have severe allergic reactions to such things as bee stings)
- ➤ Gauze and compress pads (one roll and a half dozen 4-inch square pads)
- ➤ Hydrogen peroxide, Betadine, or iodine
- ➤ Matches or pocket lighter
- ➤ Moleskin
- ➤ Sunscreen
- ➤ Water purification tablets or water filter (see "Water," on page 6)
- ➤ Whistle (it's more effective in signaling rescuers than your voice)

## Hiking with Children

No one is ever too young for a nice hike in the woods or through a city park. Parents with infants can strap on little ones with the popular Snugli device. Be careful, though: it's probably best to opt for flat, short trails when hiking with an infant. Toddlers who have not quite mastered walking can still tag along, riding on an adult's back in a child carrier.

Children who are walking can, of course, follow along with an adult. Use common sense to judge a child's capacity to hike a particular trail. Always rely on the possibility that the child will tire quickly and have to be carried.

When packing for the hike, remember the needs of the child as well as your own. Make sure children are adequately clothed for the weather, have proper shoes, and are properly protected from the sun with sunscreen and clothing. Kids can dehydrate quickly, so make sure you have plenty of fluid for everyone.

Depending on age, ability, and the hike's length and difficulty, most children should enjoy the shorter hikes described in this book. To assist you in determining which trails are suitable, a list of hike recommendations for children is provided on page xi.

## The Business Hiker

Whether in the San Antonio–Austin area on business, as a resident, or as a visitor, you'll find many quick getaways perfect for a long lunch escape or an evening hike to unwind from a busy day at the office or convention. Instead of staying cooped up inside, head out to one of the many parks and conservation areas on the fringes of the metro area, and combine lunch with a relaxing walk.

## Ticks

Ticks like to hang out in the brush that grows along trails. July is a peak month for ticks, but you should be tick-aware during all months of the spring, summer, and fall. Ticks, actually arthropods and not insects, are ectoparasites, which need a host for the majority of their life cycle in order to reproduce. The ticks that light on you while hiking will be very small, sometimes so tiny that you won't be able to spot them. The two primary varieties, deer ticks and dog ticks, both need a few hours of actual attachment before they can transmit any disease they may harbor. I've found ticks in my socks and on my legs several hours after a hike that have not yet anchored. The best strategy is to visually check every half hour or so while hiking, do a thorough check before you get in the car, and then, when you take a post-hike shower, do an even more thorough check of your entire body. Ticks that haven't latched on are easily removed but not easily killed. If I pick off a tick in the woods, I just toss it aside. If I find one on my person at home, I make sure to dispatch it down the toilet. For ticks that have embedded, removal with tweezers is best.

## Poison Ivy, Oak, and Sumac

Recognizing and avoiding contact with poison ivy, oak, and sumac is the most effective way to prevent the painful, itchy rashes associated with these plants. Poison ivy occurs as a vine or shrub, with 3 leaflets to a leaf; poison oak occurs as either a vine or shrub, with 3 leaflets as well; and poison sumac flourishes in swampland, with each leaf containing 7–13 leaflets. Urushiol, the oil in the sap of these plants, is responsible for the rash.

Within 12–24 hours of exposure, raised lines and/or blisters will appear, accompanied by a terrible itch. Refrain from scratching because bacteria under fingernails may cause infection. Wash and dry the rash thoroughly, applying a calamine lotion to help dry it out. If itching or blistering is severe, seek medical attention. If you do come into contact with one of these plants, remember that clothes, pets, or hiking gear can transmit the oil to you or someone else, so wash not only any exposed parts of your body but also clothes, gear, and pets, if applicable.

*Hill Country Cougar Canyon Trek (see page 247)*

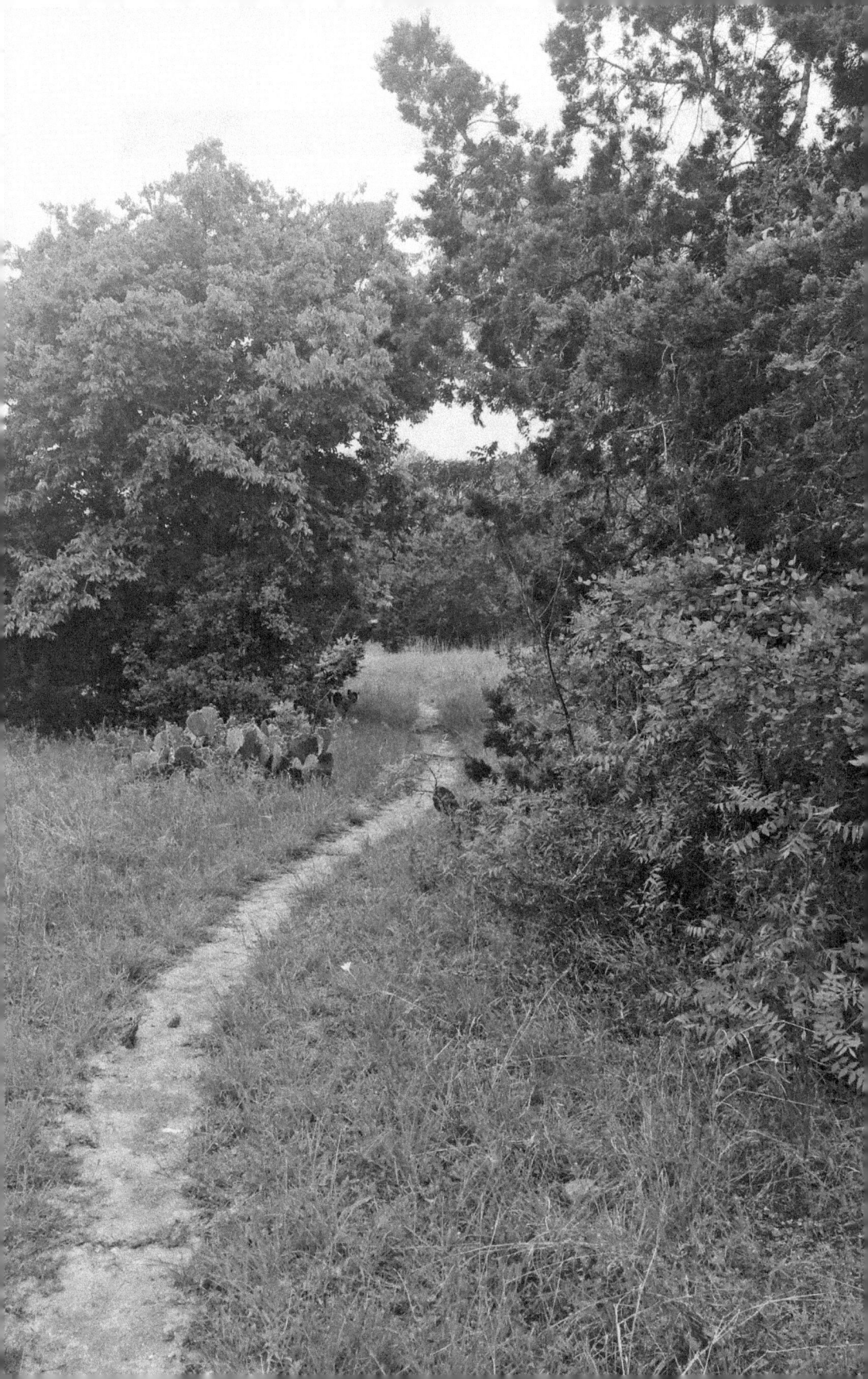

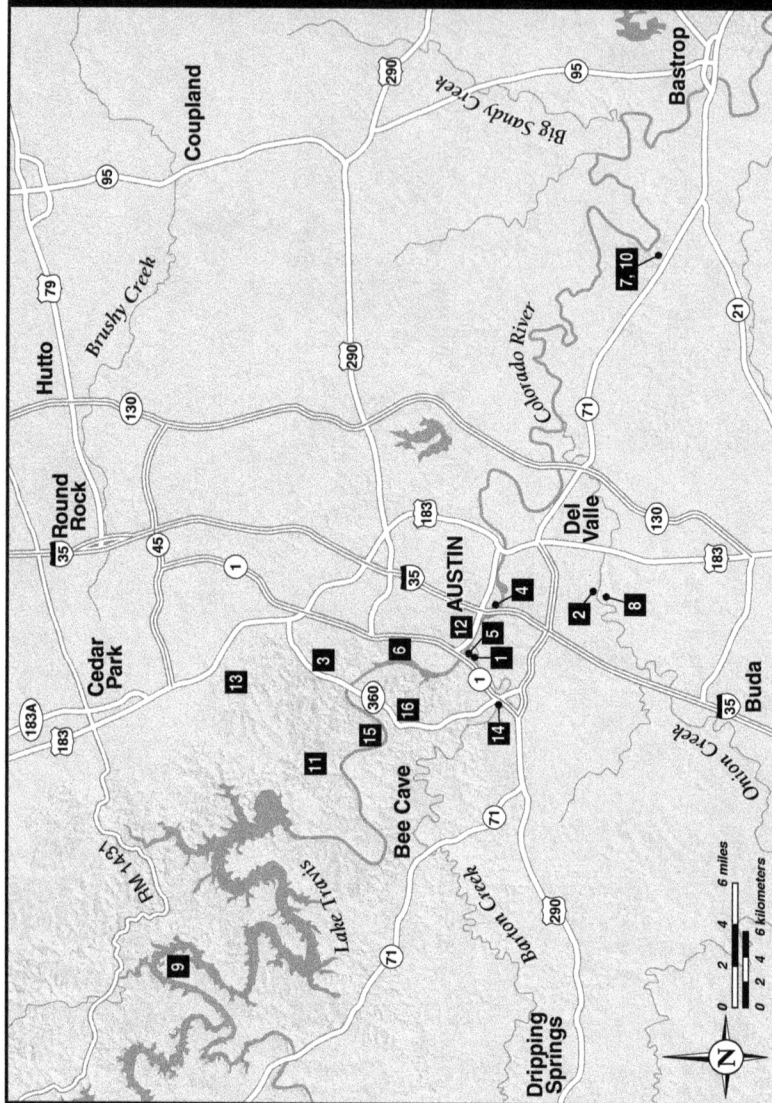

# Austin (Hikes 1–16)

Coupland

Bastrop

Big Sandy Creek

290

95

95

Hutto

79

Brushy Creek

130

290

Colorado River

7, 10

21

Round Rock

35

45

130

71

1

183

AUSTIN

Del Valle

130

183A

Cedar Park

183A

183

13

3

35

183

6

12

5

1

1

4

2

8

Buda

35

360

16

15

14

Onion Creek

11

Bee Cave

71

FM 1431

9

Lake Travis

71

Barton Creek

71

290

Dripping Springs

N

6 miles

6 kilometers

0    2    4

0    2    4    6 kilometers

# AUSTIN

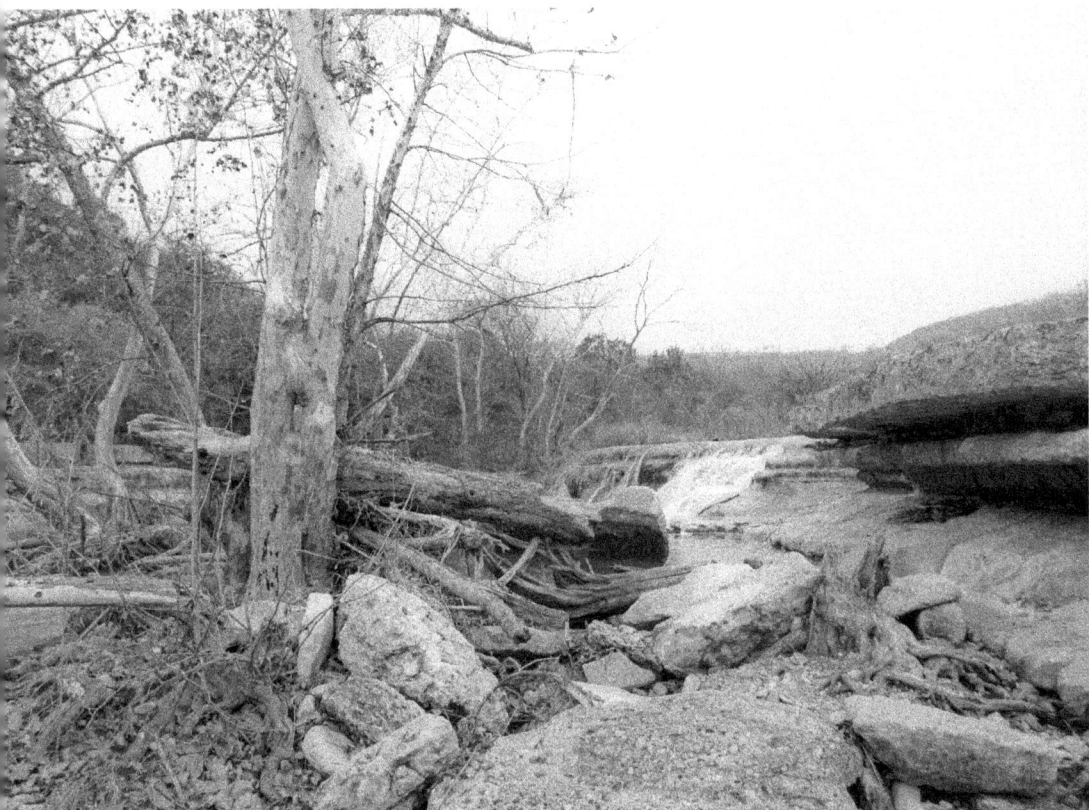

*Inga VanNynatten Memorial Trail (see page 23)*

# 1 Barton Creek Greenbelt (East)

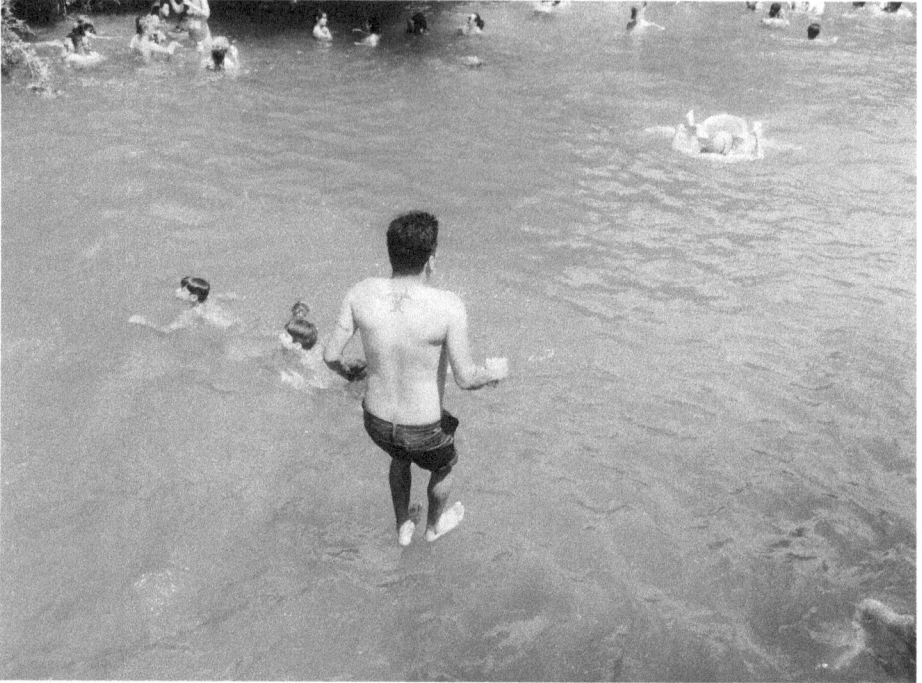

*Twin Falls*

## In Brief

This lengthy out-and-back hike travels up the Barton Creek canyon from Zilker Park to Twin Falls. You will see rock bluffs overlooking a clear blue stream bordered by riparian hardwood forests as well as drier woods of cedar. The beautiful canyon has deep swimming holes, beaches, and cascading falls. The high cliffs are popular with rock climbers.

## Description

There really aren't enough superlatives for the Barton Creek Greenbelt, home to some of the best urban hiking in America. It's gratifying that this wild canyon has been preserved in an Austin that has expanded so much over the last few decades. The water has cut a deep canyon in the limestone, putting the area's geological history on display along the rock walls. Sycamore and elm grow tall in the riverside forest. Live oak and cedar thrive

| | |
|---|---|
| **LENGTH:** 11.2 miles | **ACCESS:** Daily, 5 a.m.–10 p.m.; $3 parking fee on weekends |
| **CONFIGURATION:** Out-and-back | |
| **DIFFICULTY:** Moderate | **WHEELCHAIR ACCESS:** No |
| **SCENERY:** River canyon, woods, creek | **MAPS:** On information board at trailhead |
| **EXPOSURE:** Mostly shady | **FACILITIES:** Restrooms, water at Barton Springs Pool |
| **TRAFFIC:** Moderate to heavy | |
| **TRAIL SURFACE:** Dirt, rocks | **CONTACT INFORMATION:** 512-974-6700; austintexas.gov/department/ parks-and-recreation |
| **HIKING TIME:** 5.5 hours | |
| **DRIVING DISTANCE:** 3 miles from the state capitol | |

on the hillsides. The roar and hum of human life is never far away but always mingled with the cardinals' calls, the insects' buzz, and the soothing sound of running water.

There is a great deal to explore up and down the greenbelt. This route covers the lower part of the watershed—the eastern part of the V shape the creek makes across South Austin between MoPac and Loop 360. Along the way you will see side trails that beg to be investigated. This hike sets a baseline by following the route shown on the map at the trailhead, which stays on the northern side of the creek until the approach to Loop 360, but there are many alternate paths to scout out at another time.

The city of Austin is currently installing stylish new marker posts; like the old ones, they appear every quarter mile. According to the post at the trailhead, this is now the beginning of the Violet Crown Trail, which, if everything goes according to plan, will eventually end up more than 30 miles south in Hays County.

Leave the trailhead and head upstream on a gravel path. The first section goes through a meadow, but shortly you will come into the recurrent shade of the riparian forest, where all manner of hardwoods grow and the underbrush is thick and leafy.

The creek to your left is a braid of pools, small cascades, gravel bars, and islands. Myriad spur trails lead to pretty places where people are sunbathing, wading, or swimming in the pools. Bicyclists whiz along the path, though this being Austin they are usually polite and careful. The greenbelt is *not* an official off-leash area, though this is a divisive issue. Unfortunately, unleashed pets do their business in the creek and degrade the water quality. If do you bring your dog, scoop the poop and please take it with you— little plastic bags beside the trail have become far too common a sight. I mention this out of respect for the stunning beauty and sheer unlikeliness of this wild canyon, so beloved by generations of Austinites. It's a jewel and needs to be treasured.

Steep bluffs and boulders appear to your right, some overhanging the trail. At 0.7 mile you pass a pretty waterfall where a feeder creek comes in on your right. It is most likely moist enough that ferns decorate the stones. Shortly thereafter the creek and trail make a dogleg to the left and then back to the right. There is often a deep pool at the bend. Sometimes bathers will jump off tall bluffs on the other side. Around the corner a

# Barton Creek Greenbelt (East)

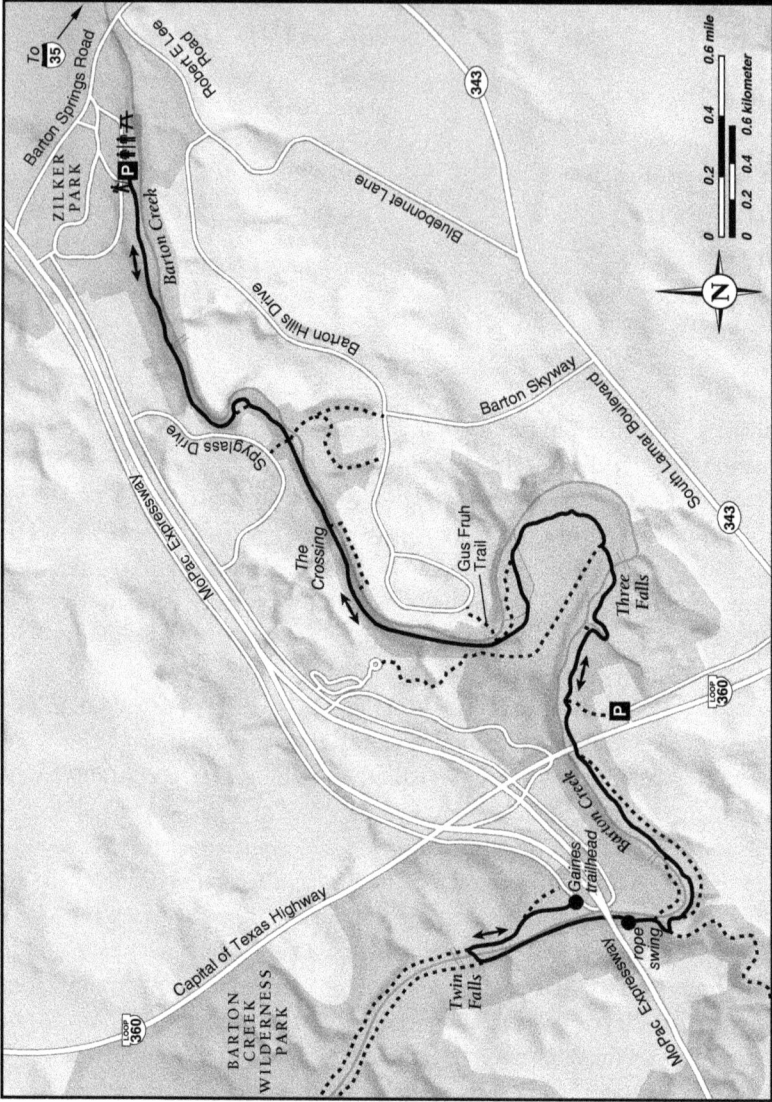

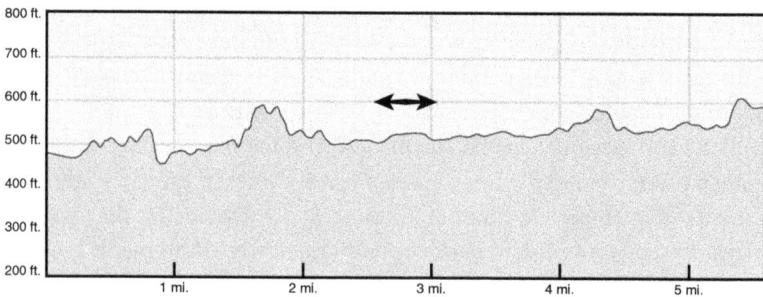

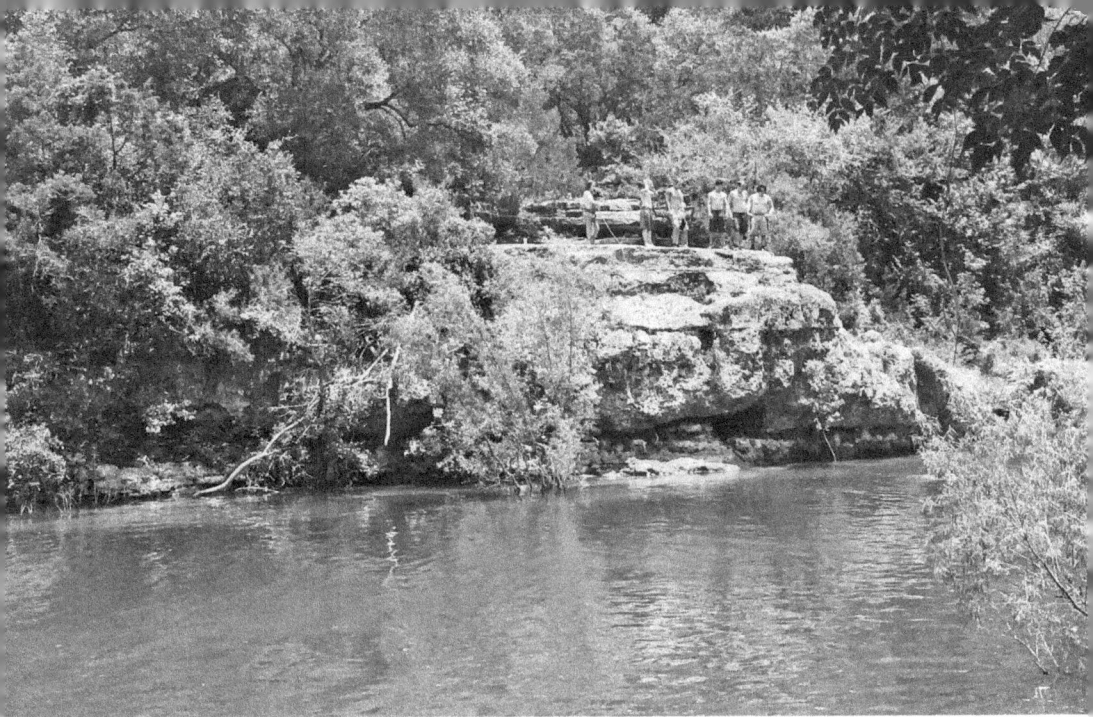

*Swimmers at Barton Creek*

series of stone slabs is popular with sunbathers and picnickers. The trail forks—one path goes by the creek and the other through cedar, but they meet up again soon, so take your pick. This splitting happens in several places, as hikers have taken differing paths over the years. In other places one route will be for bikers and the other for hikers. It's hard to get truly lost because the canyon will keep you on course.

At 1.2 miles the Spyglass Access Trail leaves to the right. A convenience store sells food and drinks at a little mall near the trailhead. On some sections of the trail the sky is visible, and on others groves of different trees provide shelter. Sometimes the path is very rocky, and sometimes it is smooth walking. At 1.6 miles look for a spur heading for a stone dam of sorts. Today you will stay on the right side of the creek, but remember this spot— on another day you can cross the creek and pick up an alternative trail on the other side of the streambed. Both options have plenty to offer.

Staying on the right side, pick your way over boulders that have tumbled down from the cliffs. Rock climbers with helmets and colored ropes might be attempting to scale the bluffs to your right. At 2.2 miles a spur to the left leads to the Gus Fruh pool, another popular swimming hole. Take this spur if you want a break and maybe a swim; otherwise keep right as the trail moves away from the main creek.

Barton Creek splits at Gus Fruh pool, and a channel that's usually dry makes a loop to the south. Pass through thick woods, and at 2.3 miles look for an arrow pointing left across this channel. Step across the streambed, and enter cedar woods. This next portion of the hike stays away from the creek, crossing the juniper-covered plateau on the inside of a large bend in the watercourse. It's likely to be the most solitary section of your walk. Cross the other end of the branch, and then at 3 miles go left at a junction and ford the multiple channels of Barton Creek, picking up the earthen path on the left side of the creek in the riparian forest.

At 3.2 miles you must walk up along a feeder branch until you find a crossing point. The trail comes back to Barton Creek by a fork in the trail. Keep left to head toward the 360 Access through thick cover, passing more spur trails. As always, if you find yourself heading away from the creek, you have left the main trail. You will start to hear the traffic on Loop 360 as you approach the highway. At 3.6 miles come to the access point and continue under the highway; then at 3.8 miles keep right at a fork. The riparian vegetation remains very thick around and above you.

At the 4-mile point a spur comes in from the right, and shortly you come to a wooden bridge over a feeder branch. The bluffs are very close to the path and the creek, and at one point a chain has been put into the cliff to keep you from falling into the creek. Stay along the bluffline through some of the greenbelt's best scenery. Overhanging rock, green ferns, deep water, and shade make this a pleasant spot on a hot day. Make your way around another side stream, and the valley widens and the greenbelt reaches a pool where there is a rope swing tied to a live oak. This makes for a good stopping spot.

Arrive at the MoPac Bridge, 4.7 miles into the hike. This bridge could be your turnaround spot. Otherwise keep on through the woods, and reach Twin Falls at 5.2 miles. Here you must cross the streambed. If there is enough water, you may want to kick your shoes off and swim or even jump off the falls into the pool below.

Pick up the trail on the eastern side of the creek, and backtrack through the slightly less lush woods on this bank. At a junction, go left, climbing the slope to reach the top of the bluff and then the Gaines trailhead. Alternatively, cross the creek anywhere after the MoPac Bridge and come to the ascent from the other direction.

## Nearby Activities

Zilker Park offers sports fields, swimming at Barton Springs, the Zilker Zephyr minitrain, refreshments, a picnic area, and a hillside theater.

### GPS TRAILHEAD COORDINATES
**N30° 15' 51.1"  W97° 46' 23.7"**

From I-35 in downtown Austin, take Exit 233, Town Lake/Riverside Drive. Cross Town Lake to reach Riverside Drive. Head west on Riverside Drive and follow it 1.1 miles to Barton Springs Road. Turn left on Barton Springs Road and follow it 1.3 miles to Zilker Park. Turn left into the park on William Barton Drive and follow it to the parking lot by the Barton Springs Pool entrance (or anywhere you can park). The greenbelt starts at the western end of the parking area. Note: The trail is sometimes closed after heavy rain. The out-and-back hike is lengthy, so consider going with a friend and leaving a car at the Twin Falls Access, the turnaround point. See "Three Falls at Barton Creek" (page 67) for directions to Twin Falls.

# 2 Homestead Trail at McKinney Falls State Park

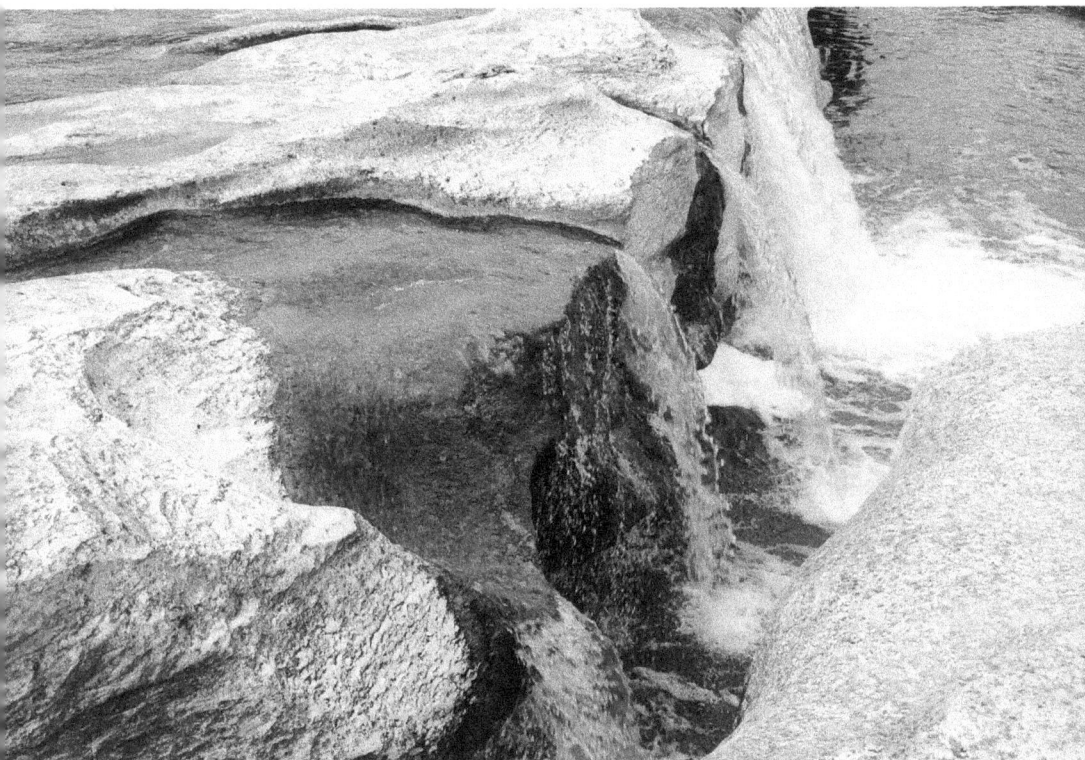

*McKinney Falls*

## In Brief

This hike travels through land once owned by Thomas F. McKinney, a frontiersman and entrepreneur who was instrumental in shaping the early history of Texas. Share the path with mountain bikers as you meander through wooded glades and pass by the ruined McKinney homestead.

## Description

Thomas Freeman McKinney was something of a go-getter. Originally from Kentucky, he and a partner helped finance the Texas Revolution, and McKinney used his own schooner

| | |
|---|---|
| **LENGTH:** 4.8 miles | **DRIVING DISTANCE:** 10 miles from the state capitol |
| **CONFIGURATION:** Loop | |
| **DIFFICULTY:** Moderate | **ACCESS:** Daily, 8 a.m.–10 p.m.; $6 entrance fee per person over age 13 |
| **SCENERY:** Thick hardwoods, the ruined homestead, and the Lower Falls | **WHEELCHAIR ACCESS:** No |
| **EXPOSURE:** Mostly shady | **MAPS:** Available at park office or at tinyurl.com/mckinneyfallsmap |
| **TRAFFIC:** Light, but watch for mountain bikers | **FACILITIES:** Restrooms, showers, picnic tables, and camping. Many stores are located nearby. |
| **TRAIL SURFACE:** Dirt | |
| **HIKING TIME:** 2 hours | **CONTACT INFORMATION:** 512-243-1643; tpwd.texas.gov/state-parks/mckinney-falls |

to capture a Mexican boat. A cofounder of the city of Galveston, he acquired 40,000 acres by the confluence of Onion and Williamson Creeks in 1839 from Mexican land speculator Santiago del Valle, either directly or through middlemen. In 1843 he divorced his first wife, Nancy, and married the 21-year-old Anna Gibbs, and in a few years the couple moved from Galveston to Travis County. McKinney settled down, built a house and a gristmill, and bred racehorses. He died in 1873, and Anna sold the property to James Smith, whose grandson donated the portion that is now the park to the state. You will pass by the ruins of McKinney's house and mill on this hike.

Getting to the trailhead can be a little tricky. After you've parked and walked across a wide sculpted rock outcrop, you'll need to cross the creek. Depending on the time of year and recent rainfall, you risk an involuntary dunking or worse. The best way is to hop along the edge of the falls. If the stepping-stones are underwater, this is the only way, unless you are prepared to swim or wade across the pool below the waterfall.

Across the creek, a sign at the edge of the woods marks the beginning of the trail. Go right toward the gristmill, walking between the treeline and the creek. Mountain bikers tend to ride this trail clockwise; hiking the other way will give you a chance to see each other and avoid collisions. The ruins are less than 200 yards from the trailhead, behind the information sign. The stones that made up the foundation are all that remain of the first working flour mill in the area. Over time, the creek has moved away from where the building stood.

Leaving the ruins, keep right at a little fork, and then very soon the trail crosses an unnamed draw, the lowest point of the hike. Climb away from the draw on sand and under cedar as the path makes a loop to the south, following Onion Creek. At 0.2 mile you pass a concrete picnic table, a good place for a secluded lunch.

Now the trail turns away from the creek to the north and begins a long climb to higher ground. Skirt a meadow where grass, cacti, and wildflowers grow. Exposed rock gives way to muddy singletrack, and dense vegetation crowds in around you. Eventually you reach the top of the rise and pass through an oak glade shading the gently

## Homestead Trail at McKinney Falls State Park

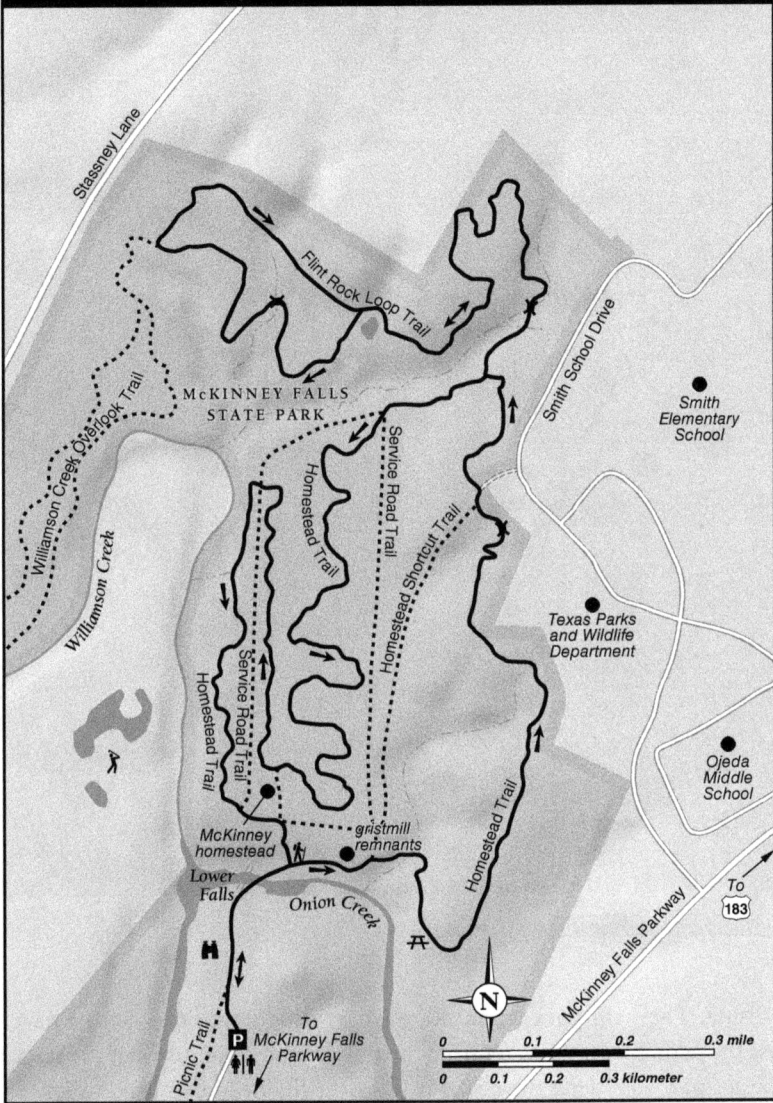

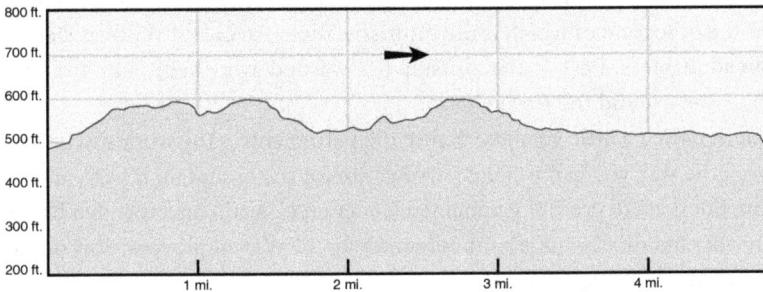

Stassney Lane

Flint Rock Loop Trail

Smith School Drive

Smith Elementary School

Williamson Creek Overlook Trail

McKINNEY FALLS STATE PARK

Williamson Creek

Homestead Trail

Service Road Trail

Homestead Shortcut Trail

Texas Parks and Wildlife Department

Service Road Trail

Homestead Trail

Ojeda Middle School

McKinney homestead

gristmill remnants

Homestead Trail

Lower Falls

Onion Creek

To 183

Picnic Trail

To McKinney Falls Parkway

McKinney Falls Parkway

N

| 0 | 0.1 | 0.2 | 0.3 mile |
| 0 | 0.1 | 0.2 | 0.3 kilometer |

800 ft.
700 ft.
600 ft.
500 ft.
400 ft.
300 ft.
200 ft.

1 mi.    2 mi.    3 mi.    4 mi.

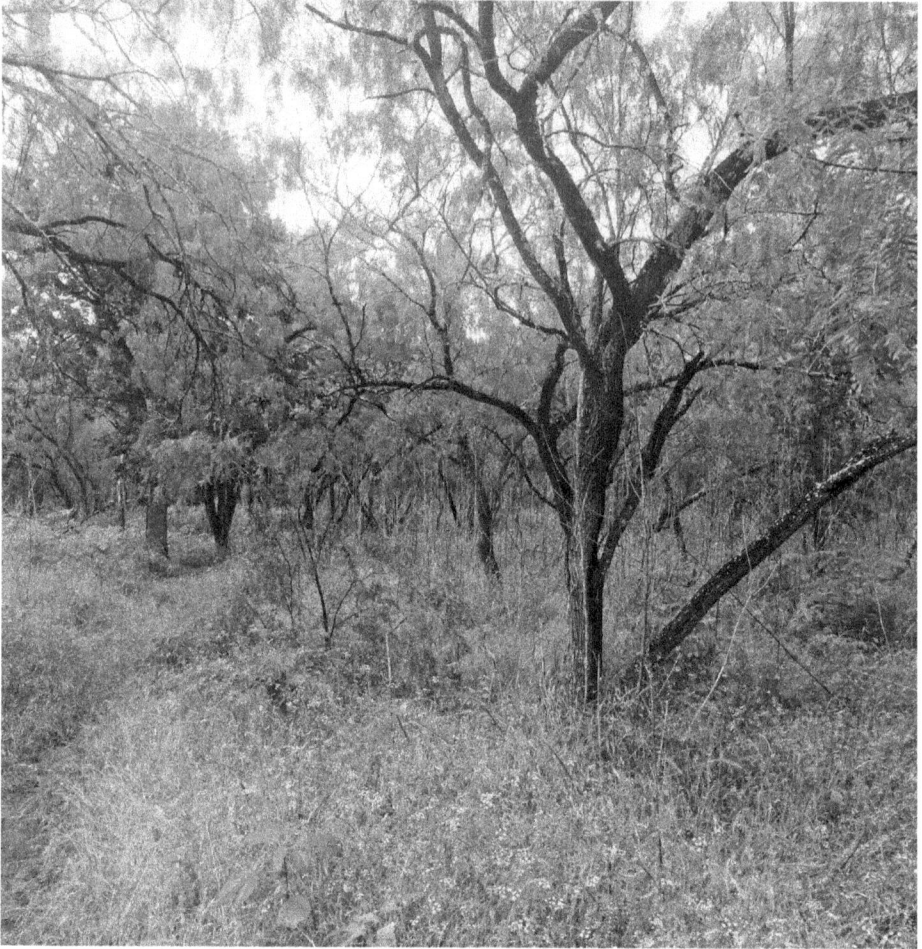

*Mesquite flats on the Homestead Trail*

sloping hillside. The path goes up and down over little drainages—berms have been built across the path, diverting water from the trail. At the 0.5-mile point the track turns left by a larger oak, following the contour line over the head of a little valley. Shortly you see glimpses of open space to your right, and then you briefly emerge onto a wide meadow, at the other end of which is the futuristic Texas Parks and Wildlife Department (TPWD) headquarters. Part of the cliffside has washed away here, and a safety fence forces a diversion around the fresh chasm.

You might notice a little sign just before the path reenters the woods, with an arrow pointing back the way you came. These arrows are for the mountain bikers, and you can ignore them. Soon you'll cross the unnamed feeder creek again on a wooden bridge, and soon see another building. This is a fitness center for TPWD employees. Stay on the trail, passing the facility on the left side. The trail curves to the left and descends. At 1 mile you

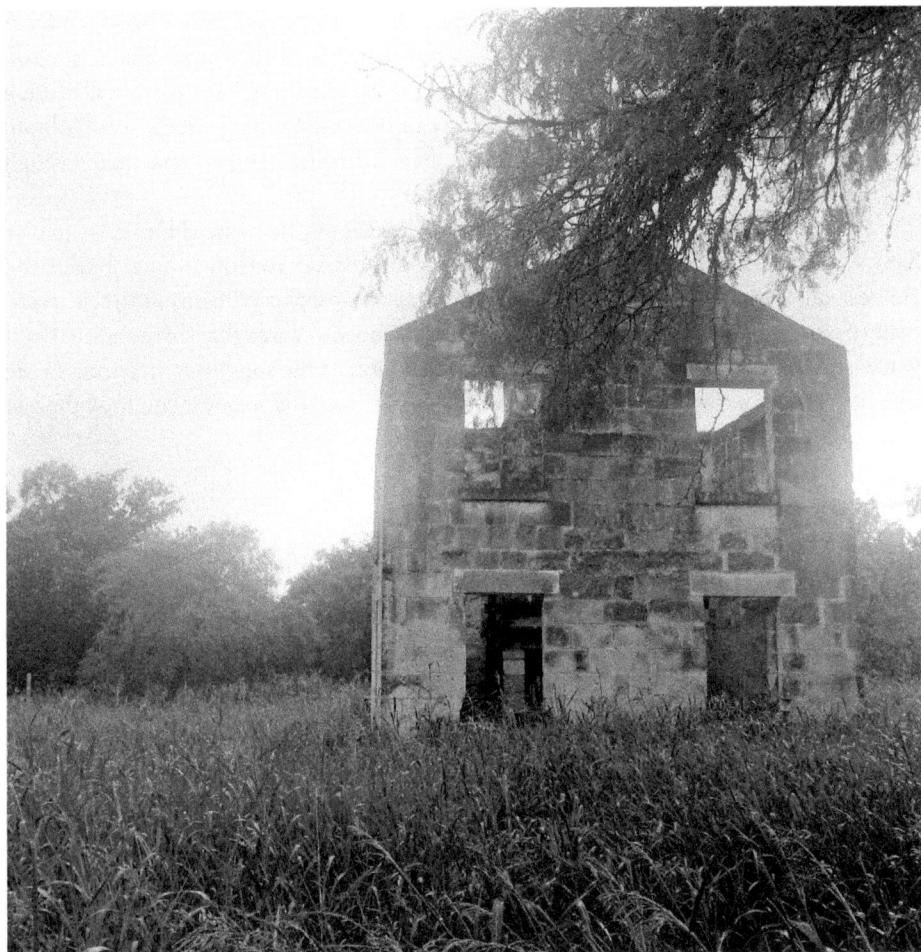

*The McKinney homestead*

arrive at the junction with the Flint Rock Loop Trail. Turn right. (Skip the Flint Rock Loop Trail to cut 2 miles from the total distance.)

This lovely balloon path goes down into a valley; crosses a feeder creek; climbs onto a plateau, where smaller walnut and cedar trees leave room for grass and cactus; drops back into the valley; and passes a pond. At the loop junction, go left. The trail winds over bridges and boardwalks through a serene and magical oak forest by Williamson Creek. At 2.1 miles a path leaves to the left, paralleling Stassney Lane into the uncharted northwestern reaches of the park. Keep right to return to the beginning of the loop, and then retrace your steps to the junction with the Homestead Trail, on the edge of the plateau.

Turn right. The path descends to the flat plain between the higher ground and Williamson Creek. At 3.2 miles you come to the apex of a V, whose stem and bar are once-cleared but now overgrown tracks leading off into the distance. The path leads straight ahead, bisecting these tracks, and shortly begins the first of several loops back and forth over the heavily wooded bottomland. Early on you will pass through a grove of mesquites. The many species of trees along this part of the trail are older and have grown taller. Blue jays and cardinals crisscross the trail, and you can hear the bunting's song, a triple-note tune that stands out from anything else in the area. Be aware of bikers speeding through this level section.

Four miles into the hike, you will glimpse the McKinney homestead through a tender hardwood glade and come to a junction. Keep right to make the longer final loop of the Homestead Trail, which backtracks north and returns closer to Williamson Creek, eventually passing the house at the southern end of the fenced-off area that surrounds it. Or, if you wish, turn left and then pass to the left of the house. At the southeastern corner of the area, go straight across the wider path—or turn right from that path, if you took the last loop—and descend to the trailhead and Onion Creek.

## Nearby Activities

This park also offers camping, picnicking, mountain biking, swimming, and fishing.

---

### GPS TRAILHEAD COORDINATES

**N30° 11' 19.6" W97° 43' 13.4"**

From downtown Austin take US 183 south and turn right onto McKinney Falls Parkway, 1.5 miles south of the junction with TX 71. After 2.7 miles turn right into the park.

---

# 3 Inga VanNynatten Memorial Trail at Lower Bull Creek Greenbelt

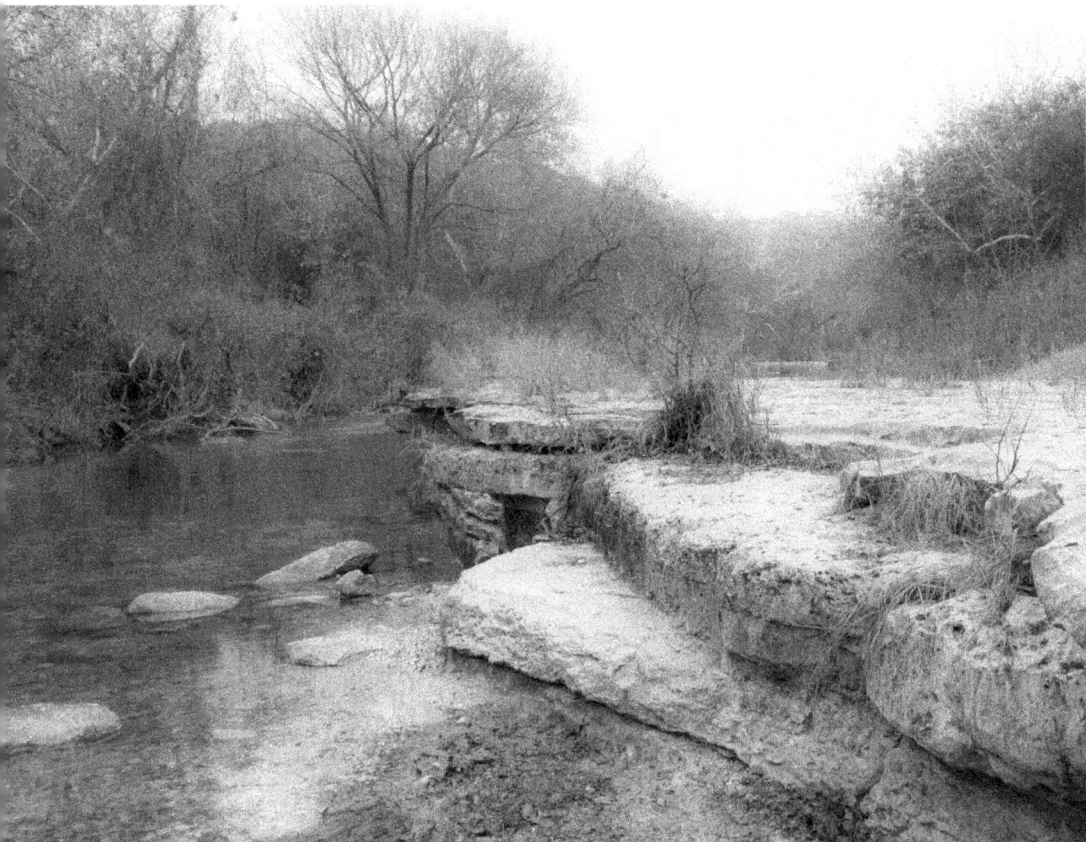

*Bull Creek*

## In Brief

If Austin didn't already have Barton Creek, this would be the feted and popular outdoor destination. By comparison, Bull Creek Greenbelt is underused. Towering bluffs and gorgeous creek scenery wait for you within a stone's throw of one of the city's busiest highways.

| | |
|---|---|
| **LENGTH:** 3.4 miles | **ACCESS:** Daily, 5 a.m.–10 p.m.; no fees or permits required |
| **CONFIGURATION:** Out-and-back | |
| **DIFFICULTY:** Easy | **WHEELCHAIR ACCESS:** No |
| **SCENERY:** Riparian woodland and water | **MAPS:** On the information board at Bull Creek District Park |
| **EXPOSURE:** Mostly shady | |
| **TRAFFIC:** Moderate–light | **FACILITIES:** Restrooms and water at Bull Creek District Park |
| **TRAIL SURFACE:** Dirt | **CONTACT INFORMATION:** 512-974-6700; austintexas.gov/department/ parks-and-recreation |
| **HIKING TIME:** 2.5 hours | |
| **DRIVING DISTANCE:** 14 miles from the state capitol | |

## Description

South of US 183, bustling Loop 360 descends into a stunning valley. This is the edge of the Balcones Escarpment, a curving line of topographic dramatics between the South and the West that was caused by countless earthquakes millions of years ago. Steep cliffs, high ridges, and Tuscan-themed architecture give the landscape an Italian feel. Neighborhoods and futuristic office buildings line the summits and slopes, but at the bottom of the valley, where Bull Creek flows past wooded banks and over limestone steps toward the Colorado River, nature still rules.

The valley is full of Austin history: It was settled in the 1800s by the Preece family, soldiers and Texas Rangers who named Bull Creek when one of their clan shot a male buffalo nearby. Mormons built one of the first roads to the northwest along the creek. Today the sound of traffic on 360 is omnipresent, but there are many spots along the creek where the view must not have changed in much more than 200 years.

The parking area overlooks a long pool between vertical rock walls. In rainy times, water tumbles between two overhanging limestone shelves. A house is perched at the top of the cedar-covered cliff across the creek. This lovely section of the creek—a free swimming pool in stunning surroundings—is very popular.

Walk along the flat, slippery rock on the western side of the stream, looking for a place to cross over. A concrete dam just beyond the 360 bridge is a good opportunity. (Alternatively, park in Bull Creek District Park, 0.3 mile south on Lakewood Drive, and ford the creek there.) Pick up the Inga VanNynatten Memorial Trail on the eastern side of Bull Creek. The trail is named after a young woman who helped establish it before her untimely passing. Some of the greenbelt is an off-leash area, so be prepared to greet enthusiastic canines. The abundance of water and dense, tangled cover provide ideal habitat for birds of all types. Cardinals are especially common, darting back and forth across the trail along the entire hike.

Head upstream. A sign points right at a fork for a short detour around an eroded section of the path. At the time of writing, much of the trail was in rough condition after

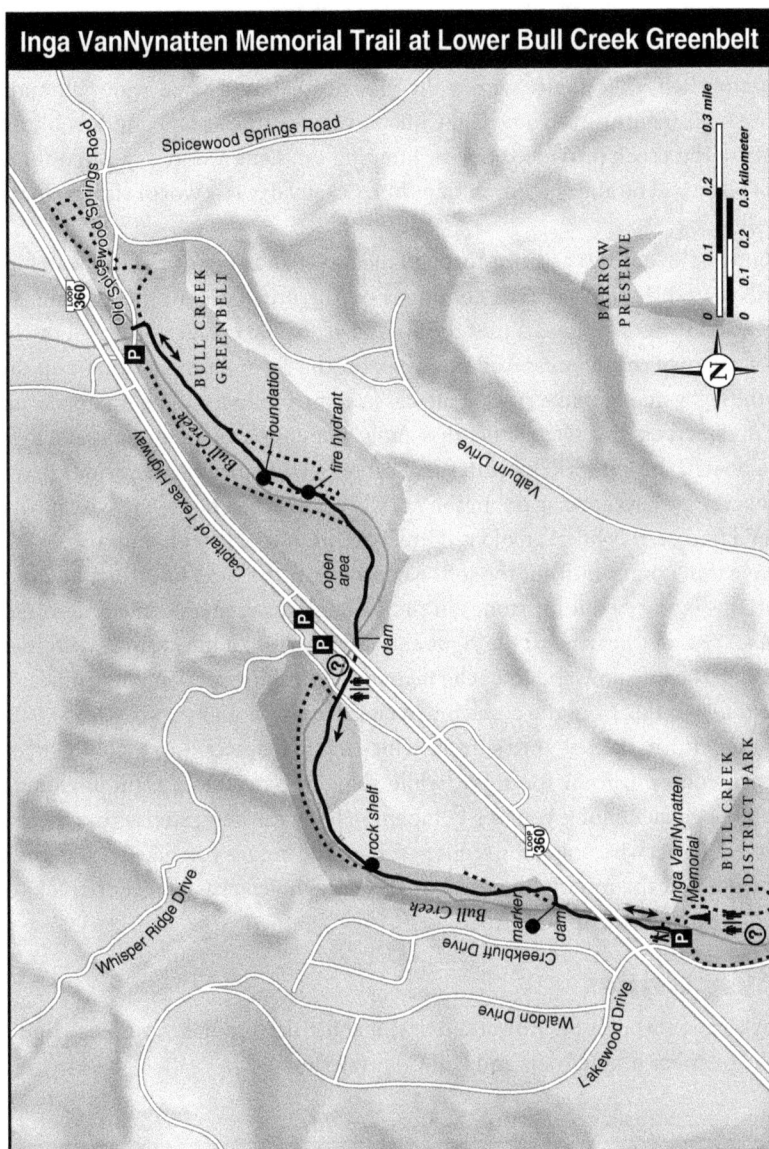

Inga VanNynatten Memorial Trail at Lower Bull Creek Greenbelt

a spring of rains and flooding. Short boardwalks have been laid across the muddiest sections. There are many spur trails leading left to the water and right to unofficial greenbelt access points. Keep forward along the creek and you won't go far wrong.

At 0.3 mile there is an unmarked fork, where you keep left; the path right leads to a private parking lot. The trail opens up a little, allowing for canyon views. At 0.4 mile you cross a drainage and come to the creek edge on a rock shelf. A feeder stream flows in from the opposite side.

The trail continues along the cracked shelf, then veers back into the woods before coming to a fork at 0.7 mile. Keep left to come to the hike's main attraction: a large *balcón,* or limestone shelf, that angles across the creek, creating a wide waterfall and a large swimming hole. There's even a beach. Cliffs tower over the scene, and low bluffs on the other side of the creek provide spots for jumping off. On a warm day when the water is high, this place will be abuzz with summer fun. On any day it is worth visiting for the view up the valley.

At 0.8 mile an access road cuts through the forest and goes over a low water crossing. Inga VanNynatten Memorial Trail continues on the other side of the asphalt. The path gets a little indistinct as it goes under the second set of 360 bridges. Just past the highway, look for a dam where you must ford the creek for the second time. (Detour up the rough path on the right side to find a rusting old car in some boulders.) The trail picks up on the left side of the creek on a plateau of grass and cedar coppices. Keep right at a fork where there is a bench; the left fork is an alternate route to Old Spicewood Springs Road. At 1.1 miles cross the watercourse again. In the middle of the creek bed stands the most curious thing you'll find on this hike: an old red fire hydrant, not of any obvious use.

A spur trail comes in from the left. Keep right at the next fork. Just before the 1.3-mile mark keep an eye out for stones in the path, all that remains of a long-disappeared structure. A narrow clearing to the right allows views into a meadow. An alternate track goes through the meadow and joins the main trail at a short section of log fence.

The trail ascends from the creek into a cedar forest, coming level with 360. Look for steps to the left, marked as Inga's Trail, which swiftly descend to a confluence. Laurel Oaks Creek comes in from the right, while Bull Creek makes a right angle under Old Spicewood Springs Road. If you or a companion left a car here, step across the creek and find your car. Otherwise enjoy the scenery for a while before you hike back to the starting point. Turn left at the top of the steps to extend the hike across a feeder creek to a trailhead on Old Spicewood Springs Road.

## Nearby Activities

Bull Creek runs through St. Edwards Park, a short drive north on Spicewood Springs Road. The park has hiking trails and Hill Country views.

### GPS TRAILHEAD COORDINATES
**N30° 22' 15.4"  W97° 47' 06.7"**

From north Austin, head south on Loop 360 and turn left at Lakewood Drive. The parking area is immediately on the left. The greenbelt is north of the Colorado River. There are several parking lots at the hike's turnaround on Old Spicewood Springs Road should you and a friend want to bring two cars and cut out the return journey.

# 4 Lady Bird Lake: Boardwalk Loop

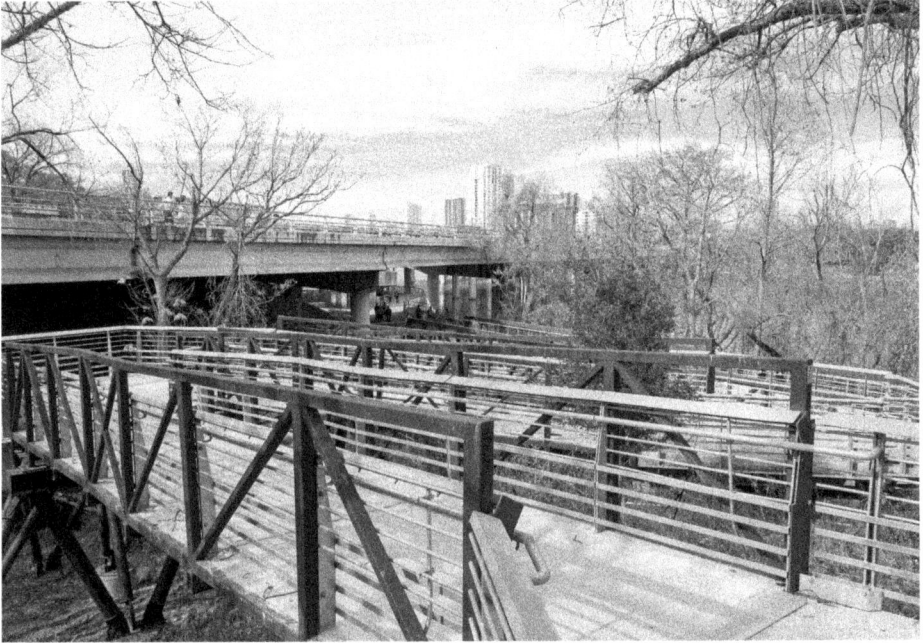

*The boardwalk along Lady Bird Lake*

## In Brief

Austin's new boardwalk, which closed a more-than-a-mile-long gap in the Lady Bird Lake loop, opened in 2014 and has proved a great success, as up to 15,000 people use this part of the trail every day. This hike takes in the eastern part of the loop, crossing Longhorn Dam and coming back via the boardwalk, where you can enjoy views of the city's skyline.

## Description

For years, the 10-mile Ann and Roy Butler Hike-and-Bike Trail had a 1.1-mile gap where topography and property lines forced trail users onto the Riverside Drive sidewalk. Closing that gap had long been a dream of many, and finally in 2006 the city of Austin gave the go-ahead for a boardwalk. The Trail Foundation, a nonprofit dedicated to improving this

| | |
|---|---|
| **LENGTH:** 3.9 miles | **DRIVING DISTANCE:** 2 miles from the state capitol |
| **CONFIGURATION:** Loop | |
| **DIFFICULTY:** Easy | **ACCESS:** Daily, 5 a.m.–midnight; no fees or permits required |
| **SCENERY:** Boardwalk, dam, parks, and neighborhoods | **WHEELCHAIR ACCESS:** Yes |
| **EXPOSURE:** Mostly exposed | **MAPS:** thetrailfoundation.org/explore/butler-trail-maps |
| **TRAFFIC:** Moderate–high | **FACILITIES:** None |
| **TRAIL SURFACE:** Gravel, sidewalk | **CONTACT INFORMATION:** 512-974-6700; austintexas.gov/department/parks-and-recreation |
| **HIKING TIME:** 1.5 hours | |

trail, raised nearly $3 million for construction, and the structure opened to the public on June 7, 2014. It extends a half mile on each side of I-35. The section you will visit on this hike, east of the highway, has three large viewing platforms, popular destinations for casual walkers. The boardwalk has also opened up access to the eastern part of the loop, previously somewhat underused, and has given impetus to businesses along Riverside Avenue east of the highway. Renting a bike and riding the trail has become a popular Austin activity, so look out for cyclists who may not be used to riding among pedestrians, or at all.

With all that to look forward to, you will start by heading east on the north side of the river, walking through Festival Beach or Fiesta Gardens—the park is known by both names. People rest at the picnic benches scattered across the lush grass, enjoying the shade beneath large pecan trees. The gravel path goes along the edge of the lake, and you might see a fisherman casting from his kayak out on the water or trying his luck on one of the fishing platforms along the bank.

At 0.5 mile there is a parking lot and lake access for boaters. Shortly the path moves away from the lake to cross a bridge over an inlet leading to a large lagoon. Once over the bridge, you'll cross some asphalt and walk by a baseball field. At the end of the first field, stay on the gravel path, bearing right to pass some batting cages. On the weekend families will be out enjoying these facilities. Step onto Riverview Street.

Across Riverview Street is a stone arch into which an artist has carved several faces. The trail goes underneath this and alongside the decommissioned Holly Street Power Plant that the city is dismantling. At this time the plant walls are decorated with graffiti of some artistry. Austin's Eastside has always had a strong Latino culture, evident in this artwork.

Come to the end of this side of the plant, and go under a square Art Deco portal. Cross the street and look for a matching structure. Go under this, passing along the north side of the construction site and through Metz Neighborhood Park, where young men often practice basketball. The path goes over some tracks and an access road, then dives down along the eastern side of the plant, but only for a few feet. A left turn takes you onto a long, narrow bar. Locals come to this bar to fish in the lagoon that it has created.

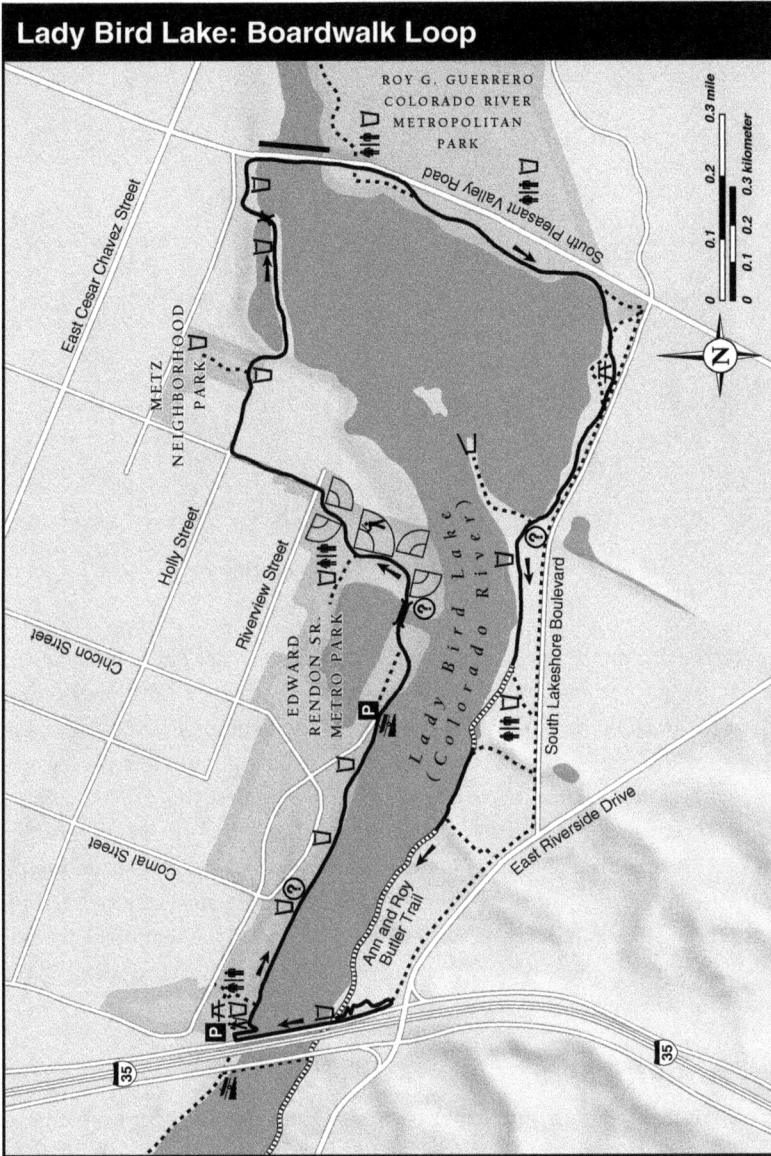

Lady Bird Lake: Boardwalk Loop

At 1.6 miles a bridge takes you back to the shore. A little plaza and metal artwork, part of the Trail of Tejano Legends, celebrates musician Roy Montelongo. From here it is a few steps to Longhorn Dam, in service since 1940. Cross the dam on the narrow pedestrian walkway, looking back for views of the lake and the city. It's an interesting gaze back in time, as there are no tall buildings in this vista.

Descend from the dam and pick up the trail as it follows the lakeshore. Across the street are the Krieg baseball fields, part of the Roy G. Guerrero Colorado River

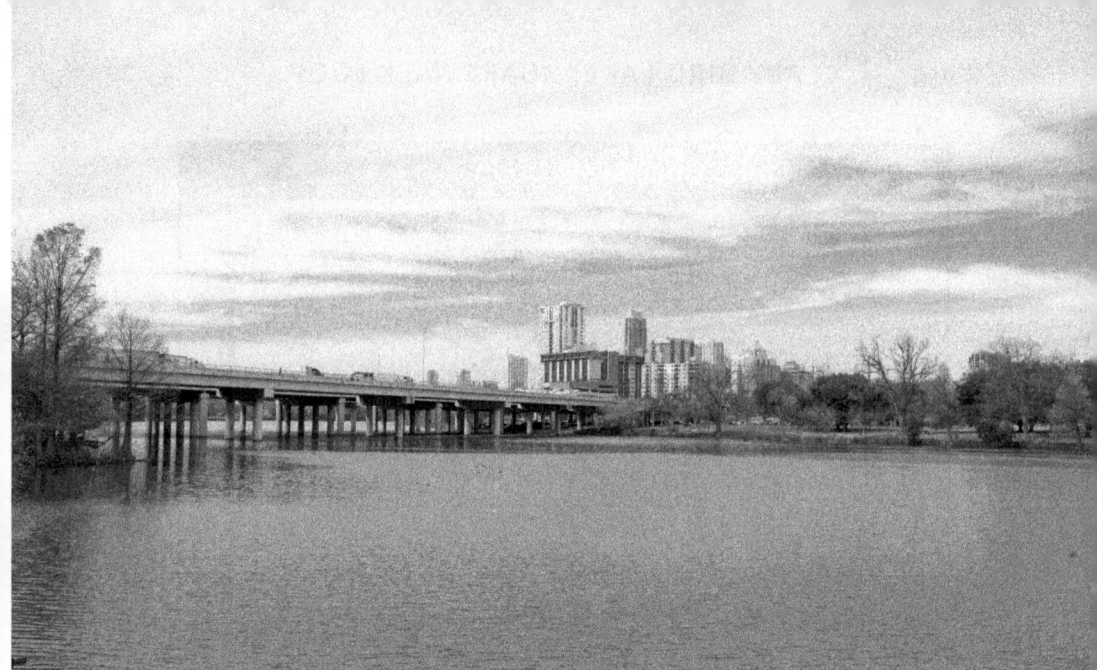

*View of downtown Austin from the Lady Bird Lake boardwalk*

Metropolitan Park, which has its own network of hiking trails. There is usually someone selling fruit from a truck in a lay-by. The path wanders between Lakeshore Boulevard and the lake's edge. At a junction a side trail goes right to a picnic area. At 2.6 miles, keep right at a fork where the trail widens. Another trail leads off right along a promontory. At 3 miles, you come to the beginning of the boardwalk. The first short piece quickly comes back to the shore, where the trail stays for another 0.2 mile before the main section of the boardwalk, with the three platforms mentioned earlier, begins. Linger on the platforms awhile for the ambience. Just before the highway, turn left onto cantilevered platforms that lead to the sidewalk, unless you wish to continue along the section of the boardwalk west of I-35. Otherwise, cross the river on the pedestrian walkway next to the traffic lanes, and walk down a ramp to return to your starting point.

## Nearby Activities

Rent a kayak or paddleboard, and explore the lake from the water, or rent a bicycle from one of the many Austin B-Cycle locations.

---

**GPS TRAILHEAD COORDINATES**

**N30° 15' 6"  W97° 44' 09.8"**

**From the junction of I-35 and Cesar Chavez Street, go south on the western frontage road. Keep straight and the road will become East Avenue. East Avenue turns left and goes under the freeway. Turn into a small parking lot. The trail goes between the parking lot and the pavement.**

# 5 Lady Bird Lake: West Loop

## In Brief

This has always been the most crowded trail in the capital city, more so now since the influx of downtown condo dwellers. It's where busy Austinites come to get their outdoor fix—bikers, joggers, and slackliners throng the trail, while kayakers and stand-up paddleboarders play in the water.

## Description

To begin this loop around Lady Bird Lake on the Ann and Roy Butler Hike-and-Bike Trail, walk east on the south side of the river, with Zilker Park on your right. The hike as described will take you all the way to I-35 and back, but on the way you will pass Lamar Boulevard, South First Street, and Congress Avenue. At any one of these bridges you can cut the loop short. The city's new attraction is the Lady Bird Lake boardwalk, which begins just this side of I-35 and continues past the highway into East Austin. That section of the loop—from I-35 to Longhorn Dam—is included in this book on page 27. (The Butler Trail is 10 miles long, all told.) The boardwalk is just one of many arresting structures, both old and new, that you will encounter on this hike. A note on Austin jargon: "the lake" means Lake Travis, not Lady Bird Lake, which longtime residents still refer to by its old name, Town Lake.

The trail is wide and easy and will stay like this all the way, the gravel surface giving way to concrete slabs at some points. Lycra-clad bodies swarm around you, chatting as they run. You'll pass some wooded drainage ponds to your right, and at 0.4 mile you'll come to the tight railroad loop at the end of the narrow-gauge track used by the popular Zilker Train. The playing fields of Zilker Park, home to the Austin City Limits music festival, open up to the right, but the path dives left down into the tree cover along the riverbank and makes a noticeable dip across a little drainage. Tall cypresses grow by the water at the bottom of the jungly bank.

At 0.8 mile you'll pass a wall of cuboid limestone blocks, where local musician Woode Wood might be strumming his guitar, and arrive at Lou Neff Point, at the confluence of Barton Creek and the Colorado River. A gazebo offers shelter while you take in the view of Austin's futuristic skyline, much-changed over the last decade. Lou Neff Point is much prettier than it used to be, the result of the work of The Trail Foundation, an organization that facilitates improvements to the Hike-and-Bike Trail. Along the way you will see signs, stone walls, plant beds, benches, and other enhancements that this foundation has provided.

Around the corner is a stretch of shoreline along which not-so-wild ducks and grackles hang around waiting to be fed. At 0.9 mile, turn left across an arched footbridge. Look right for the view up Barton Creek, though the famous swimming pool can't quite be seen from

| | |
|---|---|
| **LENGTH:** 6.9 miles | **DRIVING DISTANCE:** 3 miles from the state capitol |
| **CONFIGURATION:** Loop | |
| **DIFFICULTY:** Easy | **ACCESS:** Daily, 5 a.m.–midnight; no fees or permits required |
| **SCENERY:** Lake, downtown, and abundant greenery | **WHEELCHAIR ACCESS:** Yes |
| **EXPOSURE:** Open–shady | **MAPS:** thetrailfoundation.org/explore/butler-trail-maps |
| **TRAFFIC:** Heavy | **FACILITIES:** Restrooms, water fountains |
| **TRAIL SURFACE:** Paved | **CONTACT INFORMATION:** 512-974-6700; austintexas.gov/department/parks-and-recreation |
| **HIKING TIME:** 2–3 hours | |

here. Turn left at the end of the bridge, and walk along a particularly leafy section of the hike toward the three Lamar bridges: road, pedestrian, and rail. At the road bridge, an Art Deco design from 1942, you will have hiked 1.5 miles. The newish Pfluger hike-and-bike bridge connects to the return trail on the north bank and to the Lance Armstrong Bikeway.

Pass under the Union Pacific rail bridge and admire the solid stone piers, and then hop onto the sidewalk to go over West Bouldin Creek, and you will be in Auditorium Shores, the location of several concerts and events each year. It's likely that construction or an event will force a detour from the shoreline to Riverside Drive, but if you can get there look for the statue of guitarist Stevie Ray Vaughan, one of Austin's favorite sons, whose career was cut short in a helicopter accident. Near him are a favorite bathing spot for dogs, a pond, another gazebo, and likely lots of other activity. There's a chance to return via the South First Street bridge; otherwise forge on under the bridge and past the Lone Star Riverboat. The trail narrows as it passes between the Hyatt hotel and the river. At 2.4 miles you come to the Congress Avenue bridge. This is your last chance to turn back before I-35, a mile away.

The smell under this bridge is guano (bat dung) from the 1.5 million Mexican free-tailed bats that live in the structure in the summer. They put on a popular show every night when they leave en masse to hunt for insects. Continue past the Austin-American Statesman building, with trees shading the path, and soon you will see the new board-walk and I-35. You used to have to continue on the sidewalk along Riverside Drive, but thanks to the city of Austin and The Trail Foundation, you now walk out over the lake on a grand metal boardwalk. Look left for another view of downtown. The boardwalk goes over a promontory at Blunn Creek, where dramatic cantilevered walkways lead up a canyon to Riverside Drive.

At 3.4 miles you go under the quadruple roadways of the interstate. Go right, climbing up more metal walkways to street level. Cross the lake next to the traffic, the least pleasant part of the hike. Under the north end of the bridges, the parking lot is a popular casual fishing spot. Continue west. The setting turns back to a more natural environment of trees and grass, and the traffic here is some of the lightest you'll encounter. At the

**Lady Bird Lake: West Loop**

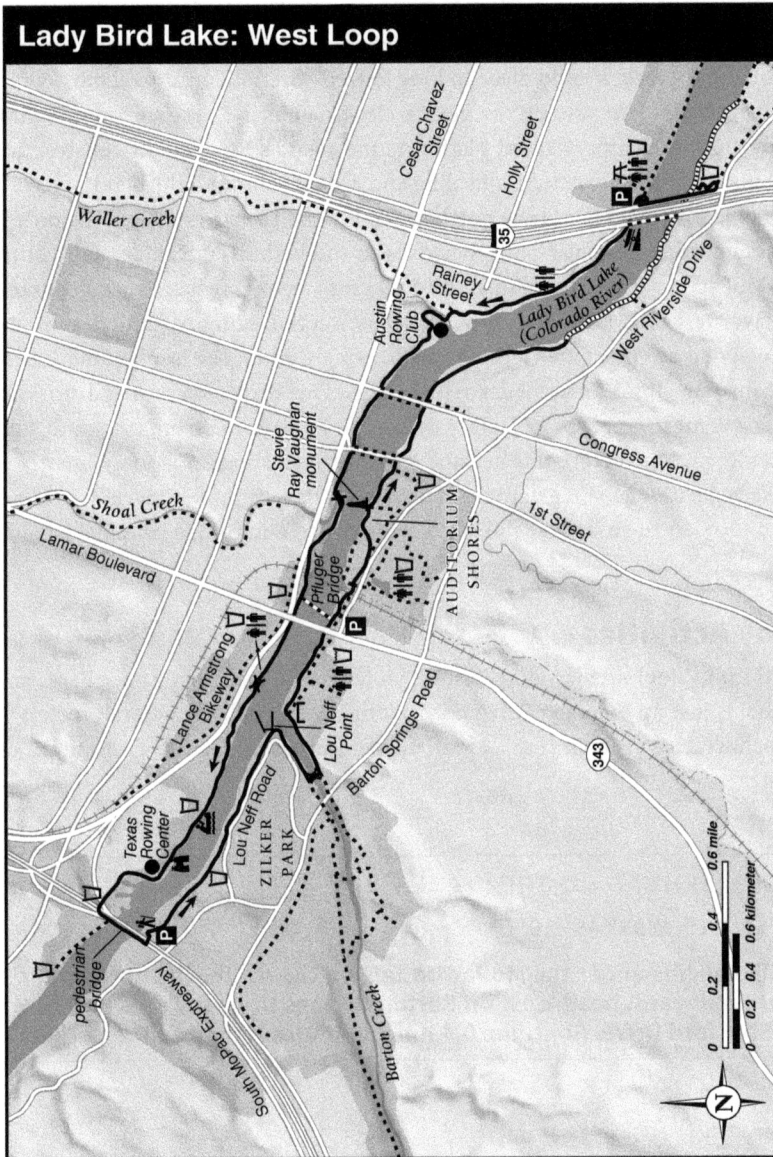

end of Rainey Street, known for its hip bars and restaurants, you'll see an arty metal restroom. There are benches at intervals and side trails to the edge of the lake. Look for a sculpture installation, part of the Trail of Tejano Legends, which celebrates local Latino musicians.

At 4.4 miles turn left at a junction to cross a bridge over Waller Creek, after which (at the time of writing) you must make a circle around some construction and walk by the handsome new home of the Austin Rowing Club, potentially a refreshment stop.

Once you've crossed under Congress Avenue again, this time on a little boardwalk, the foot and bike traffic increases. At 5.2 miles you cross a bridge onto the bar at the mouth of Shoal Creek, a good place to look for red-eared slider turtles, mostly red-eared sliders, who slip into the water if you get too close. Come up a little rise onto Cesar Chavez Street by an odd round, covered platform, and take in the view of construction, new apartments, and possibly a train squealing and groaning around the bend.

At 5.4 miles you come to the northern end of the Lamar bridges, a major trail junction. Pass under the circular path that rises to the pedestrian bridge, and continue on toward MoPac. A succession of small bridges cross feeder creeks. Cross a concrete spillway, a favorite canoe-launching spot. This last section is more natural and gets quite thickly wooded as you come to the Texas Rowing Center, the last landmark before the tennis court and the MoPac pedestrian bridge. The large concrete and iron tower by the rowing center was part of a facility used to ferry clay over from the south side of the Colorado River, long before this became a recreational area. Look for palmetto palms in the dense vegetation as you go around a final cove. Pass by tennis courts on the sidewalk, and then turn left to cross over the lake on the pedestrian bridge, and make your way to your car.

## Nearby Activities

Barton Springs Pool–the jewel in Austin's violet crown–is across Zilker Park, and Deep Eddy Pool is just up Veterans Drive north of the river. Both are natural, spring-fed, and very much worth a visit. Or rent a kayak or stand-up paddleboard, and venture out onto the lake.

---

### GPS TRAILHEAD COORDINATES

**N30° 16' 22"  W97° 46' 19.5"**

**The hike begins under the MoPac bridge, on the south side of the river. From Lamar Boulevard, head west on Barton Springs Drive 0.9 mile and turn right onto Stratford Drive. Continue 0.4 mile, and turn right into the parking area.**

---

# 6 Mayfield Park and Preserve

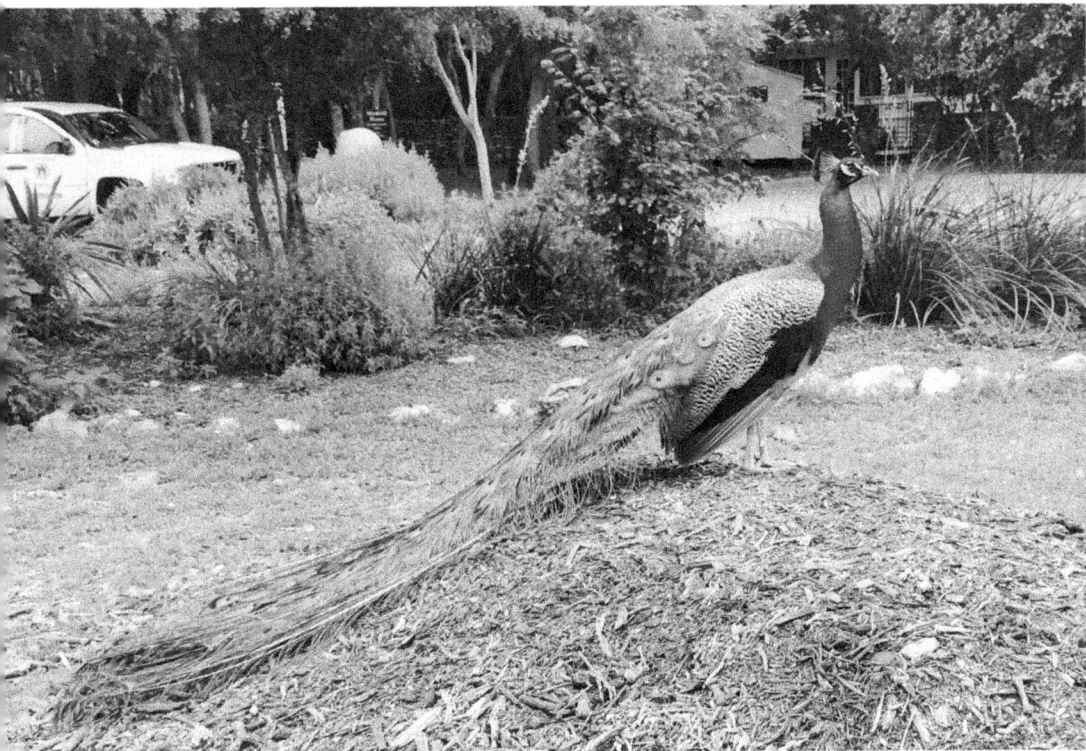

*A peacock at Mayfield Park and Preserve*

## In Brief

This walk takes place at Mayfield Park and Preserve, site of the Mayfield-Gutsch Estate. Inspect the homesite and backyard gardens, and then explore multiple trails through the woods around Taylor Slough and along the banks of Lake Austin.

## Description

Tucked away at the north end of Tarrytown next to a water treatment plant, Mayfield Preserve has a lot of Texas packed into its 21 acres. Creeks and deep canyons, trees and thick brush, birds and animals are all here, waiting for you to spend an hour or so in their company. There are marked trails that you can follow, but there are also many short trails that crisscross the preserve, sometimes leading to precarious canyon edges or dead-ending at iron gates—or simply emerging to the street. Your start and end point is the parking

| | |
|---|---|
| **LENGTH:** 1 mile | **DRIVING DISTANCE:** 5 miles from the state capitol |
| **CONFIGURATION:** Multiple inter-connected trails | **ACCESS:** Daily, 5 a.m.–10 p.m.; no fees or permits required |
| **DIFFICULTY:** Mostly easy | |
| **SCENERY:** Formal gardens, creek gorge, lake | **WHEELCHAIR ACCESS:** Yes |
| | **MAPS:** Signboard map at trailhead |
| **EXPOSURE:** Mostly shady | **FACILITIES:** Picnic area, restroom at trailhead |
| **TRAFFIC:** Moderate–busy | |
| **TRAIL SURFACE:** Concrete, dirt, rock | **CONTACT INFORMATION:** 512-974-6797; mayfieldpark.org |
| **HIKING TIME:** 1 hour | |

area; where you go in between is largely up to you. The following is just a suggestion for exploring the park. Don't worry—there is no way to be lost for more than a few minutes because the park is bounded on all sides by houses, 35th Street, and Lake Austin.

The first order of business is to admire the Mayfield-Gutsch house. This charming white villa is set in beautifully tended ornamental gardens surrounded by a stone wall. Allison Mayfield, Texas secretary of state from 1894 to 1896 and then railroad commissioner from 1896 to 1922, purchased the property in 1909. A small cottage was already here, dating from the 1870s. Mayfield used this getaway primarily as a summer cottage. In 1922 he bequeathed it to his daughter, Mary, and her husband, Milton Gutsch, and the couple began to develop gardens around the house. They kept at it for nearly 50 years, building ponds, stone walls, and outbuildings and enlarging the house itself. In 1971 the property was bequeathed to the city of Austin for use as a park, and in 1994, it was listed on the National Register of Historic Places.

Leave the parking area and take the visitor entrance to the house and gardens. An iron gate allows passage beyond the stone wall. Pass by the front of the house, noting the native Texas palms, which lend a tropical look. Head down the driveway around to the back of the house. Four concrete ponds lie around a smaller center pond, and benches overlook them. Various small gardens, lovingly tended by volunteers, grow between the ponds and the back stone wall. Stroll among the gardens, noting the varied plant species. Look over the back wall of the backyard, set against the edge of the canyon formed by Taylor Slough. You will undoubtedly see and hear the peacocks that roam the yard, and most likely the children following the peacocks as well. My guess is that most people limit their visit to the house and its immediate surroundings, but naturally you will want to explore a little farther.

Leave the gardens through the gate in the northeastern wall, where a bell hangs beneath an arbor. It might as well be the portal to Narnia, the transition is so abrupt. Nature grows in all shapes and sizes. A tangle of cedar and live oak branches obscures the sky, and thick brush hides the ground. This, the Bell Trail, descends steep earth steps

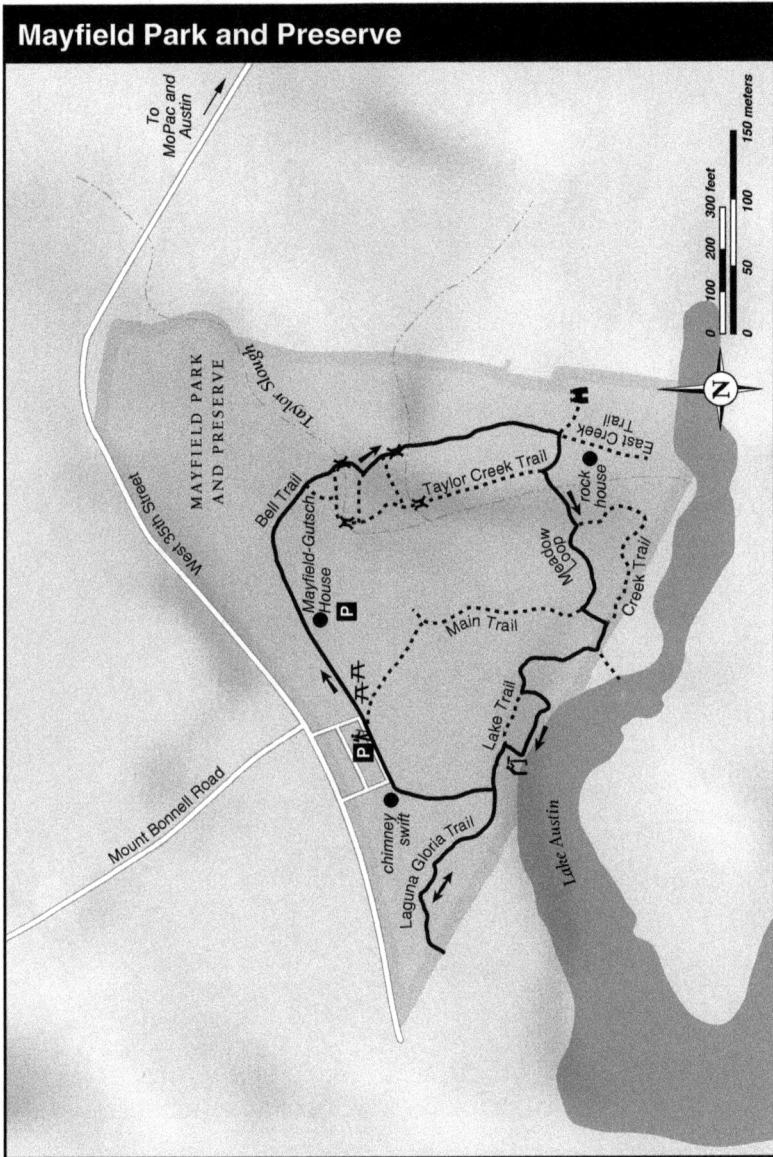

Mayfield Park and Preserve

toward a creek feeding into Taylor Slough, meeting the Taylor Creek Trail in a lush glade full of palmettos. Keep left to walk down to the creek.

The multitude of trails soon becomes evident. All the paths are short, so you can quickly backtrack. Hop over Taylor Slough and take a left, and you will come to a trail that leads into the overgrown northern end of the preserve, where the creek runs through a deep canyon. Or work south along this same canyon past high bluffs toward Lake Austin, trying not to let the dense woods and numerous trails confuse you. Several

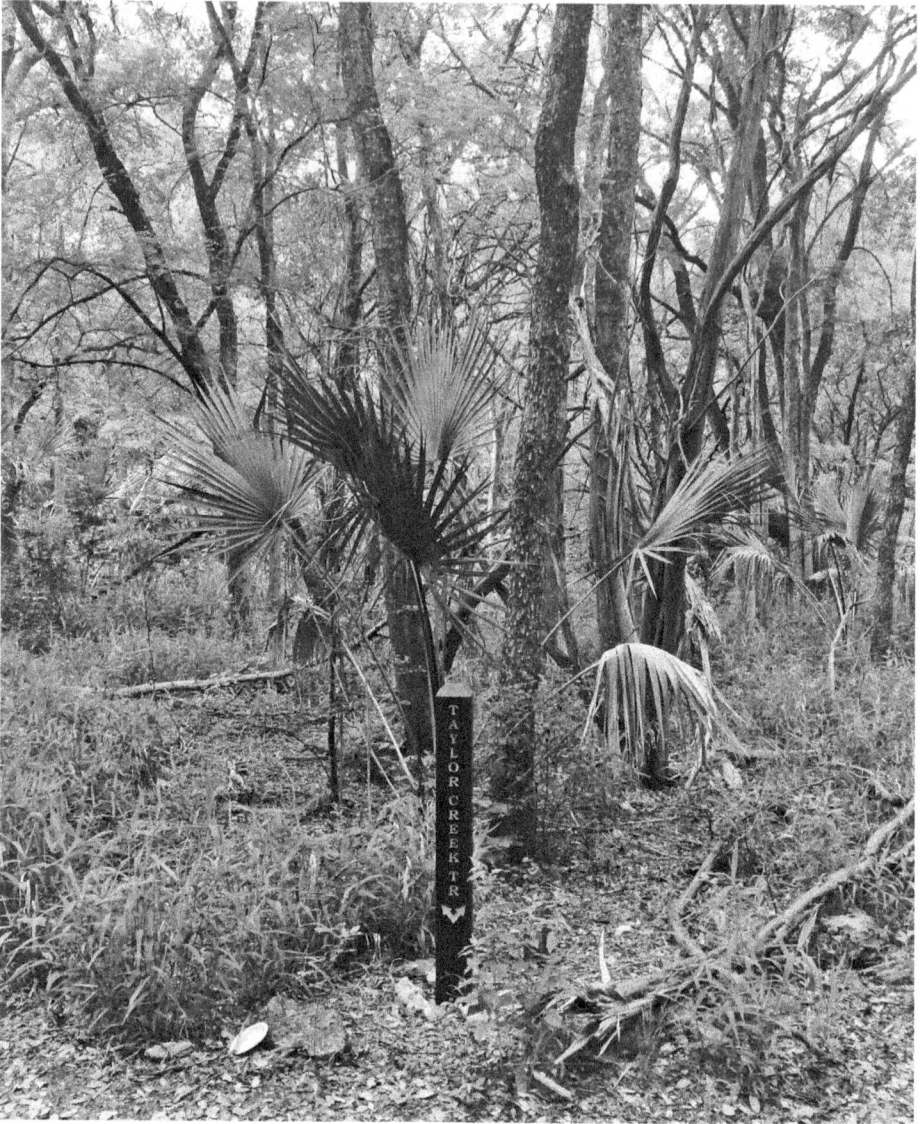

*Palmettos grow along Taylor Slough.*

paths scramble up the cliffs. Remember that Taylor Slough leads toward the lake. Pick up the easy Meadow Trail, and take a left to find the Lake Trail, from which several spurs take you to the water's edge. One leads to a short boardwalk. You can look across the quiet inlet to the boathouses and mansions on the other side. Continue west along a nice mulch trail with a rock border, and pass Laguna Gloria to end up on Old Bull Creek Road. Turn back, and look for the sign pointing left, back to the chimney swift tower and the parking area.

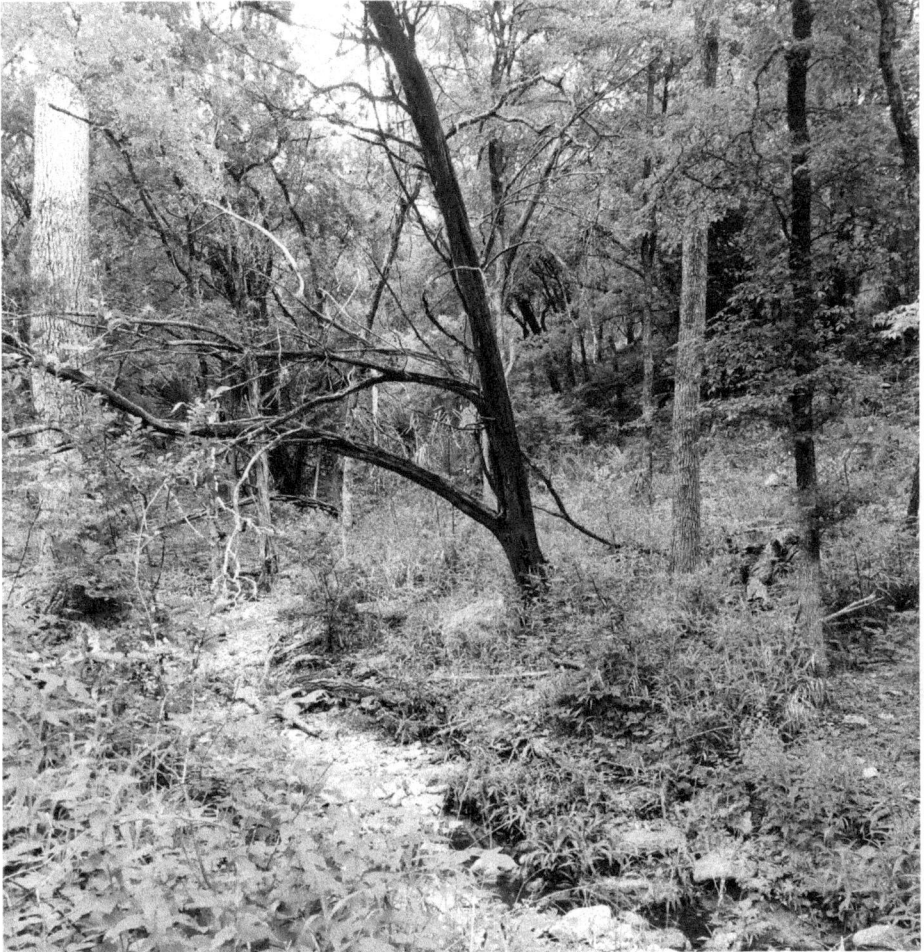

*Thick woods in Mayfield Park*

## Nearby Activities

Tour the Austin Museum of Art next door. For more information, visit thecontemporary austin.org. The Mayfield-Gutsch house and gardens can be rented for special events.

**GPS TRAILHEAD COORDINATES**

**N30° 18' 46.4" W97° 46' 17.7"**

From MoPac (Loop Road 1 in Austin) take 35th Street west 0.6 mile and prepare to veer left just past Balcones Street, staying on 35th Street 0.2 mile farther. Turn left into the small stone-gated entrance on your left, just after the turn to Mount Bonnell Road.

# 7 McKinney Roughs Nature Park: Bluffs and Bottoms

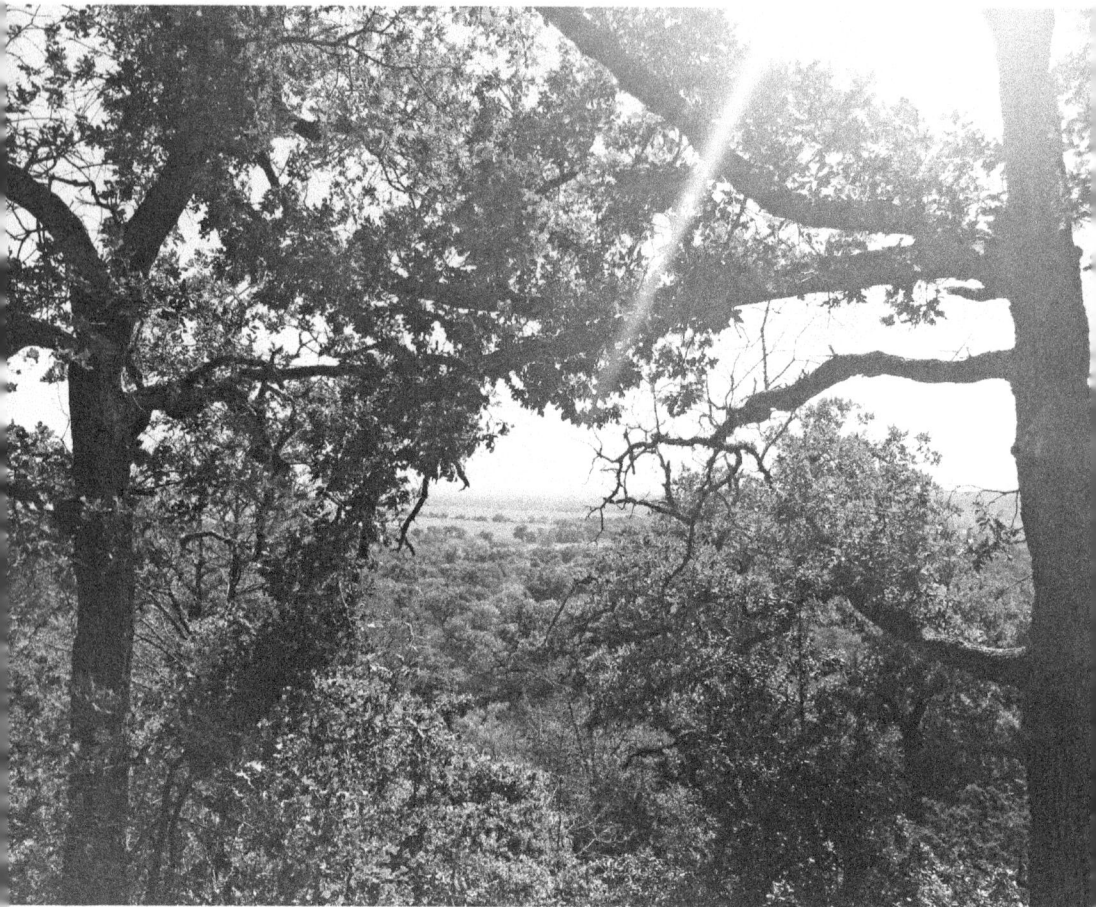

*View of the Colorado River valley from McKinney Roughs*

## In Brief

With 18 miles of hiking trails, McKinney Roughs could keep an avid hiker occupied for quite a while. This 4.5-mile, figure-eight hike offers some of the best of the park: valley views from the rim of the Colorado River valley and cool shade under the huge pecan trees in the river bottoms.

**LENGTH:** 4.5 miles

**CONFIGURATION:** Figure eight

**DIFFICULTY:** Moderate–difficult

**SCENERY:** River and valley vistas, woods, river bottom

**EXPOSURE:** Mostly shady

**TRAFFIC:** Moderate

**TRAIL SURFACE:** Pea gravel, rocks, dirt

**HIKING TIME:** 3 hours

**DRIVING DISTANCE:** 24 miles from the state capitol

**ACCESS:** Daily, 8 a.m.–sunset; $5 entrance fee per person over age 13

**WHEELCHAIR ACCESS:** Yes, first 0.5 mile of hike (Ridge Trail)

**MAPS:** tinyurl.com/mrnatureparkmap

**FACILITIES:** Picnic area, restroom at park office

**CONTACT INFORMATION:** 512-303-5073; tinyurl.com/mrnaturepark

## Description

As mentioned, there are several miles of trails in this park, all of them worth your time. Some of them are short, and they all interconnect. You'll explore eight named paths on this hike. There is much to see: views of the Colorado River valley, rich savanna, the river itself, and the river bottomland with pecan trees of staggering size. Bring the map—you'll need it. Be aware that the hike travels both hiker and hiker/equestrian trails, and also know that, if there has been rain, this route gets muddy and very difficult. Call the McKinney Roughs hotline at 512-578-7427 for trail status.

Leave the trailhead by the silo and pick up the Ridge Trail. This level, all-access path of pea gravel travels along the rim of the Colorado River valley. After only 0.1 mile you will come to the first of several short spur trails leading to overlooks with benches for contemplation. It's worth the short diversion to take in this view across the wide green valley. Return to the path and continue on through the cedars and oaks. The tangled underbrush allows only for glimpses of the hills. The Woodland Trail soon leaves left; this will be the return route. At just over 0.5 mile the Valley View Trail leaves right, and ahead is yet another junction. Dead ahead is a vista point and the end of the Ridge Trail.

Take in the marvelous view across the Colorado River valley to the fields of Wilbarger Bend, one of the last vistas around the capital city without a subdivision. Then turn back and go left, dropping onto the Bluff Trail Loop, which very soon splits. Stay right and keep downhill on a rocky trail with many switchbacks amid scattered cedars and oaks. Mesquite shrubs, grasses, and cacti thrive in small open areas, alive with birdsong and pink rock roses on my visit. The trail follows a spur, swings left to enter a valley, and follows that down to the river. Just before the 1-mile mark, you'll bisect the Bluestem Trail beneath log portals.

Ahead, the Bluff Trail Loop features consecutive fenced overlooks, each better than the last. A shortcut to the Bluestem Trail joins at the last overlook. Stay with the Bluff Trail Loop beyond the fourth overlook, and continue the ascent to meet the Bluestem Trail yet again. Now turn right onto this trail and drop off the hill you just climbed to reach the Riverside Trail down in the bottomland, rife with hardwoods and lush grasses.

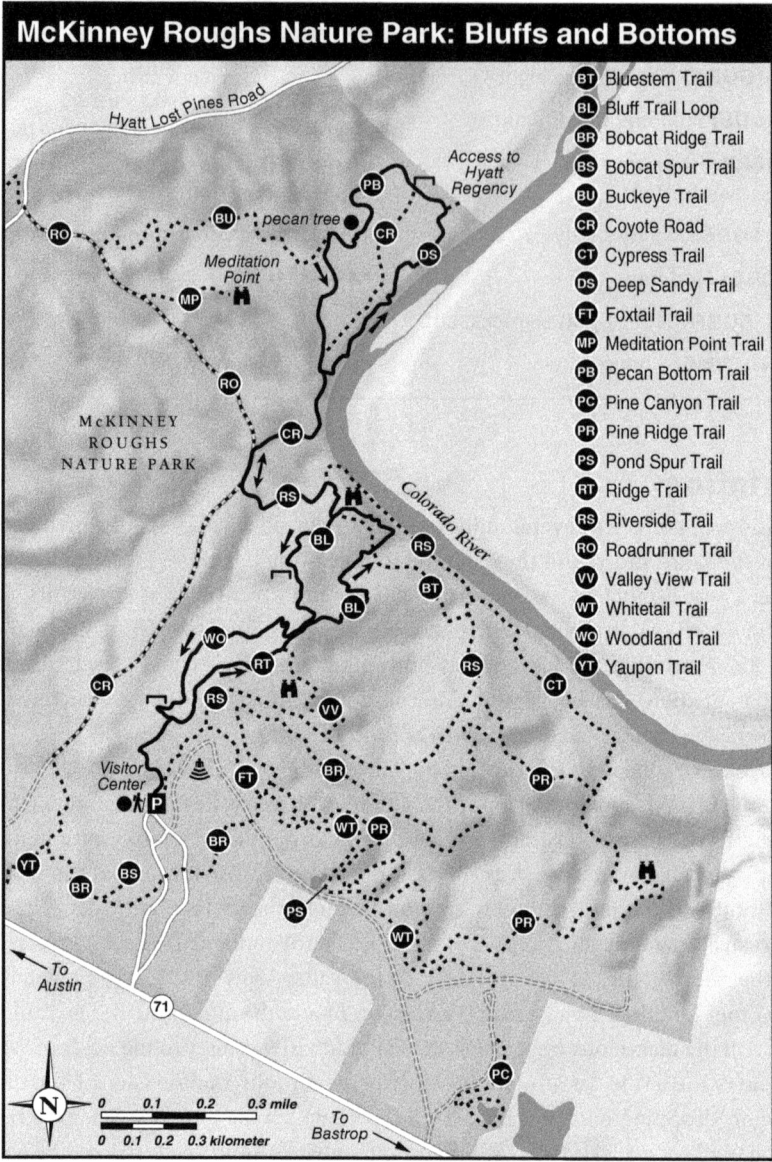

## McKinney Roughs Nature Park: Bluffs and Bottoms

- **BT** Bluestem Trail
- **BL** Bluff Trail Loop
- **BR** Bobcat Ridge Trail
- **BS** Bobcat Spur Trail
- **BU** Buckeye Trail
- **CR** Coyote Road
- **CT** Cypress Trail
- **DS** Deep Sandy Trail
- **FT** Foxtail Trail
- **MP** Meditation Point Trail
- **PB** Pecan Bottom Trail
- **PC** Pine Canyon Trail
- **PR** Pine Ridge Trail
- **PS** Pond Spur Trail
- **RT** Ridge Trail
- **RS** Riverside Trail
- **RO** Roadrunner Trail
- **VV** Valley View Trail
- **WT** Whitetail Trail
- **WC** Woodland Trail
- **YT** Yaupon Trail

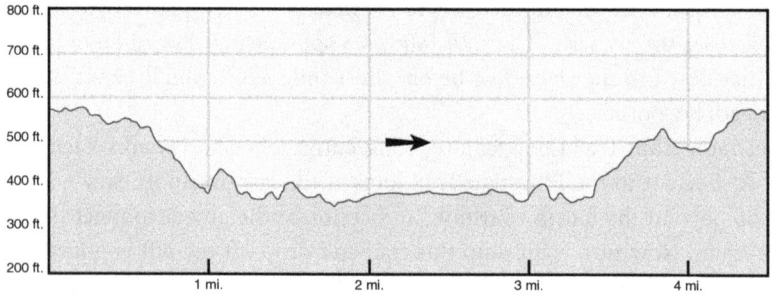

Turn left onto the Riverside Trail, working away from the river and around a wet-weather drainage through more open woodland with tall grassy underbrush. At 1.4 miles reach Coyote Road, a jeep track. Turn right here, cross the creek, and keep with Coyote Road as the Roadrunner Trail leaves left. Coyote Road, open overhead, turns left at the river, where big cottonwoods grow. You'll reach yet another junction at 1.7 miles. Turn right onto the Deep Sandy Trail. It comes even closer to the water, rolling gently amid hackberry trees, tall sycamores, and tangled vines. Pass a little shortcut to Coyote Road. The Deep Sandy trail bed is indeed soft and sandy underfoot.

Shortly before mile 2, you will see a large grass-and-gravel bar across the river, possibly occupied by fishermen. Access to the water is difficult, even where you can get to it, given the slippery mud banks. The Deep Sandy Trail makes a short, steep climb away from the river, making a sharp left as it passes access to the neighboring Hyatt resort, then meeting the end of Coyote Road, where you will find a bench. Continue straight across onto Pecan Bottom Trail.

Pecan bottoms like this one are Texas's version of the redwood forests of California—massive trees left to grow in undisturbed splendor. At 2.5 miles you will find the 200-year-old pecan tree marked on the trail map. It's unmissable, as it would take at least two people with arms stretched to reach around it. Drift back toward the hillside, passing the junction with the Buckeye Trail, before returning to Coyote Road at 2.9 miles. At this point, you will be backtracking a bit before covering new territory. Take Coyote Road, passing Roadrunner Trail and returning to Riverside Trail. Take the Riverside Trail and leave bottomland for good at the Bluestem Trail. Take the Bluestem Trail back to the Bluff Trail Loop. Turn right here, at the 3.5-mile mark, and begin covering new terrain, working sharply uphill as you pass some stunning views. One bench in a small meadow on top of a spur features sweeping views of Wilbarger Bend and beyond.

The Bluff Trail Loop ends to meet the Woodland Trail and the Ridge Trail. Take the Woodland Trail as it dips into the thickets of cedar and brush along the side of the ridge. This short trail would be a great introduction to Hill Country hiking for a novice. Another fantastic vista with a bench is reached just before the intersection with the Ridge Trail at 4.3 miles. Turn right here and backtrack a short distance to the trailhead.

## Nearby Activities

The Mark Rose Environmental Learning Center offers a variety of educational programs about the outdoors in general and McKinney Roughs in particular. It has meeting facilities, a large dining room, and dorms. The park also offers a multitude of outdoors programs.

---

**GPS TRAILHEAD COORDINATES**

**N30° 8' 26.5"  W97° 27' 33"**

From the Austin airport take TX 71 east 13.2 miles to reach McKinney Roughs Nature Park, which is on your left after the Hyatt resort.

# 8 Onion Creek Trail at McKinney Falls State Park

## In Brief

Bikers, joggers, and hikers share this loop around McKinney Falls State Park as it rambles past the shady banks of Onion Creek and the remains of Thomas McKinney's ranch.

## Description

State senator, rancher, horse breeder, trader, and privateer—Thomas McKinney was all of these, securing himself an enduring place in Texas history. He came from Galveston with a new, young wife to live on his ranch by Onion Creek in 1846, though he had purchased the land long before. McKinney Falls State Park was created from the portion of this tract donated to the state in 1971 by the Smith family, who had bought the ranch from McKinney's widow. Like the Homestead Trail, Onion Creek Loop lies within this park.

The 682-acre park contains signs of the activity that once took place here. Although the gristmill and homestead ruins are found on the Homestead Trail, the remains of McKinney's horse trainer's cabin and lines of stone fence can be seen from this path, even marking part of the park's boundary.

The hike begins by the Smith Visitor Center, currently closed due to damage from the 2013 flood. Walk away from the building and the parking lots down a short incline, toward the creek, which here tumbles or trickles over the upper falls, a popular swimming and wading area. Onion Creek is undammed, and these and the lower falls can be either a rushing torrent or a dry expanse of rock. Turn left here to begin the loop. The surface is asphalt for the entire loop and makes for an excellent short bicycle ride as well.

Watch for cyclists as you walk into the green and shady picnic area. The trail is several yards from the creek, and there are picnic tables arranged at intervals under the tall trees. The first 0.4 mile snakes through the picnic and primitive camping areas of the park. Leaving these areas, the woods thicken as the path wanders closer to the creek, glimpsed through dense greenery. Keep an eye out for painted buntings—small, colorful songbirds that nest in the park through the summer. More abundant on the Homestead Trail, they can also be seen here.

The trail passes a stone embankment on the left that was built to prevent further erosion of the hillside. An unofficial foot trail to the right ventures farther along the creekside; stay on the main path as it turns left to make a steep climb away from the water. At the top of the rise, a park bench offers a place to sit and rest or watch the birds. Cardinals are everywhere. From here on, the scenery is the familiar mix of oak and cedar, with each predominating in turn. Open meadows break up the woodlands covering this plateau.

| LENGTH: 2.7 miles | ACCESS: Daily, 8 a.m.–10 p.m.; $6 entrance fee per person over age 13 |
|---|---|
| CONFIGURATION: Loop | |
| DIFFICULTY: Easy | WHEELCHAIR ACCESS: No |
| SCENERY: Onion Creek, wildlife, wildflowers, and birds | MAPS: tinyurl.com/mckinneyfallsmap |
| EXPOSURE: Shady | FACILITIES: Restrooms, showers, picnic tables, and camping. Many stores are located nearby. |
| TRAFFIC: Moderate | |
| TRAIL SURFACE: Asphalt | CONTACT INFORMATION: |
| HIKING TIME: 1 hour | 512-243-1643; tpwd.texas.gov/state-parks/mckinney-falls |
| DRIVING DISTANCE: 10 miles from the state capitol | |

After the steep incline away from the creek, the path descends slightly, then rises again, climbing 100 feet in the next quarter of a mile. About 1.3 miles into the hike, you'll see a stone wall, dating from the mid-1800s, that once served as the land's boundary. The trail forks at 1.8 miles. Turn left and you will end up in the RV campsite area, so take the trail right and continue a gentle descent. At the fork a wooden bench allows for a rest and a chance to watch birds. In the spring, large sections of the grassy areas are occupied by deer birthing their fawns. Attentive hikers can spy the fawns hiding under the bushes or hear them calling to their mothers. These babies are not lost and should be left alone.

More of the rock wall appears 2.3 miles along the path, just after a little creek crossing. The wall still serves as the park boundary. Another bench located near here lets you sit and watch passersby as well as the deer and birds. The park headquarters is visible through the trees to the right, as are the campsites to the left. The trail crosses the park road at 2.4 miles. Directly across the road are the ruins of the cabin that belonged to John Van Hagen, McKinney's horse trainer. Cross the road to get a better look, keeping an eye out for traffic in this busy park. The last section of the hike goes through taller hardwoods, which you'll exit at 2.6 miles onto the parking lot next to the Smith Visitor Center. Avail yourself of the opportunity to cool off in the creek.

## Nearby Activities

McKinney Falls State Park offers camping, picnicking, mountain biking, swimming, and fishing.

### GPS TRAILHEAD COORDINATES

**N30° 11' 2.1"  W97° 43' 32.3"**

From downtown Austin take US 183 south and turn right onto McKinney Falls Parkway, 1.5 miles south of the junction with TX 71. After 2.7 miles turn right into the park.

## Onion Creek Trail at McKinney Falls State Park

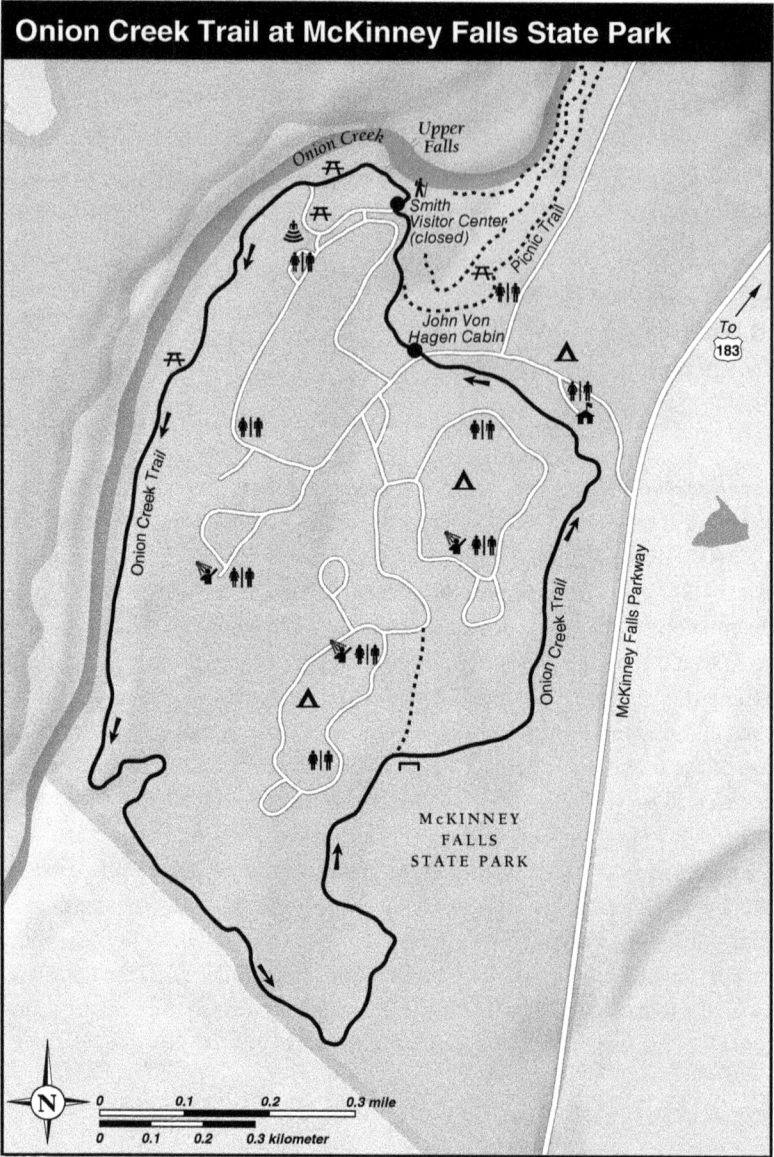

Onion Creek

Upper Falls

Smith Visitor Center (closed)

Picnic Trail

John Von Hagen Cabin

To 183

Onion Creek Trail

Onion Creek Trail

McKinney Falls Parkway

McKINNEY FALLS STATE PARK

N

| 0 | 0.1 | 0.2 | 0.3 mile |

| 0 | 0.1 | 0.2 | 0.3 kilometer |

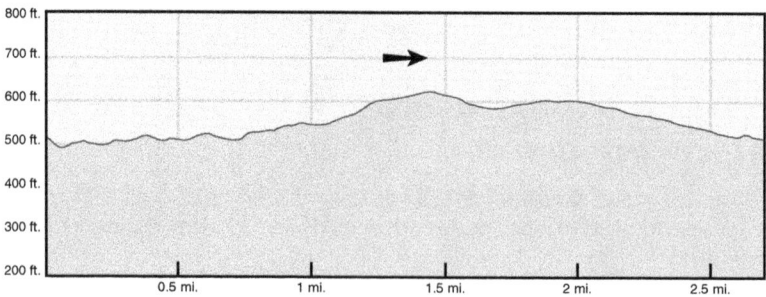

# 9 Pace Bend Park

## In Brief

The boat ramps are popular, but other than that, this laid-back park on a Lake Travis peninsula is often largely empty. Multiuse trails crisscross the central area (a wildlife preserve) and you'll likely have them to yourself—though several, designed more for off-road cycling than hiking, are a draw with that crowd.

## Description

Spicewood, the nearest town to Pace Bend Park, is home to Willie Nelson's Luck, Texas, ranch, and has retained traces of an older, kinder Austin in which men with gray ponytails pause to greet each other in run-down grocery stores. Pace Bend has been infused with some of that spirit; the park has a kind of laid-back, time-has-passed-me-by feel. Though trucks rumble along the park's main loop road to the boat ramps and beaches, if you get away from the shoreline the solitude and peace might surprise you, though there is nothing new or dramatic about the scenery for experienced Hill Country hikers. A mix of juniper and oak covers limestone knobs and rocky washes, where the brush grows thicker. Our route wanders around the eastern slopes of Pace Bend, returning via a high ridge at the park's center. Enough of the hike takes place between stands of trees to warrant a hat and sunscreen.

The chance to see wildlife is one of the attractions of this hike. Lake Travis, which surrounds the peninsula, is a natural draw for both mammals and waterfowl. Bring your binoculars and look for everything from titmice to pelicans, depending on the time of year. One other feature merits a mention: the spiders, who like to build large webs spanning the trails. Keep an eye out for them in the air ahead, and on the ground below, as tarantulas are prevalent.

Start at the North Trailhead, halfway along the stretch of Ranch Road 2322 that goes roughly east–west. Note that there are two trailheads along the road. This hike starts from the second one, if you are traveling west to east, catty-corner to the Highland Lakes Baptist Encampment.

Walk away from the road and immediately come to a five-way junction and an information sign in a clearing. The most obvious path, Powerline Trail, goes off at a slight diagonal to the left. As the name suggests, it runs dead straight and follows a line of pylons. Take the rougher path to the right of this, leaving the signboard to your left. Immediately make another left. According to the map, this should be the Pancho Trail, but when I visited the signs said PACK TRAIL. At 0.3 mile you will come to the junction with the Lefty Trail. Turn right, staying on the Pack Trail. At 0.3 mile you will come to the junction with the Lefty Trail. Turn right, staying on the Pancho Trail. The path narrows to a singletrack through scrubby cedar, then widens out.

| | |
|---|---|
| **LENGTH:** 6.1 miles | **DRIVING DISTANCE:** 34 miles from the state capitol |
| **CONFIGURATION:** Balloon loop | |
| **DIFFICULTY:** Moderate | **ACCESS:** Daily, sunrise–sunset; $10 day-use fee per vehicle |
| **SCENERY:** Lake, woods, and grasslands | **MAPS:** tinyurl.com/pacebendparkmap |
| **EXPOSURE:** Moderate | **FACILITIES:** Restrooms |
| **TRAFFIC:** Light | **CONTACT INFORMATION:** 512-264-1482; parks.traviscountytx.gov/find-a-park/pace-bend |
| **TRAIL SURFACE:** Dirt | |
| **HIKING TIME:** 3 hours | |

At 0.6 mile the Chicken Foot Trail leaves right. Keep left, staying on the Pancho Trail. At 0.9 mile there is another junction. A steep, rocky trail leads down to the left. Take this, and in 120 yards turn right at the T-junction onto Well Road Trail. Thick juniper pushes up against this wide jeep road, which crosses a drainage and bends left, heading south. Three trails come in from the right at this point, though they are indistinct and not signed. You will return by the last one, which comes back to the Well Road Trail down another rocky slope.

At 1.2 miles (at marker post 700) Wookiee Way dives off to the left. (Props to whoever named these trails.) Wookiee Way, a narrow singletrack for its entire length, makes a 3-mile series of squiggles through woods and ravines and over plateaus. It joins the Abby Road Trail, which meets Well Road at its southern end. (You could choose to amble down Well Road and pick up this route again at that point, making for a much shorter hike.) Wookiee Way is undoubtedly a lot of fun on a mountain bike, and some hikers might get frustrated at the endless twists and turns that rob you of a sense of moving toward a destination. But take it and you will have the reward of a more challenging hike that brings you closer to the nature and wildlife in the park and presents views of the park's western coves and the houses and docks of Lago Vista across the lake.

There are several forks along the earlier part of Wookiee Way, and it doesn't really matter if you make different choices than those listed here, as the paths will rejoin. At 1.4 miles, go left at the first one. You'll soon start making a succession of crossings of a little creek. At 1.7 miles an alternate path comes in from the right, and from a clearing you'll get the first of the vistas over the lake. At the next fork, at 2 miles, turn right. A path comes in from the left. Here the trail is quite close to the park road, and there are more views.

At the 2.9-mile mark, you come into the open at an old quarry, crossing the topmost of descending terraces. Keep left at the junction, following the sign that says SOUTH QUARRY. The path descends through the quarry on a section that really does cry out for an off-road bike, especially when you come to a banked wooden bridge. At 3.9 miles the Rock Garden of Greatness Trail leaves left and shortly thereafter returns from its journey. At 4.1 miles come—at last—to Abby Road, and turn right, following a creek and crossing

# Pace Bend Park

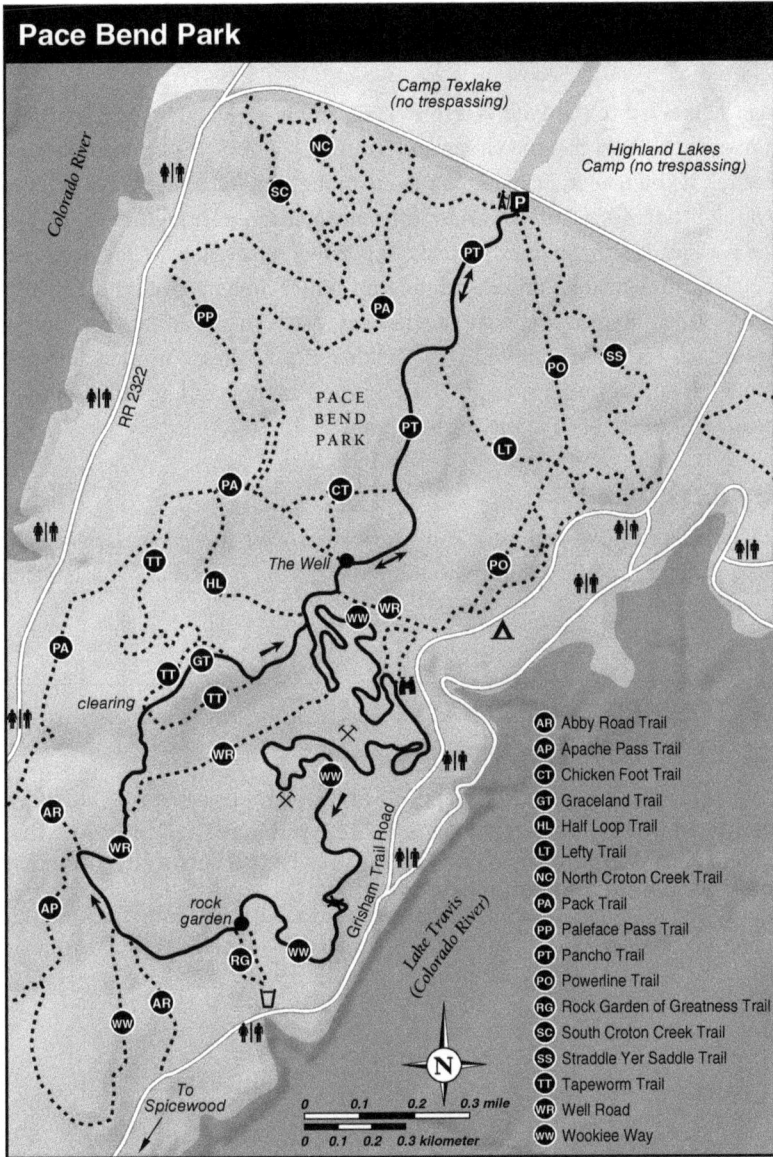

*Camp Texlake (no trespassing)*

*Highland Lakes Camp (no trespassing)*

*Colorado River*

*RR 2322*

PACE BEND PARK

*The Well*

*clearing*

*rock garden*

*Grisham Trail Road*

*Lake Travis (Colorado River)*

*To Spicewood*

| | |
|---|---|
| AR | Abby Road Trail |
| AP | Apache Pass Trail |
| CT | Chicken Foot Trail |
| GT | Graceland Trail |
| HL | Half Loop Trail |
| LT | Lefty Trail |
| NC | North Croton Creek Trail |
| PA | Pack Trail |
| PP | Paleface Pass Trail |
| PT | Pancho Trail |
| PO | Powerline Trail |
| RG | Rock Garden of Greatness Trail |
| SC | South Croton Creek Trail |
| SS | Straddle Yer Saddle Trail |
| TT | Tapeworm Trail |
| WR | Well Road |
| WW | Wookiee Way |

0   0.1   0.2   0.3 mile
0   0.1   0.2   0.3 kilometer

N

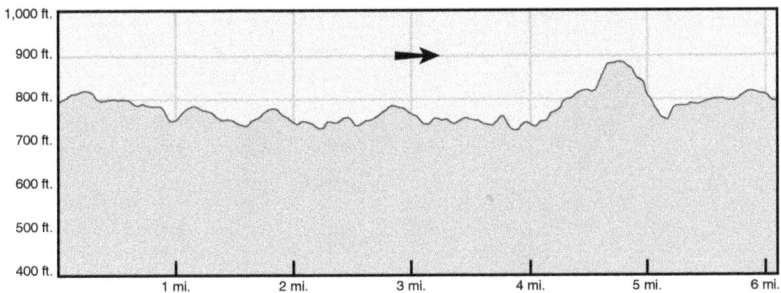

the power line. At 4.3 miles look for a fence to your right. Turn right and go alongside this fence, which prevents access to some infrastructure, and come to the southern end of Well Road.

A sign points left to the Well Worth It Trail, and it is indeed if you have the stamina. (Recent maps now label this the Graceland Trail.) This track leads up to the ridge mentioned earlier. If you take it, keep left at the next junction, 0.1 mile farther. In another 0.1 mile go straight, across a little clearing, into more cedar, continuing on the Graceland Trail. The path leads onto an open plateau. At 908 feet, you reach the highest point of this hike. Keep left at the next junction, and the trail comes to the top of the steep hill leading down to Well Road. Before you make the descent, pause to take in the view one last time. When you reach the main trail you will have hiked 5.1 miles. Turn left, retracing your steps, going left and right again to get back on the Pancho Trail. At the 6-mile mark, be sure to turn right to get back to the starting point.

## Nearby Activities

The park offers primitive camping and a few improved sites that usually need to be reserved in advance. Poodie's Hilltop Roadhouse, on TX 71, has that old Austin ambience and live music.

---

### GPS TRAILHEAD COORDINATES
**N30° 27' 57.2"  W98° 0' 55.2"**

From the intersection of Ranch to Market Road 620 and TX 71, take TX 71 west 10 miles to RM 2322. Turn right on RM 2322 and travel 5.2 miles to the park entrance. From there, follow the road 3 miles to the second trailhead, opposite the sign to Kate and Johnson Coves.

# 10 Pine Ridge Loop at McKinney Roughs Nature Park

## In Brief

This hike explores the McKinney Roughs from top to bottom and back again. Start on a high plateau and trace a wild ravine, reaching a crow's-nest promontory with far-reaching views. Descend to the Colorado River and walk through the woods along the water's edge. Look for relics of the land's ranching days along the way.

## Description

In 1995 the Lower Colorado River Authority acquired the land now known as McKinney Roughs and built a first-rate environmental education facility to complement the 1,100-acre preserve situated on the Colorado River between Austin and Bastrop. The park has 18 miles of hiking and equestrian trails that explore its rugged folds, known as roughs because the steep ravines made agriculture difficult. They also provided refuge for frontier outlaws. This trail follows and then descends into one of these long, winding wooded canyons.

Ecologically the park is an unusual blend of swaths of oak savanna, pine woods, and grassy blackland prairie—all in addition to the overgrown riparian zone. Loblolly pines like those in nearby Bastrop and Buescher State Parks flourish in the sandier soils found in the area. The cedar trees in the park are eastern red cedar and not the Ashe juniper of the Hill Country.

The park trailhead is beside the dining hall, which is past the metal silo next to the park office. Find the marked Riverside Trail and step into the thick brush on a wooded plateau. At nearly 0.2 mile you'll reach an intersection with the wooden portals that mark many trail junctions at McKinney Roughs. Cross the wider trail, suitable for horses as well as hikers, and keep forward, now on the Pine Ridge Trail, which is pedestrian-only. (Foxtail Trail leaves to the right; Riverside Trail continues left and will be your return route.) Blackjack oaks and cedars grow tall over the thriving shrubbery. At this junction you are close to the western end of the ravine that is the main feature of the first part of the hike, though the thick underbrush means you can only guess at the surrounding topography.

More portals await you at the junction with the Bobcat Ridge Trail at 0.3 mile. Cross the Whitetail Trail at 0.5 mile. This trail, predominantly for equestrians, shadows the Pine Ridge Trail as it heads to the TX 71 trailhead. You'll notice pine trees replacing the cedar,

| | |
|---|---|
| **LENGTH:** 3.7 miles | **DRIVING DISTANCE:** 24 miles from the state capitol |
| **CONFIGURATION:** Loop | |
| **DIFFICULTY:** Moderate | **ACCESS:** Daily, 8 a.m.–sunset; $5 entrance fee per person over age 13 |
| **SCENERY:** Steep ravines, pine–oak woodlands | **WHEELCHAIR ACCESS:** Yes, at start of hike |
| **EXPOSURE:** Mostly shady, some exposed | **MAPS:** tinyurl/mrnatureparkmap |
| | **FACILITIES:** Picnic area, restroom at park office |
| **TRAFFIC:** Moderate | |
| **TRAIL SURFACE:** Natural surfaces | **CONTACT INFORMATION:** 512-303-5073; tinyurl.com/mrnaturepark |
| **HIKING TIME:** 2.25 hours | |

and to your left the ravine getting deeper. Astonishingly tall trees are growing in the wild, earth-banked canyon. The trail winds back and forth around side valleys, passing the Pond Spur Trail, which leads to an old stock pond at the edge of the park, the first piece of ranching history on this hike. Meadow areas open up on the plateau to your right.

At 0.9 mile there is a high outcrop with a picnic table and a bench, which overlooks a confluence of green wooded valleys, something more like Oregon than Texas. One spindly pine sticks up above all the others in the distance. A sign explains that, since the wildfire of 2008, with less vegetation to suck it up, water has flowed constantly into the stream below, no doubt fueling the expanse of greenery before you.

Come around the top of the second side canyon, and pass the remains of a few old sheds. At 1.3 miles walk through a meadow where an old barn is still standing, and then cross over a dam at the end of the third side canyon. A jeep track comes in from the right. The trail emerges from the woods along the canyon and heads across the bluestem grass–covered plateau. It traverses a knife-edge ridgeline that widens to a little knob standing over the sea of green. Keep right to circle around this high point to find a contemplation bench and a far-reaching view of Wilbarger Bend and the river valley. This is the 2-mile point. Take in the vista before beginning your descent toward the Colorado River by switchbacks on cedar steps.

Reach a streambed and follow it a bit through a jungle of branches and creeper. Cross the branch on a wooden bridge, and then ascend to the intersection with the Cypress Trail at 2.2 miles. Look for clay erosion-created ravines on the way up. Turn right onto Cypress Trail, and head down from the spur to the shady riparian forest in which sycamore, cottonwood, and hackberry thrive. The trail heads upstream along the Colorado on the bank that slopes down to the river. Despite the trail's name, there are no cypresses here.

At 2.6 miles go down steps to the river's edge, coming to the end of the Riverside Trail. Horses have churned up the trail getting to the water. Go under a wooden portal to continue along the Cypress Trail for a little bit; it soon rejoins the Riverside Trail. Turn

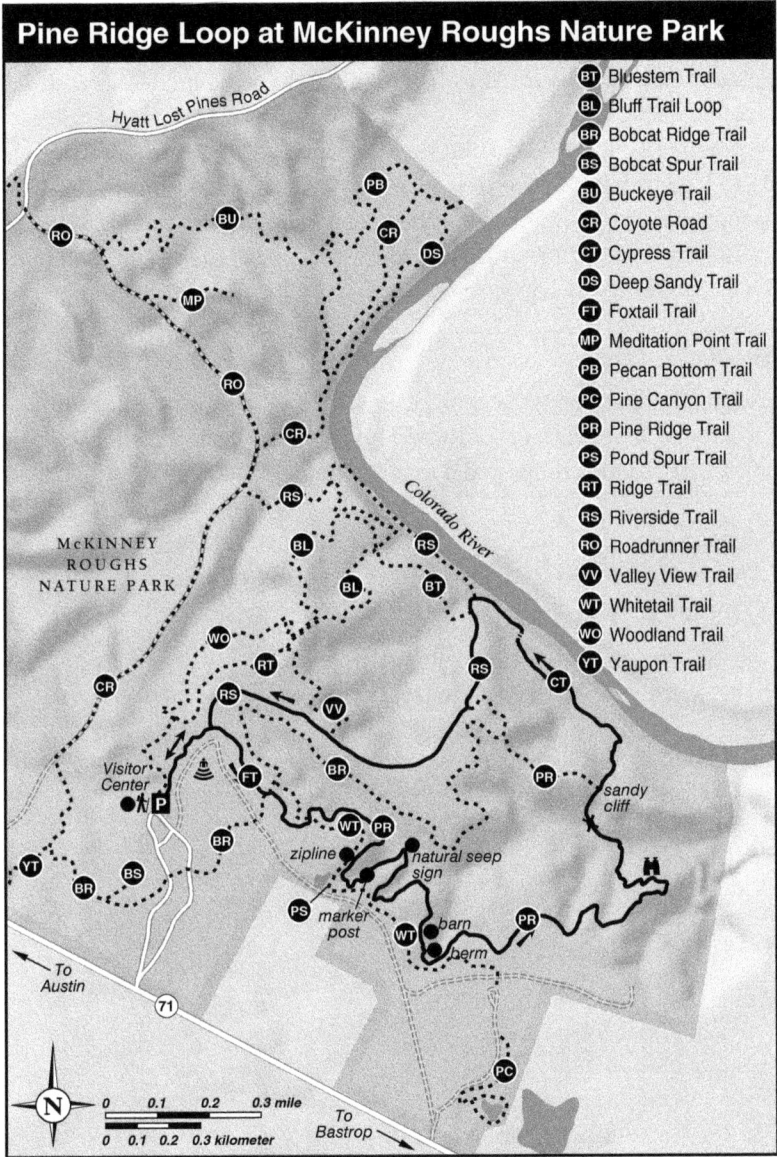

## Pine Ridge Loop at McKinney Roughs Nature Park

BT Bluestem Trail
BL Bluff Trail Loop
BR Bobcat Ridge Trail
BS Bobcat Spur Trail
BU Buckeye Trail
CR Coyote Road
CT Cypress Trail
DS Deep Sandy Trail
FT Foxtail Trail
MP Meditation Point Trail
PB Pecan Bottom Trail
PC Pine Canyon Trail
PR Pine Ridge Trail
PS Pond Spur Trail
RT Ridge Trail
RS Riverside Trail
RO Roadrunner Trail
VV Valley View Trail
WT Whitetail Trail
WO Woodland Trail
YT Yaupon Trail

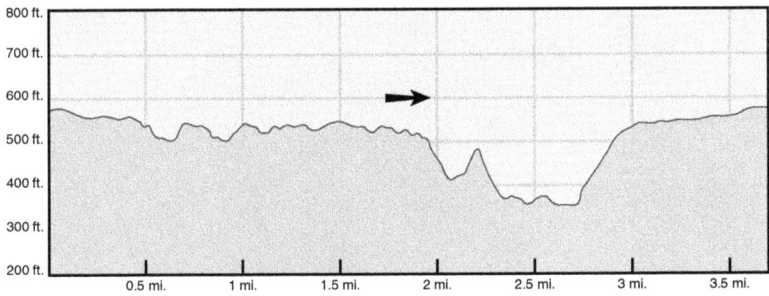

left onto the wider trail, passing the Bluestem Trail coming in from your right. Climb the hill away from the river, turning around to enjoy more views of the lands across the Colorado. The path stays exposed for the climb and for the mile-long walk across the plateau back to the trailhead.

Bobcat Ridge Trail comes in from your left when you reach the level savanna. Keep forward as the path makes its way through grassy clearings and scattered brush and cedar coppices topped with oaks. Valley View Trail comes in from your right at 3.3 miles. Reach a final trail junction at 3.5 miles, turning right to stay on Riverside Trail, and retrace your steps to return to the trailhead.

## Nearby Activities

The Mark Rose Environmental Learning Center offers a variety of educational programs about the outdoors in general and McKinney Roughs in particular. The park also has meeting facilities, a large dining room, and dorms and offers a multitude of outdoors programs.

---

**GPS TRAILHEAD COORDINATES**

**N30° 8' 27.9"  W97° 27' 31.5"**

From the Austin airport take TX 71 east 13.2 miles to reach McKinney Roughs Nature Park, on your left after the Hyatt resort.

---

# 11 River Place Nature Trail

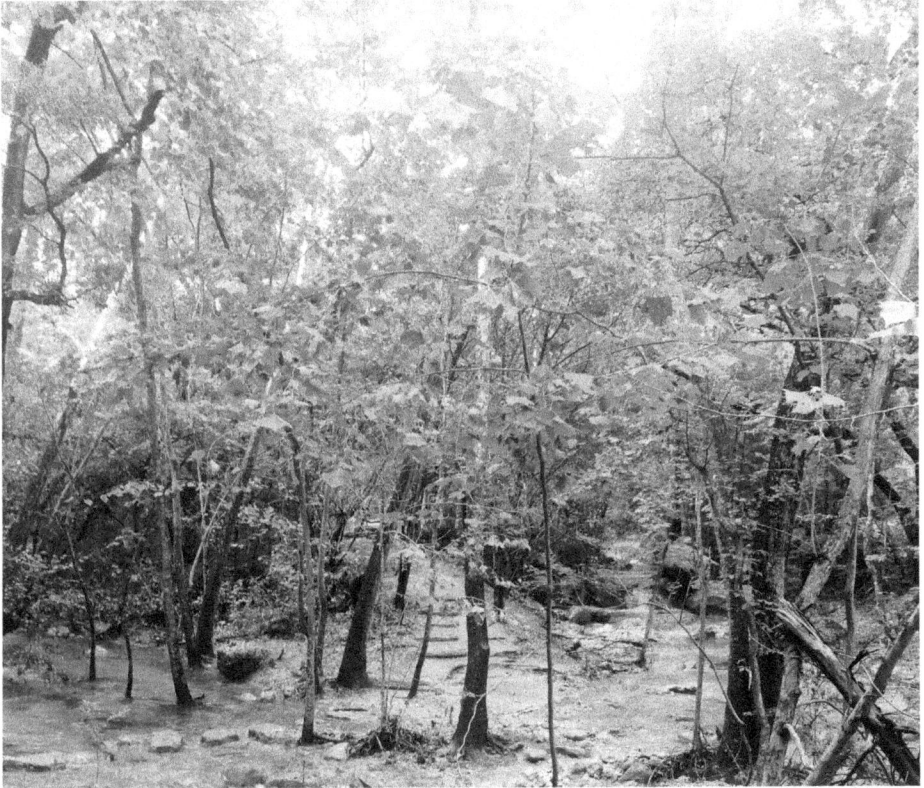

*Panther Hollow Creek*

## In Brief

Urban planning at its best, this rugged hike down the deep Panther Hollow Creek canyon is getting a great reputation, thanks to its mix of accessibility, natural beauty, and technical challenge.

## Description

Reopened in 2014 after some squabbling between the River Place MUD, the city of Austin, and the U.S. Fish & Wildlife Service, this well-maintained and increasingly popular trail is some of the best hiking in Austin for those who like a little challenge with their nature. It might be better named the Trail of a Thousand Steps because the first mile of the hike goes up and down countless steep stairs. Overall the first section drops down 300

| | |
|---|---|
| **LENGTH:** 5.4 miles | **DRIVING DISTANCE:** 15 miles from the state capitol |
| **CONFIGURATION:** Out-and-back | |
| **DIFFICULTY:** Difficult | **ACCESS:** Daily, sunrise–sunset; free |
| **SCENERY:** Cedar breaks, creek canyon | **WHEELCHAIR ACCESS:** No |
| **EXPOSURE:** Mostly shady | **MAPS:** On information board at trailhead and downloadable via QR code |
| **TRAFFIC:** Moderate–heavy | |
| **TRAIL SURFACE:** Natural surfaces | **FACILITIES:** None |
| **HIKING TIME:** 3–4 hours | **CONTACT INFORMATION:** 512-246-0498; riverplacehoa.org/mud |

feet through wild ravines and cedar breaks into the Panther Hollow valley. Apparently the creek got its name because ranchers kept finding dead goats in a hollow, though no one ever saw a panther or mountain lion.

Like many Austin hikes, River Place Nature Trail gives quick access to the kind of wild nature that you might think you would have to drive to Bandera, if not Colorado, to experience. But west Austin has spread over some of the prettiest topography of the Hill Country; between the subdivisions, the green valleys retain their charm and profuse vitality. Kudos to the River Place planners for including this trail through one of the most beautiful of those valleys.

From the trailhead, the path winds north and west through the cedar-covered slopes at the top end of the vale, coming to the upper reaches of Panther Hollow Creek after a strenuous mile of hiking. Another mile brings you into the leafy, shady creek bottom, where the trail might be muddy but descends more gently until it ends at a boardwalk overlooking a pond. After rainfall, the music of water dripping, splashing, and falling, overlaid with birdsong, will accompany the sound of your steps.

Step from the sidewalk into the juniper forest—as mentioned, an instant transition—and come to a signboard crammed with lots of information about the hike, including a map. The steps begin immediately. The trail angles northeast along the side of a hill, heading toward four ravines that it will traverse before coming to the main valley. At nearly 0.2 mile a bench overlooks the first ravine, a narrow, steep chasm where trees and bushes proliferate. The trail crosses the drainage under a steep drop-off. To the right, rocks and moisture combine to make a little grotto. Steep steps lead up away from this crossing. You'll come to the quarter-mile marker, which is a sign denoting this as the Canyon Trail and giving the mileage to both ends of the trail. These signs appear every quarter mile in both directions, another example of the planners' thoughtfulness.

Occasionally views open up of houses, the golf course, and green ridges as the trail marches up and down the steep hillsides. At 0.7 mile cross a fainter path at right angles on a descent. The left path leads to the golf course; a sign marks it as the first of two emergency exits. At 0.9 mile a short spur goes right to the Upper Creek Wall, and then you come to the steps leading down into the wooded Panther Hollow Creek valley. The rest of the hike stays almost entirely under the shady tree canopy as it follows the stream

## River Place Nature Trail

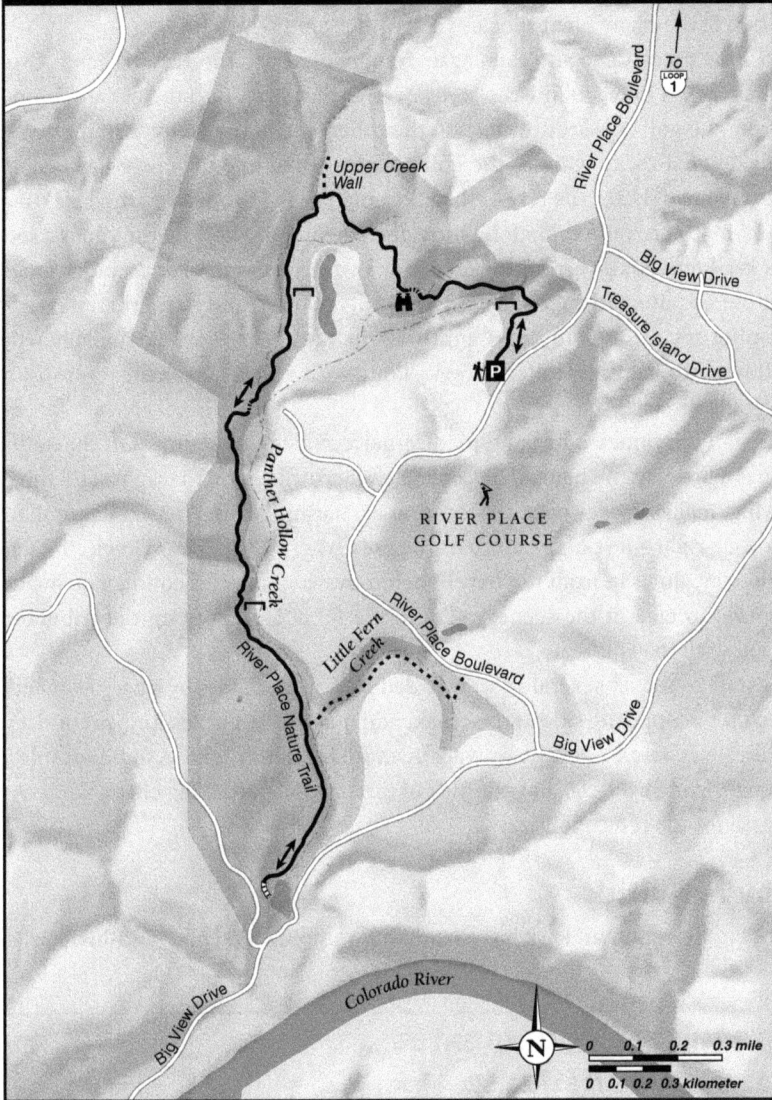

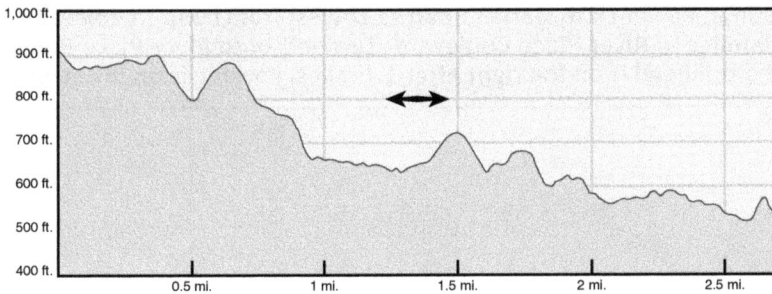

Upper Creek
Wall

River Place Boulevard

To
LOOP
1

Big View Drive

Treasure Island Drive

P

Panther Hollow Creek

RIVER PLACE
GOLF COURSE

Little Fern Creek

River Place Boulevard

River Place Nature Trail

Big View Drive

Big View Drive

Colorado River

N

| 0 | 0.1 | 0.2 | 0.3 mile |

| 0 | 0.1 | 0.2 | 0.3 kilometer |

1,000 ft.
900 ft.
800 ft.
700 ft.
600 ft.
500 ft.
400 ft.

0.5 mi.    1 mi.    1.5 mi.    2 mi.    2.5 mi.

downhill almost to the confluence with Lake Travis. Feeder creeks come in from left and right, and someone has set benches at the prettiest spots. Inland sea oats and milkweed are just two of the many plant species you will see along the path.

Cross the creek once and then again, coming back to the eastern bank. Cross once more; then, at 1.4 miles follow the steps over a spur, back into the cedar. You may hear voices from the golf course, now just on the other side of the creek. Another emergency exit leads down a rocky wash to the golf course. Come to a tall chain-link fence, which will stay to your right for the rest of the hike, and then to more steps that lead to a feeder creek crossing. The trail keeps along the right side of the valley. Below you is a set of falls.

The trail moves away from the creek for a while, passing over a sudden small opening where mesquite and cactus have seized their opportunity and then descending an almost spiral set of steps to cross another tributary. There are larger falls where this stream flows into Panther Hollow Creek, along with a view across the treetops to a bluff and the golf course.

The trail continues down the picture-perfect glen, sometimes on the valley floor, sometimes a little up the bank. The canyon wall crowds in on the right, and the creek, if it is flowing, makes its way over a succession of charming falls. At 2.3 miles look for a fern bluff on your right—just one feature of the area where Little Fern Creek, in fact quite a large tributary, flows in from the left. Benches overlooking this confluence make a good resting place to take in the scenery. The Little Fern Trail goes up the tributary valley, should you wish to explore it.

The trail goes over several short boarded platforms, passes by a narrow meadow that opens up on the opposite side of the creek, and makes a last little climb around a wooded flank to arrive at a smart new boardwalk overlooking a little lake. A fountain splashes and a swan might glide by. Relax in your pick of three wooden rocking chairs while you catch your breath for the return journey.

## Nearby Activities

Emma Long Metropolitan Park has swimming, camping, and hike-and-bike trails.

### GPS TRAILHEAD COORDINATES
**N30° 22' 25.6"  W97° 51' 23.8"**

In Austin, take Ranch to Market Road 2222 west from Loop 1 (MoPac Expressway) 9 miles to River Place Boulevard. Turn left onto River Place Boulevard, and the trailhead is on the right after 1.7 miles. Parking is on the street.

# 12 Shoal Creek Greenbelt

## In Brief

From the high-rises of downtown to a deep pool under an overhanging bluff, this ribbon of greenbelt—once the town's western boundary—is popular with moms and kids, dog lovers, and athletes. Informative signs add historical background to the city scenery, trail architecture, and natural surroundings.

## Description

Though it is true that an urban hike can only get so woodsy, and the sound of traffic on Lamar Boulevard will accompany you for the duration of this walk, there are some surprisingly tranquil spots along the way. There is also a sense of going back in time and seeing the land as it was before and during the development of the settlement that became our capital. The Parks Department has put up a few signs that tell some of the stories of this transformation—snapshots of the history of Austin and Texas. Despite the noise, concrete, and construction, perhaps you can see this place as it once was, a pretty valley with freshwater and shade, and allow the city to grow up around you in your mind's eye.

Stand on the pedestrian bridge, and take a look up and down Shoal Creek. This spring-fed stream is 9 miles long. Construction has closed off the part of the trail that joins the Lady Bird Lake Loop, so this is the starting point for now. This first section from Third to Ninth Street is definitely set in the modern world, under the towering presence of Austin's increasingly Dubai-like skyline. The creek banks have been shored up to support the weight of the condominiums that line them, and though there are trees shading the path, most of the time nature trickles through a setting that is designed to restrain it. Even here, though, you can catch birdsong above the city noise.

Go down a few steps and follow the path north along the channel. Continue around a bend, and the way forks; go right, down a slope to the creek bed. A concrete boardwalk leads under West Avenue, past some willow trees, and then gives out. You must step down onto a little cement dam, the hike's lowest point, to cross to the other side of the creek.

Crunch along a rocky bar on the eastern side, and find a very short section of sidewalk. Almost immediately you must make your way back across the creek over some stones. Go under Fifth Street. Next is the Sixth Street bridge, the first historic landmark of the hike. Austin's oldest bridge is a beautiful structure of three masonry arches that was built in 1887, allowing developers access to land west of Shoal Creek.

At the Ninth Street bridge, a more modern design, the boardwalk crosses to the eastern side of the creek and the path emerges into the sunlight along the edge of grassy Duncan Park. The southern portion of this park used to be an unofficial BMX zone, but the riders and skateboarders now use a new facility next to House Park. You might hear

| | |
|---|---|
| **LENGTH:** 6.4 miles | **DRIVING DISTANCE:** 1 mile from the state capitol |
| **CONFIGURATION:** Out-and-back | |
| **DIFFICULTY:** Moderate | **ACCESS:** Daily, 5 a.m.–10 p.m.; no fees or permits required |
| **SCENERY:** Wooded city parks, urban creek, scattered forest | **WHEELCHAIR ACCESS:** Yes |
| **EXPOSURE:** Partly sunny, partly shady | **MAPS:** None |
| **TRAFFIC:** Moderate–heavy | **FACILITIES:** Water fountain, restroom at Pease Park |
| **TRAIL SURFACE:** Rock, pea gravel, dirt | **CONTACT INFORMATION:** 512-974-6700; austintexas.gov/department/ parks-and-recreation |
| **HIKING TIME:** 2.75 hours | |

laughter through the trees from the deck of the Shoal Creek Saloon. At the end of 11th Street a short spur angles back down to the creek.

Cross under the 12th Street bridge and look north, across 15th Street. The line of hills that marks the edge of Judges' Hill and West Campus can now be visualized as the eastern side of the Shoal Creek valley. To your right are the skateboarders and the House Park stadium, built in 1939 on land donated by Edward M. House, a diplomat who served under President Woodrow Wilson.

The concrete path continues north and goes under the low Lamar Boulevard bridge and then the high 15th Street roadway, a structure that spans the entire valley. For a brief stretch you are on the Lamar Boulevard sidewalk. At 1.2 miles turn left into Pease Park, crossing the creek on an arched iron trestle bridge. Look right for a view up the leafy watercourse. Pease Park was established in 1875 on land bought by the sitting Texas governor, Elisha Pease. These days it is home to one of Austin's most iconic activities: the annual Eeyore's Birthday festival. The disc golf course that was such a draw for youth has been moved to Roy G. Guerrero Park.

Turn right onto a wide gravel path when you enter the park. The bottom end of the park is full of playgrounds, volleyball courts, and long concrete picnic tables. The trail goes up a wooded hill and over a bluff, from which there is a good view north. Descend into the more natural north end of Pease Park, where you can pause and enjoy the shade of some trees at one of the picnic tables. Perhaps General Custer enjoyed the same shade. A sign says that his troops bivouacked here during the winter of 1865–1866. Many of the men perished from cholera, and their bodies were uncovered by later flooding.

The surface changes to rocks for a stretch once you go under 24th Street, and the going can be rough. Houses of the Pemberton Heights neighborhood are visible at the top of the wooded bluff to your left. A grove of large oak trees lies between the trail and the creek. From here to 29th Street is an off-leash area for dogs and is correspondingly popular with their owners. At 2.2 miles you pass Dog Park on your left and then come to the parking area at Shoal Creek Boulevard and Gaston Avenue. Notice that the Shoal Creek valley has narrowed at this point.

## Shoal Creek Greenbelt

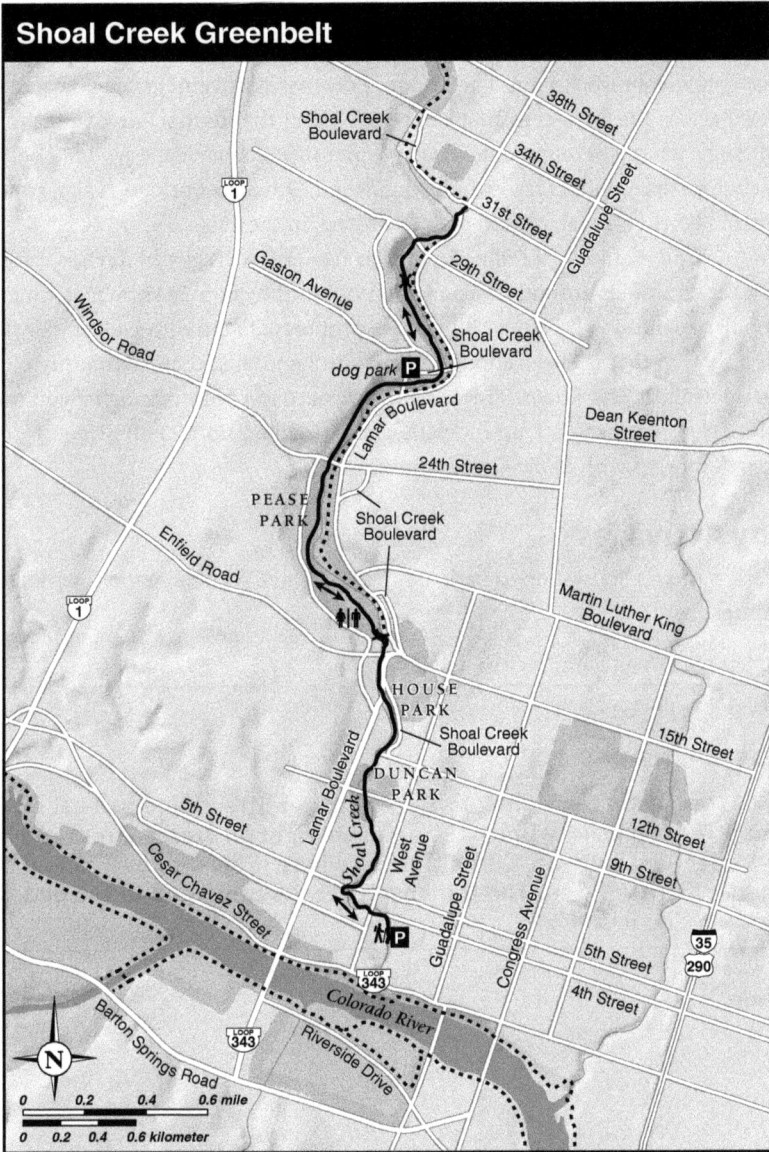

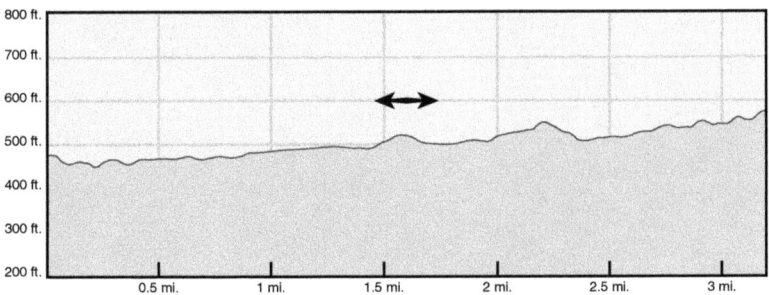

Cross Shoal Creek Boulevard again, and climb through a wooded area, one of the prettiest sections of the hike. At 2.7 miles the concrete walkway veers right to cross the creek just below Split Rock Pool. The bridge, a recent improvement, is dedicated to Janet Long Fish, whose idea it was to build this path along the disappearing Comanche Trail roadbed. Some exercise equipment sits on a wider piece of bank at a wooded bend in the river just before the architecturally undistinguished 29th Street bridge. A sign commemorates Austin's brief outbreak of gold rush fever back in the 1890s.

Past this bridge, there's a dramatic shift in scenery. A craggy bluff rises to the right, and the path scrambles around it. The wide pool in the creek is known as Blue Hole, a once-popular swimming hole now on private property. The trail travels under the overhang on a section that is sheer enough to require handrails, then summarily ejects you onto the sidewalk at 31st Street. This is a good turnaround point, though if you walk west along 31st Street you can pick up the path again as it goes up to 38th Street. From there the bike trail merges with Shoal Creek Boulevard.

## Nearby Activities

Pease Park is the most developed park along the Shoal Creek Greenbelt, with play areas and picnic tables.

---

**GPS TRAILHEAD COORDINATES**

**N30° 16' 2"  W97° 45' 2.2"**

From I-35 in Austin take Exit 234, Cesar Chavez Street, and go east on Cesar Chavez Street 4 blocks to Brazos Street. Turn right on Brazos Street and left on Third Street. Continue on Third Street to where it dead-ends at Shoal Creek, and park where you can. The trailhead is at the other end of the pedestrian bridge over Shoal Creek.

# 13 Spicewood Valley Trail

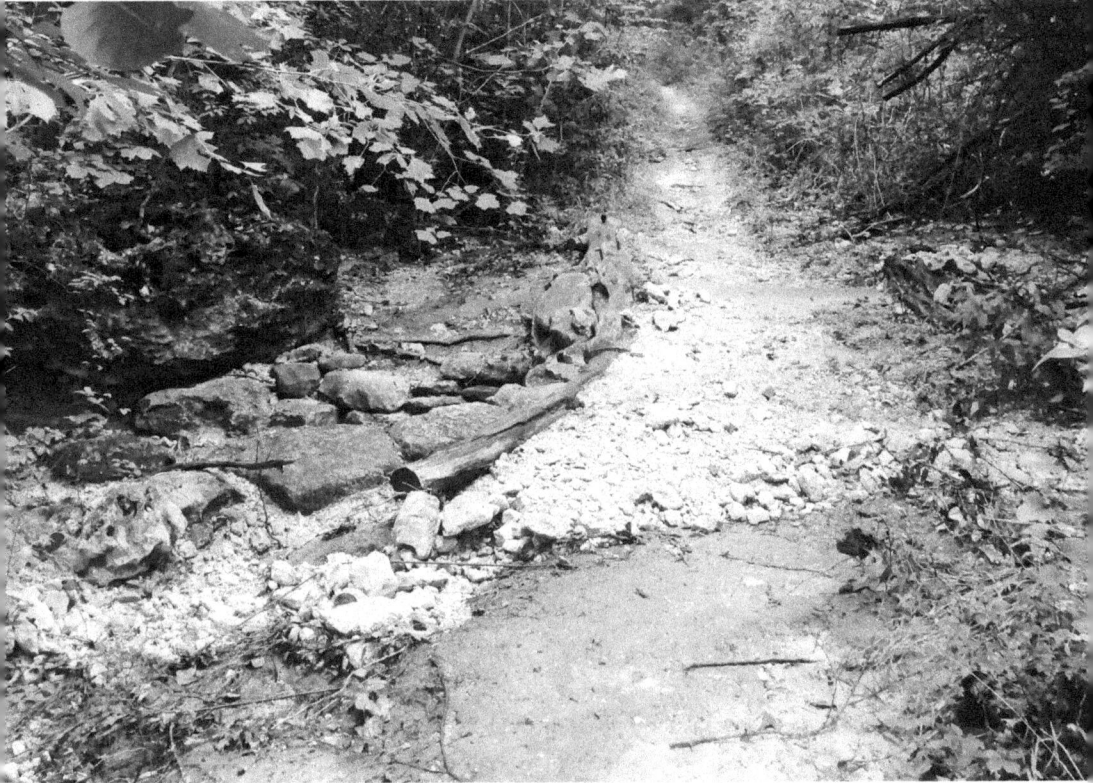

*A rough patch along the trail*

## In Brief

This suburban trail is tucked away in a deeply wooded canyon through which a tributary of Bull Creek flows. The shady trek goes up the bluff-bordered forest corridor, passing by spring branches, big trees, and an old homesite. At the end there are high cascades.

## Description

This green trail corridor in the suburban hills of north Austin is so hidden from view that I bet many nearby residents don't even know it's there. The Spicewood Valley Trail, built by Austin YouthWorks Environmental Corps in late 2005, isn't well marked or publicized but serves as an example of how to integrate quality wilderness-type paths into a populated area.

**LENGTH:** 2.6 miles

**CONFIGURATION:** Out-and-back

**DIFFICULTY:** Easy

**SCENERY:** Wooded creek valley

**EXPOSURE:** Shady

**TRAFFIC:** Moderate

**TRAIL SURFACE:** Gravel, natural surfaces

**HIKING TIME:** 1.5 hours

**DRIVING DISTANCE:** 17 miles from the state capitol

**ACCESS:** Daily, 5 a.m.–10 p.m.; no fees or permits required

**WHEELCHAIR ACCESS:** None

**MAPS:** N/A

**FACILITIES:** Nearby Mountain View Park has a short path, restrooms, and picnic areas.

**CONTACT INFORMATION:** 512-974-6700; austintexas.gov/department/ parks-and-recreation

The hike traces a tributary of Bull Creek as it cuts a startlingly steep-sided canyon. Cedars shade the path for much of the way. Along the creek, tall hardwoods and thick brush shut out the sun. You will find relics of a small ranch, including the home's foundation, a spring, and a small tributary dam. Nearby, a field is slowly surrendering to the trees reclaiming the flat land. Many springs feed the main tributary. As you approach the end, the canyon closes in and rock bluffs squeeze the path, which finally ends downstream from a watery cascade, just below the Balcones Country Club lake.

On this upper end of the trail, there are two alternate trailheads, a good thing because the main trailhead on Scotland Well Drive has limited parking. If the Scotland Well lot is full, continue on Scotland Well Drive 0.6 mile to Westerkirk Drive. Turn right on Westerkirk Drive and follow it to a parking area on the left at Mountain View Park. From here, you pick up the trail by walking east through the small park to Callanish Park Drive. Look for the trail descending east between two houses on Callanish Park Drive.

From the Scotland Well trailhead, begin your trek by joining the sidewalk uphill 300 feet along Scotland Well Drive and then bearing right at two white metal posts into a tunnel of cedar. Continue on a wide gravel track. Step over a succession of intermittent drainages on the well-shaded, steep slope. Many of the crossings have been paved. Stone and cedar supports keep the trail level and prevent erosion. Climb to a high point at 0.3 mile, where a user-created track cuts south, back to the parking lot. Stay left, and the path opens to a meadow. At the half-mile point, the trail meets the tributary. The valley closes in, and trees, including sycamores and live oaks, block the sky. The streams keep flowing down from the high ground to the left. At 0.6 mile, pass a concrete box protecting a spring on your left. It is surrounded by a tumbledown log fence. Look for the foundation of a house next to the spring. This homesite was well placed, near level land and on the west side of the canyon, protecting it from the heat of the long Texas summer. Vegetation spills down the canyon banks, pushing in on the rooty path, which continues past a stone dam that spans the clear stream.

At 0.9 mile the trail doglegs right around the meadow—it won't be that long before this grassy area will be completely covered in trees—and continues upstream, traveling

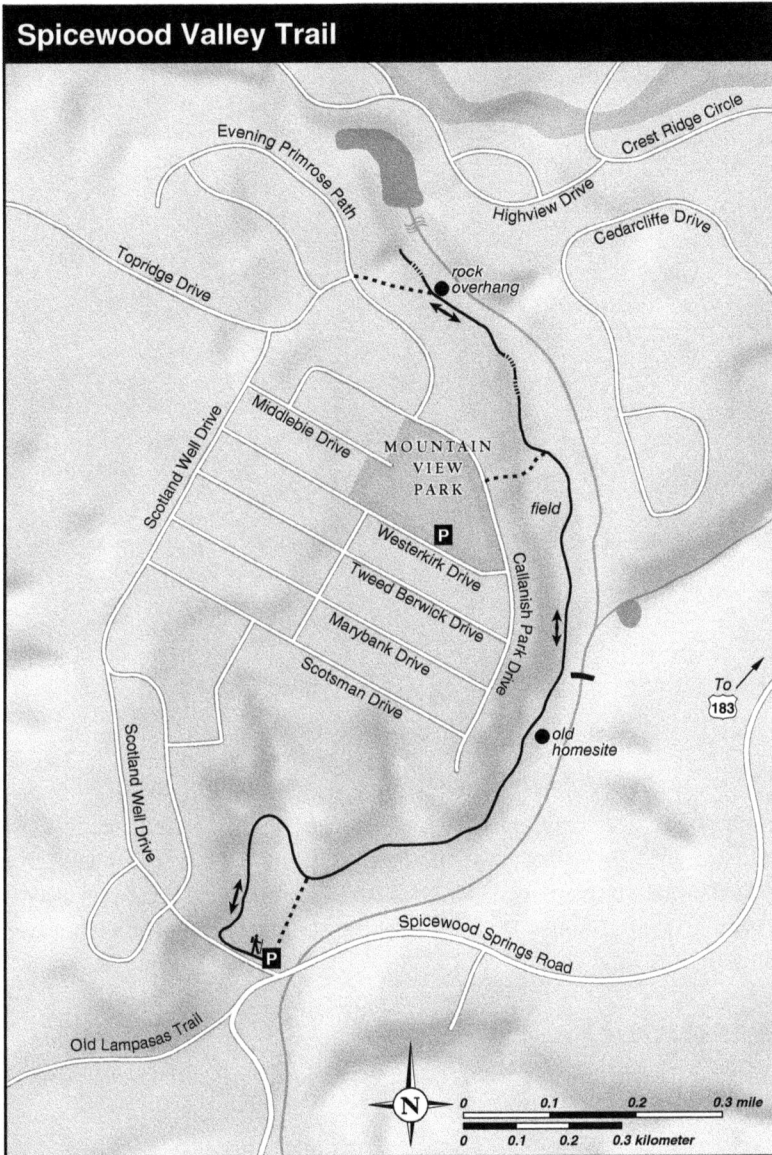

**Spicewood Valley Trail**

the margin between the stream and meadow. At 1 mile you'll reach a trail junction, marked by a tiny menhir (standing stone). The spur trail goes left, angling up through rocky bluffs to the alternate access at Callanish Park Drive. The main path keeps straight, crossing more spring branches flowing from the rugged terrain on the left. Steps climb up the left side of the bluffs, and stone supports maintain the trail's integrity. Pass by rock overhangs, squeeze between the bluff and a fallen rock, and then reach another trail junction at 1.3 miles. Stone steps lead left to an overgrown path that emerges at the

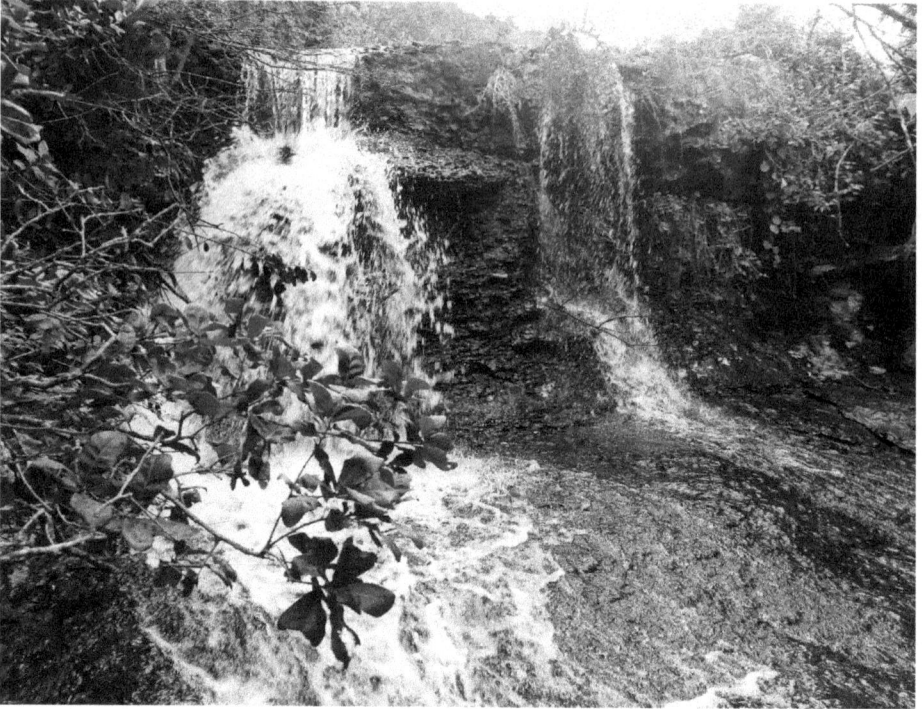

*The waterfall at the end of Spicewood Valley Trail*

intersection of Topridge Drive and Evening Primrose Path. The trail keeps forward and ends at the side of a high waterfall, where the cliffs drop suddenly into the wooded valley. You may be tempted to clamber across the falls and look into the section of canyon that is between you and the Country Club lake, where the valley has been engineered into a wide spillway.

## Nearby Activities

Mountain View Park has shaded picnic facilities; a short, hard-surface trail; tennis courts; and playgrounds.

---

**GPS TRAILHEAD COORDINATES**

**N30° 25' 22.5"  W97° 47' 37.8"**

From US 183 north of Loop 360, north of downtown Austin, take Spicewood Springs Road west 1.8 miles to Scotland Well Drive, which is at the bottom of a hill. Turn right on Scotland Well Drive, and the small parking area is immediately on your right.

---

# 14 Three Falls Hike at Barton Creek Greenbelt

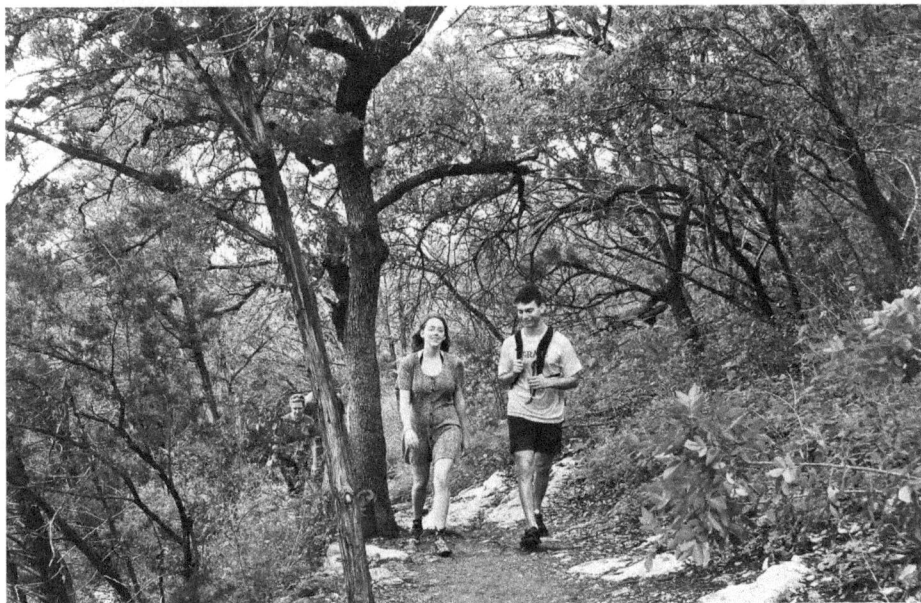

*Hikers on the Barton Creek Greenbelt*

## In Brief

This out-and-back hike begins midway along the Barton Creek Greenbelt. Leave the busy Twin Falls–Gaines Access, and descend into the creek canyon. Then head upstream, passing Twin Falls, Sculpture Falls, and finally Bench Falls at Lost Creek. I recommend saving this hike until after a good rain, when the falls become attractive swimming holes.

## Description

The Barton Creek Greenbelt is one of the best urban wildernesses in the world and is routinely cited as a reason to move to or stay in the capital city. It is enjoyed not only by hikers but also by rock climbers, mountain bikers, swimmers, and teenagers, who often take over Twin Falls on summer afternoons. That and the two other enticing swimming holes make this particular section of the Greenbelt very popular. In fact its lower reaches are surely among the busiest stretches of trail in this guidebook. Try to visit during the week, and in the morning would be even better. The trail cruises along the rim of a deep

| | |
|---|---|
| **LENGTH:** 6.8 miles | **DRIVING DISTANCE:** 6 miles from the state capitol |
| **CONFIGURATION:** Out-and-back | |
| **DIFFICULTY:** Moderate | **ACCESS:** Daily, 5 a.m.–10 p.m.; no fees or permits required |
| **SCENERY:** River canyon, waterfalls, woods | |
| **EXPOSURE:** Mostly shady | **WHEELCHAIR ACCESS:** No |
| **TRAFFIC:** Very heavy | **MAPS:** tinyurl.com/bartongreenbeltmap |
| **TRAIL SURFACE:** Dirt, rock | **FACILITIES:** None |
| **HIKING TIME:** 3–4 hours | **CONTACT INFORMATION:** 512-974-6700; austintexas.gov/department/ parks-and-recreation |

canyon before angling down toward Barton Creek. The first waterfall, Twin Falls, is shortly upstream. Travel beneath a tall tunnel of woods to find Sculpture Falls, another wide drop over a rock shelf. Continue another mile to Bench Falls, and from there, if you wish, explore onward to the end of the trail.

Pass the signboard at the trailhead and walk past a bench and table. Take a few steps to the rim of the canyon, looking across the green valley. A familiar geometry of cedar trunks and branches shades the dirt path. Head right, upstream, though Barton Creek is far below. At 0.2 mile begin to descend on a rocky graded trail, reaching the canyon bottom in another 0.1 mile. The trees are thick and tall here in the riverine woodland. If there has been rain, Barton Creek flows on your left. After a downpour the water is brown and turbulent.

Continue upstream. The heavily used path braids into numerous tracks cut by multiple users. Twin Falls is just ahead. You may hear music and laughter mixed in with the sound of rushing water as you approach. The pool closest to the trailhead is very popular with teenagers and college students looking to while away a summer afternoon.

Keep upstream through big trees, and soon pass a gray and tan bluff at 0.5 mile, its color the result of fairly recent erosion. Look for precarious overhangs and crumbling grottoes in the bluff walls. The sound of small riffles and shoals accompanies your hike. Live oaks and cedars grow seemingly everywhere but the trail, forming a tunnel over the path. Pass a normally dry feeder branch, the first of many branches that flow into Barton Creek from either side. The valley widens out, tall trees growing in the shelter of the high bluff to your right. The level path makes for easy hiking.

At just under a mile, you will see a 5.5-mile marker, which notes the distance from the trailhead at Zilker Park. Another creek comes in from the right. Shortly you will come to a large oak tree, also to your right. Look for stone ruins. Local legend has it that these rock formations were part of a failed Spanish mission from the early 1700s. Leaving the oak tree, dip down to cross another dry feeder, and continue through more towering trunks. The sky is a patchwork between tree branches.

Though there has continued to be some braiding in the trail, at 1.4 miles there is a more serious split. Keep to the left, along the flat earthen path by the stream. Short spurs lead left to the creek.

# Three Falls Hike at Barton Creek Greenbelt

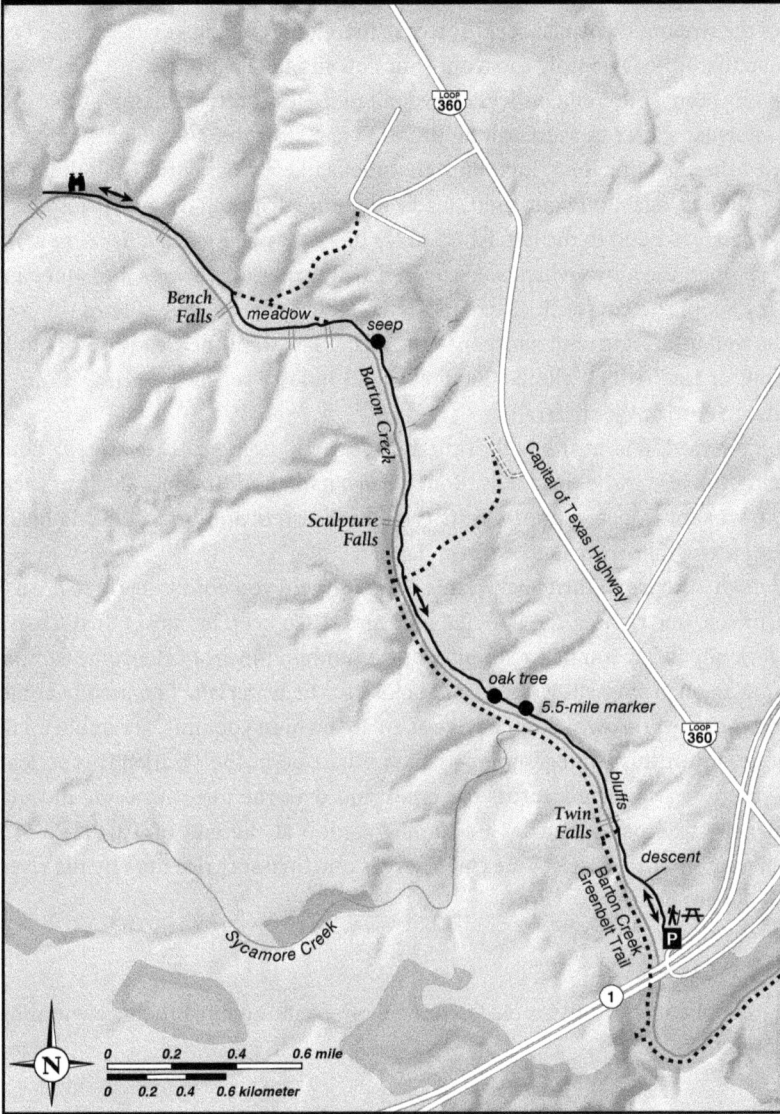

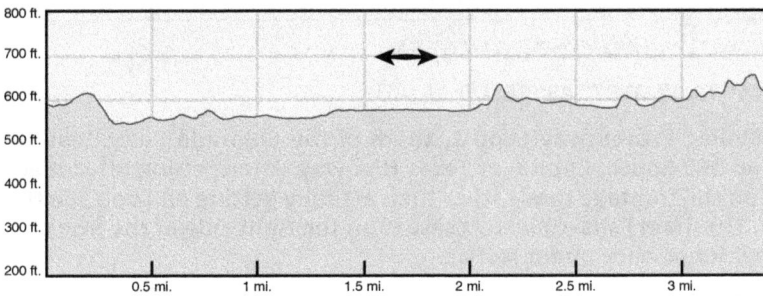

LOOP 360

Bench
Falls    *meadow*        *seep*

Barton Creek

*Sculpture
Falls*

Capital of Texas Highway

*oak tree*
*5.5-mile marker*

LOOP 360

*bluffs*

*Twin
Falls*          *descent*

Barton Creek
Greenbelt Trail

*Sycamore Creek*

1

N

| 0 | 0.2 | 0.4 | 0.6 mile |
| 0 | 0.2 | 0.4 | 0.6 kilometer |

800 ft.
700 ft.
600 ft.
500 ft.
400 ft.
300 ft.
200 ft.

0.5 mi.    1 mi.    1.5 mi.    2 mi.    2.5 mi.    3 mi.

Reach Sculpture Falls at 1.6 miles. Barton Creek descends over a dimpled shelf of rock. A long, deep pool forms below the low, wide drop. The rock shelf continues on the far side of the stream. If you can rock-hop over there, the shelf makes an excellent spot for lunch or sunbathing. Or simply toss your shoes off and take a dip.

Past this point, the trail gets less crowded but no less pretty. You start to find various small, somewhat secret treasures along the way. Just after the 2-mile mark, look to your right to see the start of a long, high bluff that looks like a worthy rock-climbing destination. At 2.1 miles, again on your right, water might be dripping down a pretty rock face. The creek starts to bend to the left. At 2.3 miles there may be a small falls, after which you come to an open meadow, which was covered with gaillardia flowers and Queen Anne's lace on my visit. You can walk closer to the creek or on the other side of the meadow, where the trail intersects with another to the right. The right fork leads up a path known as the Trail of Life, which climbs 300 feet in 0.3 mile to reach the Camp Craft Access trailhead on Scottish Woods Trail.

Keep forward, and at the end of the meadow you come to Lost Creek, flowing in from the right. Here is the third falls, Bench Falls, named for its single stair of rock. This lesser-known spot is just as pretty as its two lower sisters and boasts a little beach area across the creek. Take a break to swim and relax.

You might choose to turn back at this point. Should you continue, there are a couple more surprises, one right at the end, 0.7 mile ahead. To keep on, cross Lost Creek. Take the left fork ahead. At 3 miles a stream comes tumbling in from the right from a steep canyon, and a small spur allows you to get close to the waterfall. The path becomes narrower and more overgrown. Soon, arrive at an area where you must scramble up the cliff to continue. From this vantage point—which might be in the Ozarks, it is so leafy and remote—there is a fine view across the creek and over the forest to some distant cliffs. Eventually the trail peters out by a pumping station at the end of Turtle Point Drive, where yet another little creek comes in. There is one final surprise here by the riverbank, which is yours to discover.

## Nearby Activities

This section of the Barton Creek Greenbelt offers mountain biking, swimming, and rock climbing.

---

**GPS TRAILHEAD COORDINATES**

**N30° 14' 38.9"  W97° 48' 36.1"**

From MoPac Expressway/Loop 1, south of the Colorado River, take the exit for Loop 360 South, Capital of Texas Highway. After getting off MoPac, keep south on the frontage road rather than actually getting on Loop 360 North or South. The Twin Falls–Gaines Access is on the right side of the frontage road before it loops back under MoPac.

# 15 Turkey Creek Trail at Emma Long Metropolitan Park

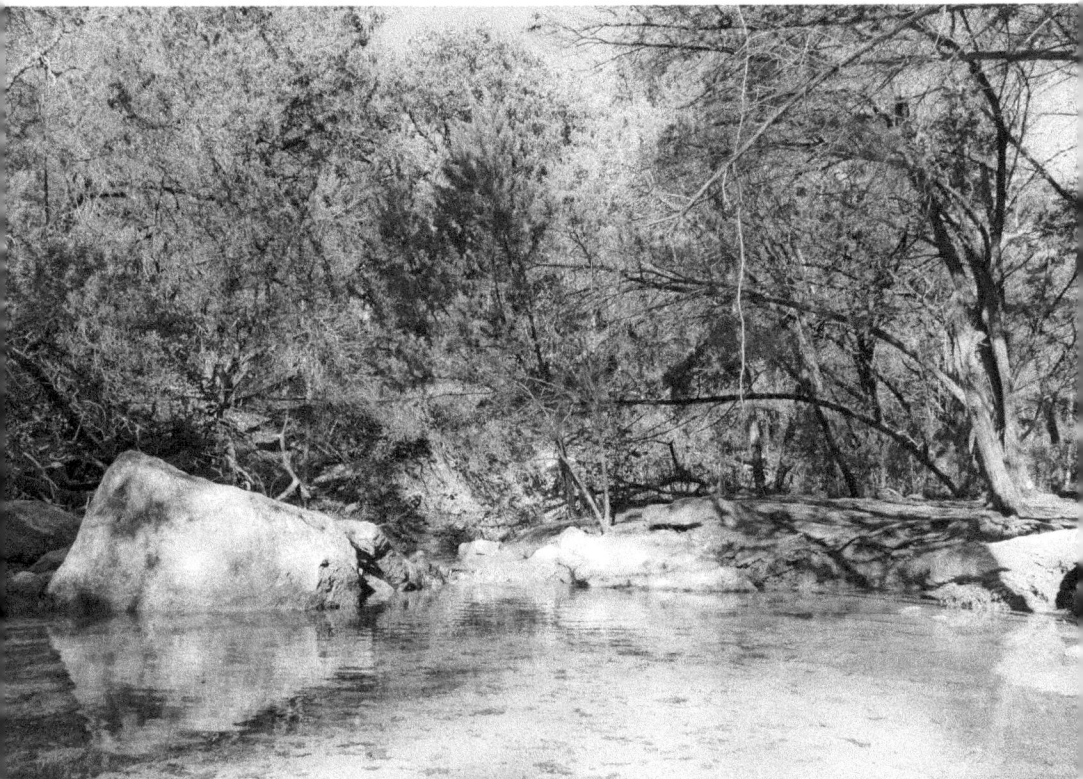

*Turkey Creek*

## In Brief

This ramble up a wild ravine in the middle of a juniper forest is one of the city's best hikes, even if it's no longer an unknown jewel. As an off-leash area, it's a favorite with dog owners, and although it is part of Emma Long Metropolitan Park, it is outside the fee area.

## Description

This trail explores the lush Turkey Creek canyon where cedars, oaks, and sycamores form a nearly continuous tree canopy. Sheer rock bluffs and sloping, wooded walls lead down to the crystal-clear creek.

| | |
|---|---|
| **LENGTH:** 2.7 miles | **DRIVING DISTANCE:** 16 miles from the state capitol |
| **CONFIGURATION:** Balloon loop | |
| **DIFFICULTY:** Moderate | **ACCESS:** Daily, 7 a.m.–10 p.m.; free |
| **SCENERY:** Wooded creek canyon | **WHEELCHAIR ACCESS:** No |
| **EXPOSURE:** Shady | **MAPS:** tinyurl.com/emmalongmetropark |
| **TRAFFIC:** Moderate–busy | **FACILITIES:** None |
| **TRAIL SURFACE:** Rocks, dirt | **CONTACT INFORMATION:** (Emma Long Metropolitan Park) 512-346-1831; austintexas.gov/department/ parks-and-recreation |
| **HIKING TIME:** 1.5 hours | |

From the trailhead, walk through cedar over a spur and down some steps to the creek, close to City Park Road. You should be able to step over the water, but if it is too high to cross, turn back, as there are 17 more crossings to make on this hike.

On the other side of the creek, the trail passes an information board and follows the stream up the pretty canyon. The scenery is wild and untamed, yet intimate. Some shafts of sunlight might penetrate the tree cover to cast light on the water. The canyon is narrow, and the creek is the center of attention. Until the point where the loop climbs up onto the rim, you are never more than a few feet from the water, which glides over wide rock flats into wider pools. Small cascades add light and sound appeal to the walk.

The fords come frequently. On most crossings, stepping-stones have been laid across the creek. Approach the fourth crossing on a rock shelf that becomes the falls where it crosses the stream, clearly demonstrating the stair-step topography of the Hill Country. The softer layers erode to leave the typical rock *balcones*.

The fifth crossing takes you back to the eastern side of the creek. A side canyon opens up to the right, and just after that, at the three-quarter-mile marker (there are markers every quarter of a mile), you arrive at the beginning of the loop. Go left, fording the creek again below the tallest and prettiest falls so far, and then cross three more times before reaching the 1-mile marker on the inside of a stream curve.

The trail climbs away from the creek at a bend, then comes back down into the bed. At the 1.1-mile point cross the streambed again from east to west, the 10th crossing. High water or flood debris might obscure the path on this section, so double-check that you are on the right track. The forest opens slightly, and the streambed is more diffuse. Rocks and boulders are sprinkled on the hillsides. In other places, the rocky canyon wall is plainly visible. Three more creek crossings lead you to the fern wall, 1.3 miles into the hike. The moist, cool canyon wall supports a fern colony, resulting in a draping green swath hanging over the creek bed. A bench allows you to sit and absorb the atmosphere. Moss growing on the horizontal branches of live oaks is more evidence of green abundance.

Beyond the fern wall, turn away from Turkey Creek to ascend the side of the canyon. The rock *balcones* are clearly visible on the ascent. The woods are no longer the lush riot

## Turkey Creek Trail at Emma Long Metropolitan Park

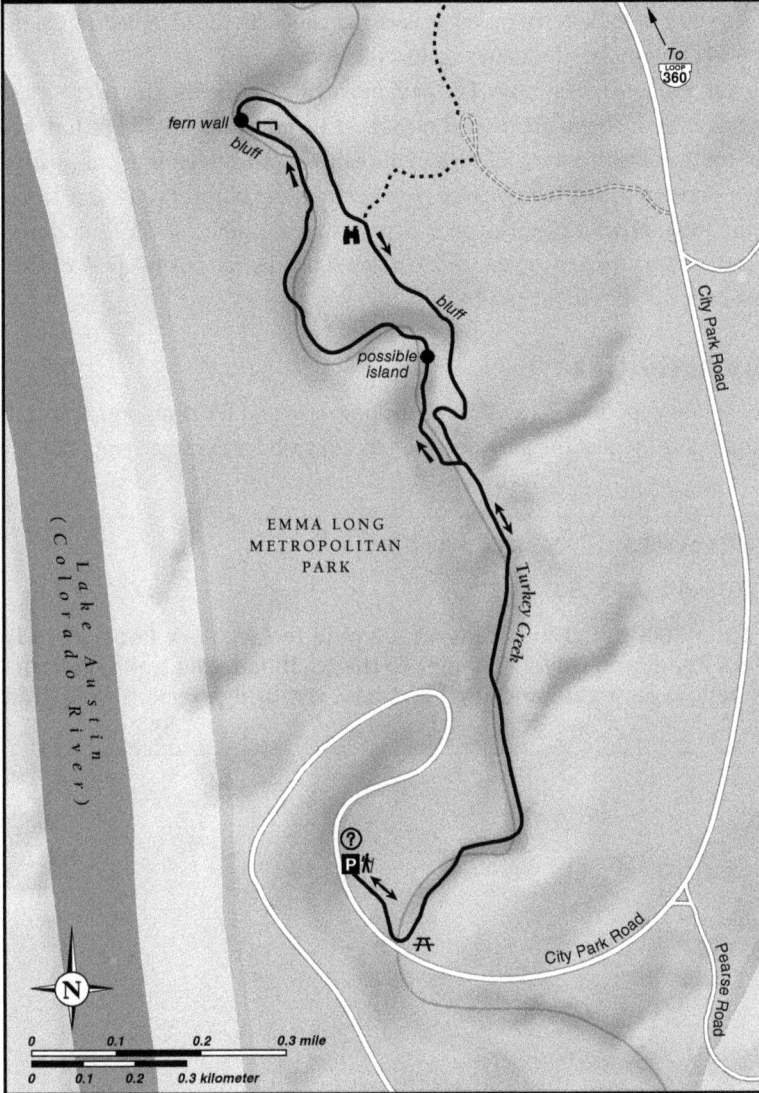

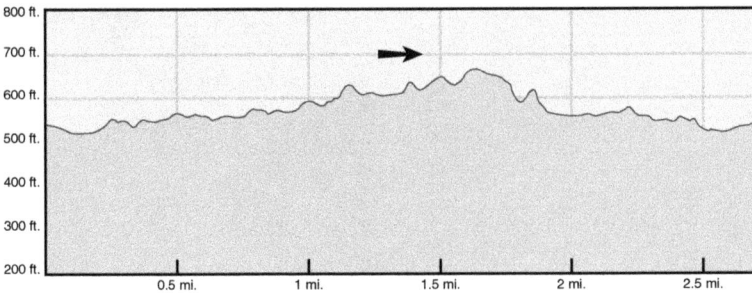

To
LOOP
360

fern wall
bluff

bluff

possible
island

EMMA LONG
METROPOLITAN
PARK

*L a k e   A u s t i n
( C o l o r a d o   R i v e r )*

Turkey Creek

City Park Road

City Park Road

Pearse Road

N

| 0 | 0.1 | 0.2 | 0.3 mile |

| 0 | 0.1 | 0.2 | 0.3 kilometer |

800 ft.
700 ft.
600 ft.
500 ft.
400 ft.
300 ft.
200 ft.

0.5 mi.    1 mi.    1.5 mi.    2 mi.    2.5 mi.

of the canyon; instead, scattered cedars grow side by side with grasses, cactus, and mesquite. The rock has eroded into sharp edges in many spots. The trail comes to the canyon rim, where you can look down on the leaves and trunks in the glen below. On the opposite ridge, treetops make silhouettes against the sky.

The trail walking is easy now. The path moves away from the rim to cross a spur that corresponds with the bend mentioned earlier. At 1.6 miles keep right at a fork in an open area. The route comes back to the edge of the canyon and descends a rocky path that zigzags down some steps to Turkey Creek. Not far from the bottom you come to the beginning of the loop, at which point you will have hiked 2 miles. Walk back downstream, making the stream crossings again. At 2.6 miles make the final of 18 creek crossings, and walk back over the spur to the trailhead.

## Nearby Activities

Emma Long Metropolitan Park offers picnicking, tent and RV camping, fishing, boating, and swimming. Note that the park does not accept cash for entrance and other fees.

---

### GPS TRAILHEAD COORDINATES

**N30° 20' 0.4"  W97° 50' 23.7"**

From Loop 360, take FM 2222 west 0.7 mile to City Park Road. Turn left on City Park Road, and travel 4.9 miles to the trailhead. The trailhead is 0.3 mile past a yellow park gate and then just past the bridge over Turkey Creek, on the right.

---

# 16 Wild Basin Wilderness Preserve

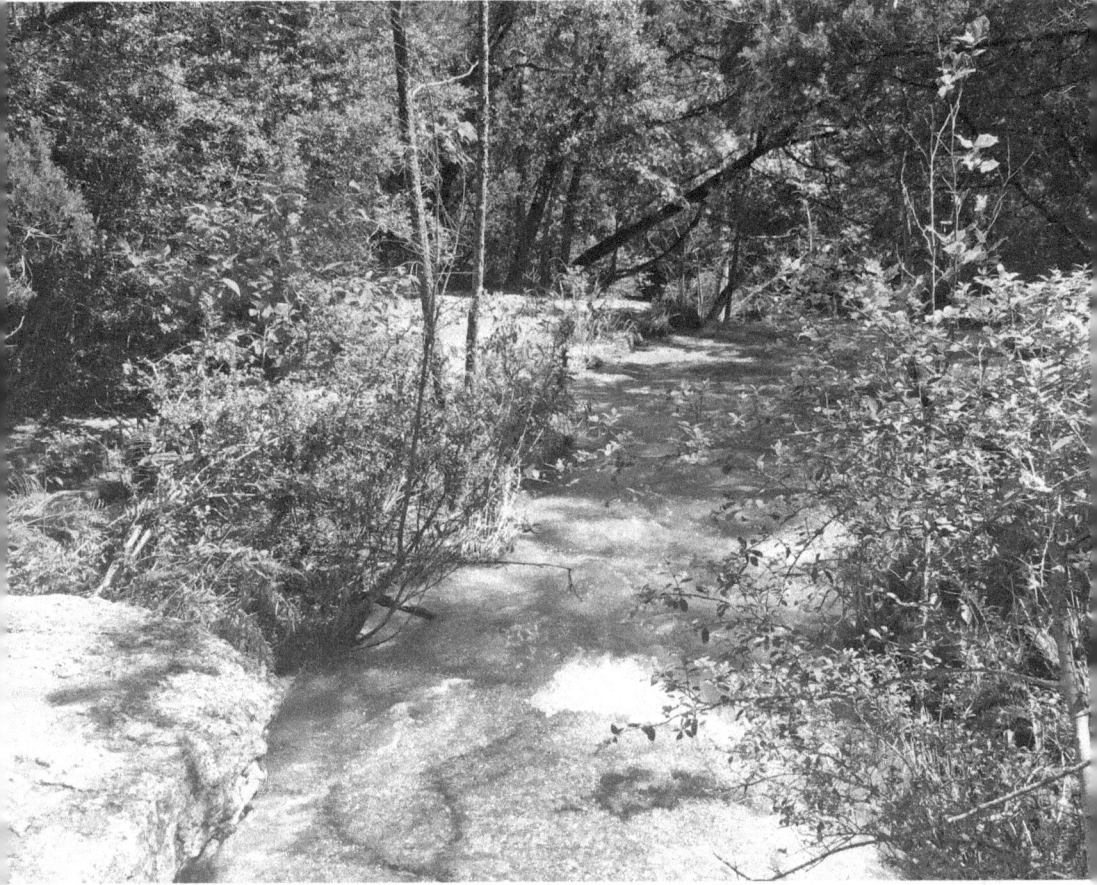

*Bee Creek at Wild Basin Wilderness Preserve*

## In Brief

Part of the Balcones Canyonlands Preserve and operated as an educational resource by St. Edward's University, these 227 acres are a rare tract of undisturbed Hill Country within the city limits. With creek access and extensive interpretive information, you could easily spend the better part of an afternoon on this hike. Please note that pets, bicycles, and picnics are not allowed.

| | |
|---|---|
| **LENGTH:** 1.8 miles | **DRIVING DISTANCE:** 10 miles from the state capitol |
| **CONFIGURATION:** Loop | |
| **DIFFICULTY:** Moderate | **ACCESS:** Daily, sunrise–sunset; $3 donation requested |
| **SCENERY:** Creek, hills, and typical Hill Country vegetation | **WHEELCHAIR ACCESS:** No |
| **EXPOSURE:** Moderate | **MAPS:** Trail map and interpretive booklet available at entrance or at tinyurl.com/wildbasintrailmap |
| **TRAFFIC:** Light–heavy, depending on time and trails | |
| **TRAIL SURFACE:** Rocks and dirt | **FACILITIES:** Restroom at parking area |
| **HIKING TIME:** 1–2 hours | **CONTACT INFORMATION:** 512-327-7622; think.stedwards.edu/wildbasin |

## Description

Wild Basin Preserve exists through the tenacity of the environmental group Now or Never. In the 1970s, members of this group lobbied the government, rallied the community, and succeeded in raising the money to purchase this land and keep it as a haven for plants and wildlife. It is now part of the Balcones Canyonlands Preserve and supports several threatened species, including local favorites the golden-cheeked warbler and black-capped vireo. The Wild Basin Creative Research Center, affiliated with St. Edward's University, is located in a building on the preserve and facilitates "research, public awareness and preservation of Austin's wildlands." Consider printing out the Self-Guided Trail Map; its entries correspond to numbered and lettered signs along the Arroyo Vista and Creek Trails.

This hike starts on a ridge and makes its way down to and across Bee Creek, looping around the far side of the creek valley, then returns via the other side of the spur. If there is water, you'll see some pretty falls on the creek on the way back. Although it has the same name, this isn't the Bee Creek that flows north through Bee Cave to reach the Colorado at Inverness Point. This creek flows east through West Lake Hills and into Lake Austin just above Tom Miller Dam.

Stand at the large map display at the end of the parking area. A short spur goes left to an observation point, where a bench looks across the steep green valley to the next ridge. The main trail passes to the left of the Creative Research Center—a white house—and travels along a level gravel path through cedar and red oak. You will see a chimney swift tower through the trees to your right. At 0.1 mile keep left at a fork, and you will be on the Arroyo Vista Loop. The trees provide scattered, dappled shade. A wooden bridge crosses a wash, and another bench allows for contemplation of the namesake vista over the arroyo.

At 0.3 mile you reach the junction with the Triknee Trail, but rather than continuing straight, go left toward the valley down some steps to an overlook, where there is yet another bench. Metal plaques set into concrete plinths give information about the Hill Country and the flora and fauna.

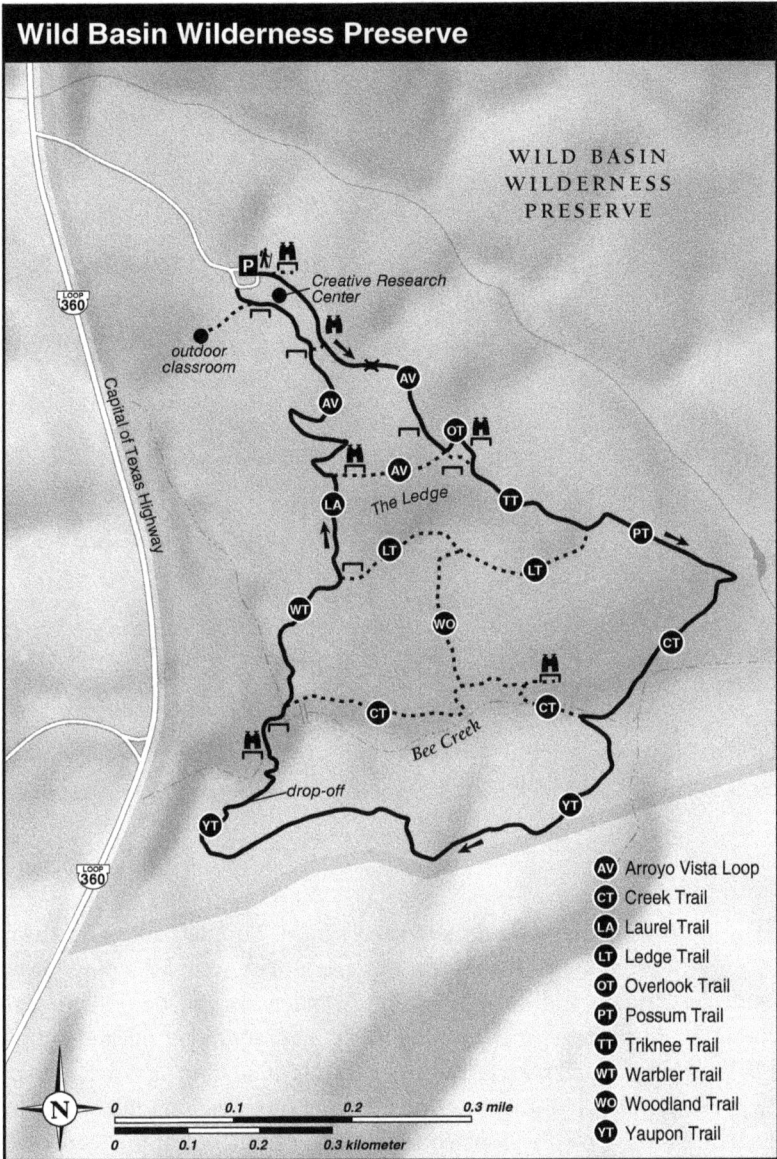

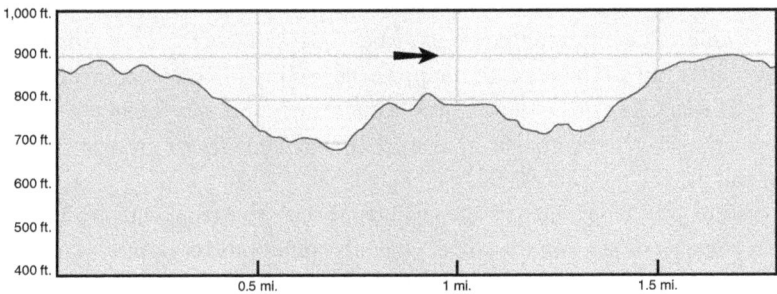

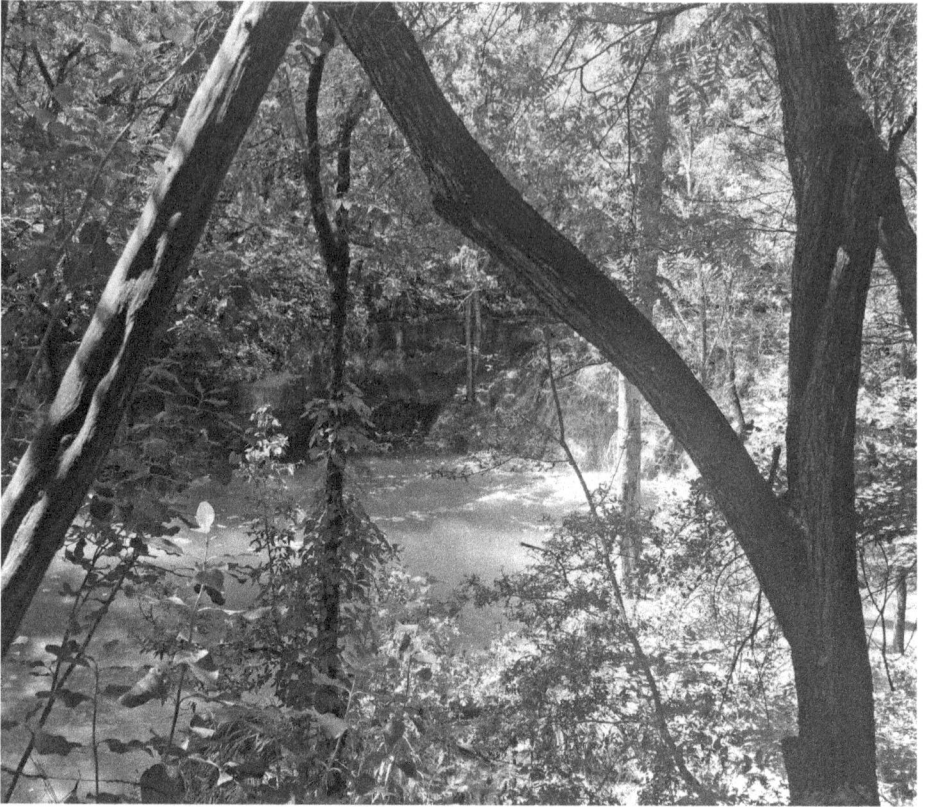

*Bee Creek at Wild Basin Wilderness Preserve*

The overlook trail takes you back to the Triknee. Turn left and start down a long series of wide steps, going down toward the creek. The scrubby juniper around you echoes with sharp tweets and trills. At 0.4 mile keep left, moving onto the Possum Trail, which continues down more steps into the valley. The woods get thicker and the shade deeper. To your left you will see a feeder creek, at this point flowing down a deep trench. The path makes a right turn (there's a no-entry sign on a fence) at the beginning of the Creek Trail and traverses a soggy patch around the confluence of the feeder creek and Bee Creek.

At 0.7 mile you will reach Bee Creek, where stones allow for a dry crossing after all but the heaviest rains. The parts of the preserve around the creek are truly delightful, especially if there has been rain. Thick woods surround the rocky streambed, and though you are less than a mile from Loop 360, you could be far away in a remote Hill Country valley.

As soon as you cross the creek, you will come to the junction with the Yaupon Trail. Turn left; steep steps lead up the slope. Once the trail finds its elevation, it follows the contour around the hillside through sparser cedar in the lea of a neighborhood. The reward comes at 1.2 miles, just after a descent—more steps—into denser cedar. A bench sits a few feet from a vertiginous cliff directly above Bee Creek. A little stream might be trickling over the edge. When you are ready to move on, follow the trail down a series of steep zigzags into the ravine and to a creek crossing. A few yards farther along the path, you will come to the preserve's main attraction, the falls on Bee Creek. Water tumbles off a rock ledge into a deep, shaded pool. Two access trails, the second with a bench, allow for closer viewing. A feeder creek coming in from the left might be splashing down its own falls to join the larger stream.

Leave the falls and follow the Warbler Trail to begin the half-mile climb back to the trailhead. Steps lead up the side of the spur. At 1.5 miles you keep left to join the Laurel Trail, and less than 0.1 mile farther, keep left to follow the other side of the Arroyo Vista loop back to the Research Center and the trailhead, passing the chimney swift tower again as you approach the center building and parking lot.

## Nearby Activities

Nearby Emma Long Metropolitan Park, off RM 2222 at the end of City Park Road, offers camping, swimming, and fishing.

---

**GPS TRAILHEAD COORDINATES**

**N30° 18' 38.1"  W97° 49' 26.4"**

**The entrance is located off Loop 360 South, west of downtown and south of the 360 Bridge.**

# North of Austin (Hikes 17–24)

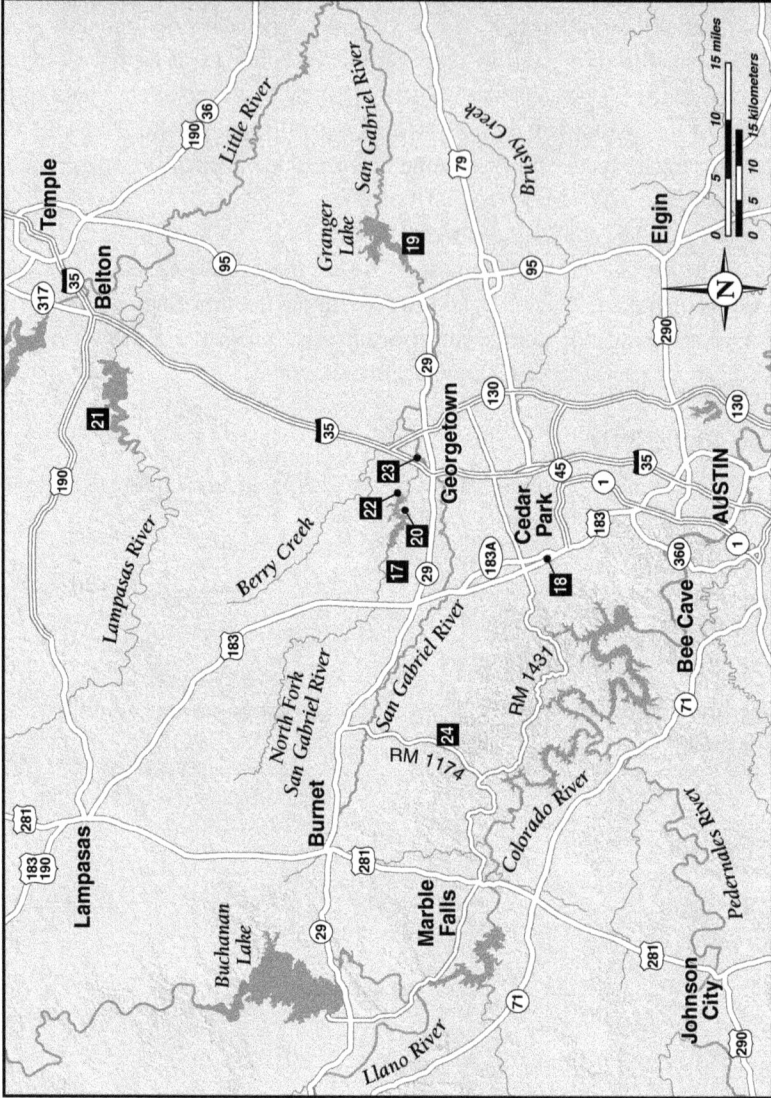

# NORTH OF AUSTIN

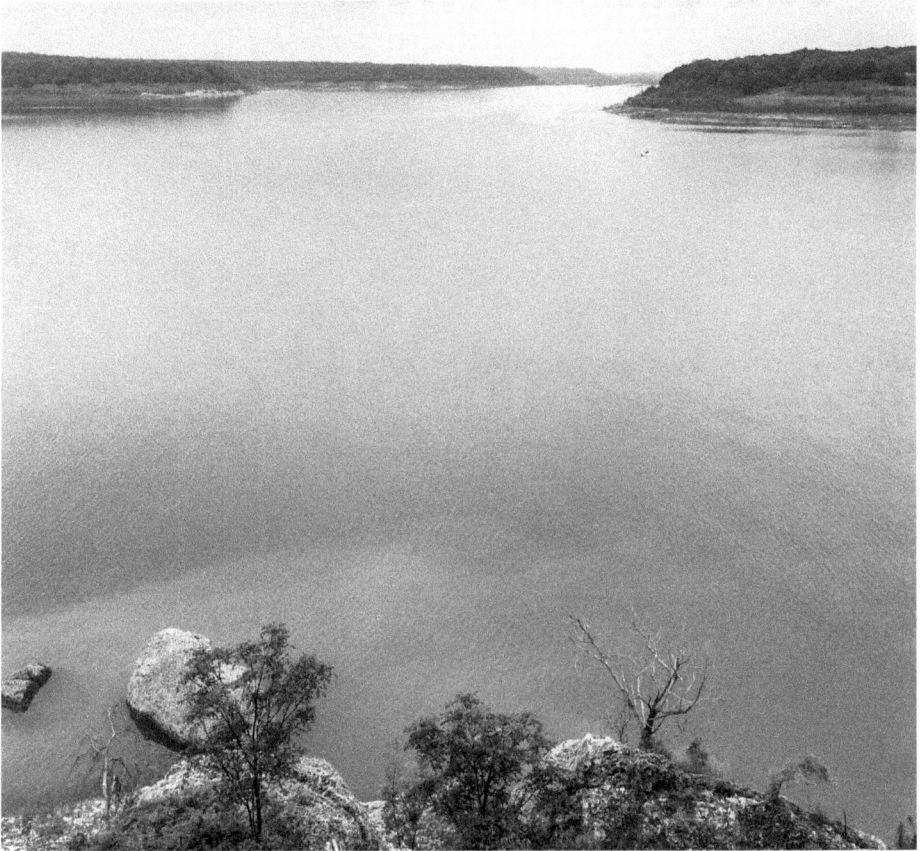

*View of Lake Georgetown from the Crockett Gardens Trail (see page 95)*

# 17 Bluffs of the North Fork San Gabriel River

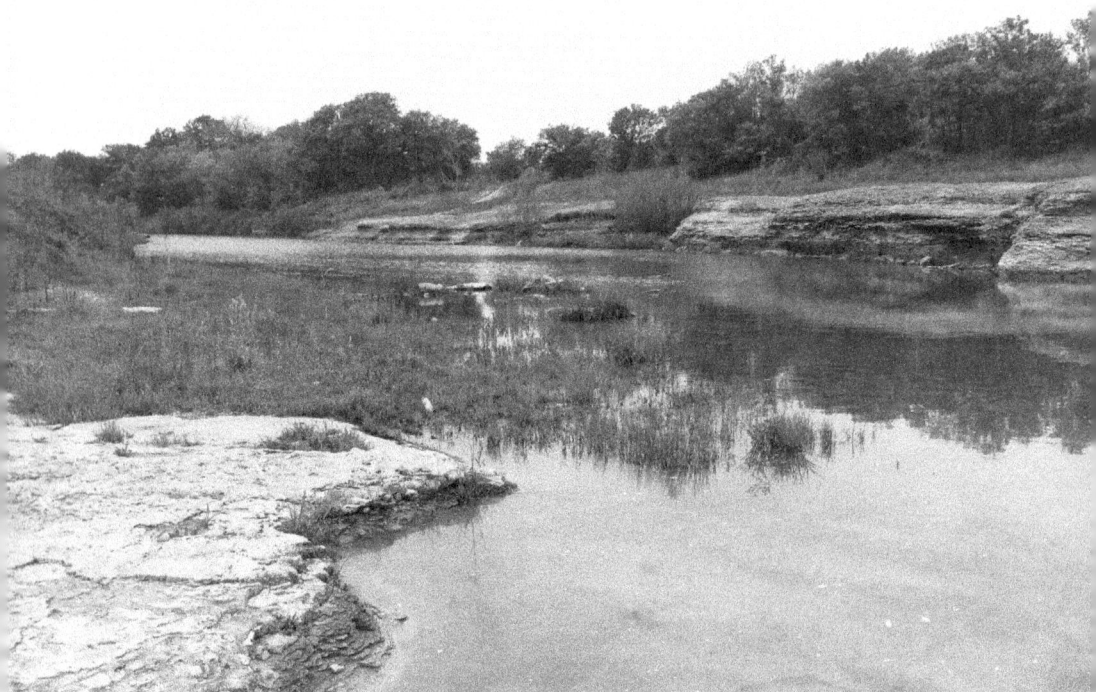

*North Fork San Gabriel River*

## In Brief

This hike traces an old roadbed along the North Fork San Gabriel River at the western end of Lake Georgetown, passing impressive bluffs on the way. It then opens to a flat meadow before reaching a sharp turn in the river, where more cliffs offer extensive views.

## Description

This hike encompasses a section of the Good Water Loop of the San Gabriel River Trail, a 28-mile trek around Lake Georgetown. For this particular walk, you travel east on the trail from the low-water crossing at Tejas Camp. The level walk leads past bluffs on the

| | |
|---|---|
| **LENGTH:** 3.6 miles | **DRIVING DISTANCE:** 36 miles from the state capitol |
| **CONFIGURATION:** Out-and-back | |
| **DIFFICULTY:** Easy | **ACCESS:** Daily, 6 a.m.–10 p.m.; $4 for day use |
| **SCENERY:** Lakeside woods and fields, bluffs | **WHEELCHAIR ACCESS:** No |
| **EXPOSURE:** Mostly open | **MAPS:** tinyurl.com/goodwaterloop |
| **TRAFFIC:** Moderate–busy on weekends | **FACILITIES:** Restrooms at trailhead |
| **TRAIL SURFACE:** Dirt, grass, rocks | **CONTACT INFORMATION:** 512-930-5253; tinyurl.com/tejaspark |
| **HIKING TIME:** 2 hours | |

north side of the North Fork San Gabriel river and then along flats to reach more bluffs on the south side of Lake Georgetown, where you can overlook the lake and the farmland north of the river.

The area around Tejas Camp was once known as West End Crossing. It was the fourth upstream river crossing from Georgetown in pre-dam days and is the only crossing between here and the town that is not now at the bottom of the lake. Hayden Hunt and his brothers settled at West End Crossing and built a log cabin, cotton gin, and cornmill. The bluffs across the river from Tejas Camp hold the family cemetery. Nowadays the river below the bridge is a popular spot for swimming, fishing, or tubing down the river to the lake.

Pick up the San Gabriel River Trail by leaving the Tejas Camp parking area and walking toward the low-water bridge over the North Fork San Gabriel River. Before crossing the bridge, turn right and begin following an old roadbed. Pass Tejas Camp on your right. For the first mile the level dirt path enjoys the shade of a ribbon of river-bottom woodland. As you make your way along the track, you will notice occasional side trails leading left toward the river. At just over 0.5 mile white and tan cedar-studded bluffs tower over the wide, grassy banks on your side of the stream. Look for winged elm, a tree with an unusual name that often grows in abandoned clearings and is easily identified by the corky "wings" running along its branches. The fiberlike inner bark of this tree was made into rope and used to tie cotton bales in the 1800s.

Hills rise in the distance, encircling a lost valley to your right behind the trees. The trail eventually emerges from the shade and descends to the riverside. Here, flat rocks give good access to the water. A wet-weather stream comes in from the right from a small ravine known as Hunt Hollow. This streamlet and the entire San Gabriel drainage are part of the Brazos River system, which enters the Gulf of Mexico near Freeport, south of Houston. The North Fork meets the South Fork and Middle Fork close to the city of Georgetown. Step over the stream and clamber up the bank to cross a wide field broken by a lone live oak. At 1.4 miles skirt around a fence at the end of the field to reach a doubletrack roadbed. Turn left here, staying on level land. Steep bluffs now rise to your right and ahead of you at a sharp bend in the river. Large boulders lie in the water at the base of the cliffs.

**Bluffs of the North Fork San Gabriel River**

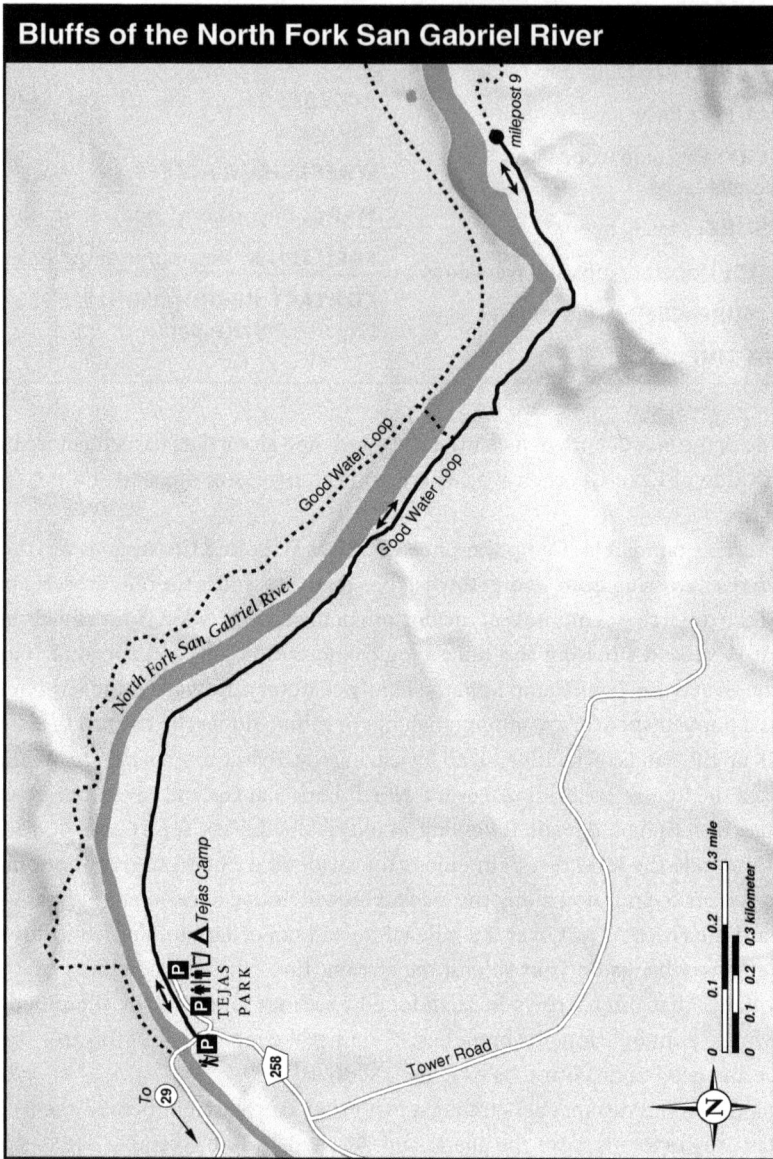

Keep forward, passing the mouth of the steep-sided Jim Hogg Hollow to your right. The San Gabriel River Trail keeps going forward, crossing the outflow from Jim Hogg Hollow. At 1.8 miles begin the steep ascent of the bluff over wooden steps. Stop on the ascent—before the path narrows and tunnels beneath thick woods—and turn to enjoy the view west. The path levels and there are views through the branches up the narrow embayment of the river. The land to the north is still wide-open cattle country, settled with only a few houses. Shortly you'll hit the 9-mile post, which is the distance from

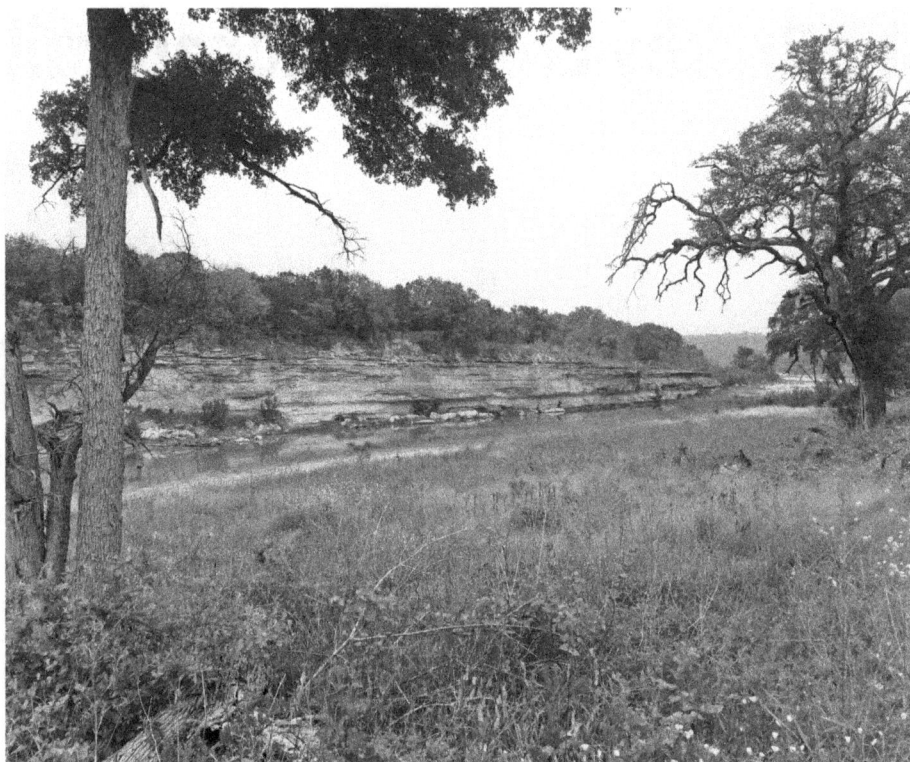

*Bluffs along the North Fork San Gabriel River*

Cedar Breaks Park and a good turnaround point. Going forward, the trail descends to flats along the river ahead. If you are feeling energetic, turn back and explore Jim Hogg Hollow or possibly scramble up through the undergrowth to where the bluffs flatten out above you. That vantage point offers extensive views of the area.

## **Nearby Activities**

Tejas Camp is a good put-in for paddlers wishing to explore Lake Georgetown.

---

### **GPS TRAILHEAD COORDINATES**

**N30° 41' 46.2"  W97° 49' 40.4"**

From Austin, head north on I-35 to Exit 261 (Taylor/Burnet, TX 29). Head west on TX 29 to reach the intersection of TX 29 and Ronald Reagan Boulevard. Head north on Ronald Reagan Boulevard 4 miles. Turn right onto County Road 258 and continue to the low-water bridge crossing of the North Fork San Gabriel River. Tejas Camp is on the right just before the bridge. This hike starts on the south side of the low-water bridge.

# 18 Brushy Creek Regional Trail

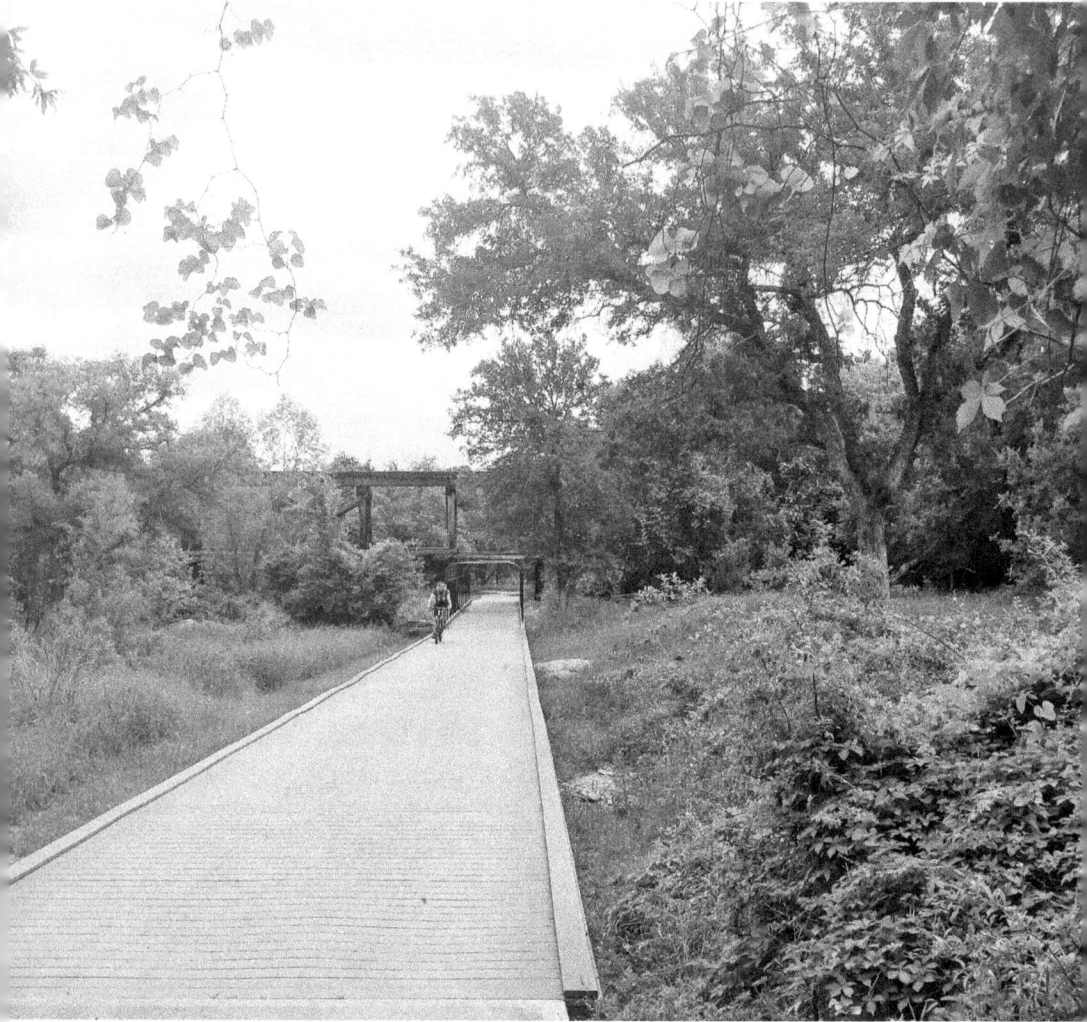

*A disused railroad bridge crossing the Brushy Creek Regional Trail*

## In Brief

This hike across the Williamson County town of Cedar Park makes use of another expanding greenway of the greater capital region. The trail travels along heavily wooded South Brushy Creek to Brushy Creek Lake and continues through three more greenbelt areas before ending at Fern Bluff, with views aplenty along the way.

**LENGTH:** 13 miles, with many shorter options

**CONFIGURATION:** Out-and-back

**DIFFICULTY:** Easy

**SCENERY:** Creek and lake

**EXPOSURE:** Partly wooded

**TRAFFIC:** Heavy on weekends

**TRAIL SURFACE:** Concrete and gravel, with some natural surfaces

**HIKING TIME:** 2–5 hours, depending on distance

**DRIVING DISTANCE:** 19 miles from the state capitol

**ACCESS:** Daily, sunrise–sunset; no fees or permits required

**WHEELCHAIR ACCESS:** Yes

**MAPS:** wilco.org/portals/0/mapside3.pdf

**FACILITIES:** Restrooms at Twin Lakes Park, Brushy Creek Sports Park, Brushy Creek Lake Park, Champion Park, and Creekside Park. Champion Park has picnic areas. Brushy Creek Lake Park has picnic areas, kayak rentals, and a sand volleyball court.

**CONTACT INFORMATION:** 512-943-1920; tinyurl.com/bctrail

## Description

The greenways of Williamson County continue to expand and improve, offering great recreation for hikers, bikers, kayakers, families, and fishermen. The ever-lengthening Brushy Creek Regional Trail now extends from US 183 to beyond Great Oaks Drive, and there are plans to link it to Brushy Creek East Trail in Round Rock and then join that to trails in Hutto to the east. This Cedar Park stretch connects eight parks and greenbelts, making a tree-lined corridor across the city. You will start by the YMCA at Twin Lakes Park; continue to Brushy Creek Sports Park and then Brushy Creek Lake Park; cross the dam to reach Champion Park; and hike through Olsen Meadows and Creekside Parks, finishing up at Fern Bluff on Hairy Man Road. With plenty of access, you can pick and choose your start and end points, or perhaps choose to cycle the whole trail, if you don't want to hike 13 miles. Much of the trail is often chock-full of joggers, cyclists, dog walkers, and chatting moms, so be prepared to share the path.

From the parking area, walk toward the YMCA parking lot along a wide concrete sidewalk, which bends to the left to follow the edge of a patch of woods. Leaving the YMCA precinct, the path dips down to cross South Brushy Creek at 0.3 mile on a nice new bridge over pretty falls. (South Brushy Creek joins Brushy Creek at Olsen Meadows.) From this short stretch you can already get the feel of the route—smooth surfaces and modern infrastructure tell you that this is an urban hike through a well-appointed suburb.

Cross the bridge and enter into woodland. The creek bottom is green with dense vegetation, and tall hardwoods press up against either side of the path. Look for the useful plaques that identify various trees and shrubs. At intervals, the concrete has been decorated with impressions of animal tracks crossing the trail. After 0.5 mile you go under the TX 183A toll road. Cedar mesas alternate with the hardwood bottoms, and at 1.4 miles you reach a meadow. The path continues along the northern edge of the meadow, and at

## Brushy Creek Regional Trail

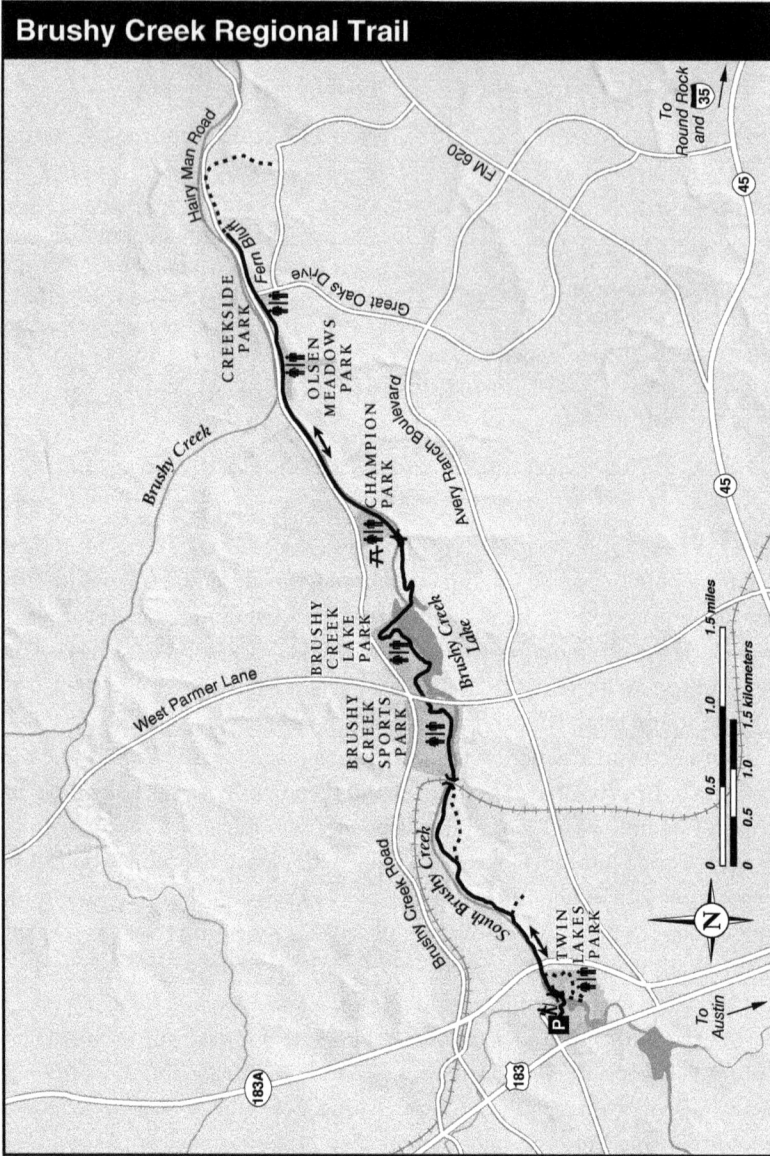

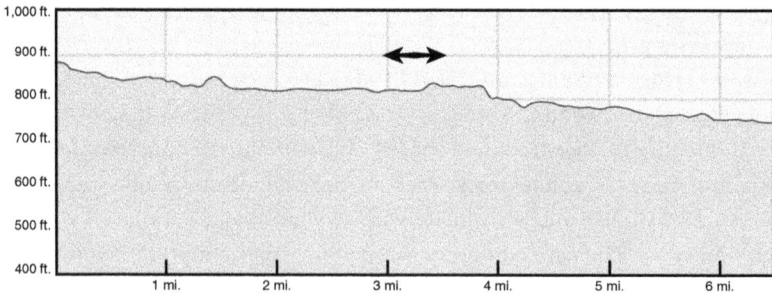

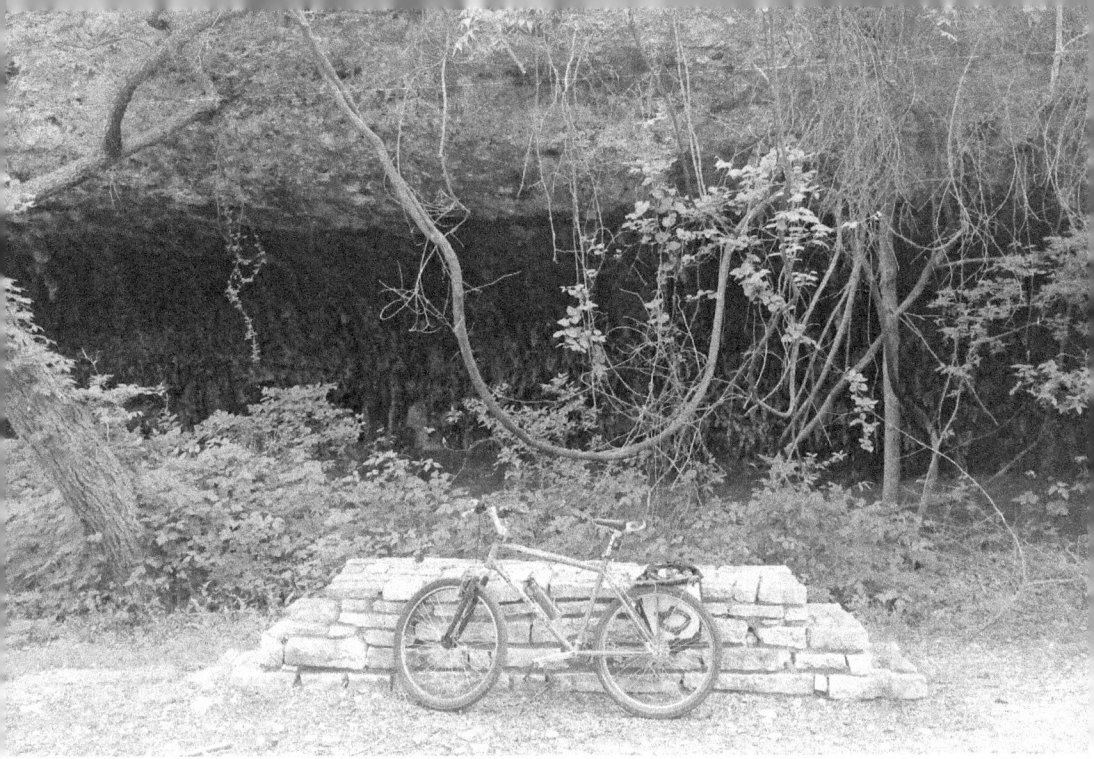

*Fern Bluff*

2 miles you will see a wooden trestle bridge in front of you. This is the old Austin and Northwestern line, used to haul granite to Austin to rebuild the capitol after the fire that destroyed it in 1881. The trail continues under the rail bridge and crosses to the north side of the water, skirting Brushy Creek Sports Park, a developed sports facility. The creek now becomes the upper end of Brushy Creek Lake. The path turns north to follow the eastern edge of the playing fields and crosses under Palmer Lane, the second and last major highway on the route. You are now in Brushy Creek Lake Park. A tenth of a mile after the highway bridge, step over a feeder creek, and turn right on a caliche trail to walk along the lakeshore. The dam is in front of you, and most likely there are fishermen on the bank and kayakers on the water.

The trail will bring you past the kayak rental outfit, through a charming oak motte, and across the access road to climb onto the dam itself, on which you cross the creek again back to the south side. Enjoy the views of the lake, Avery Ranch Golf Club, and the neighborhoods of Cedar Park. After the dam, the path zigzags down into woodland, and after 0.5 mile you emerge at Champion Park, with numerous facilities—picnic tables and a children's play area—and a few short trails of its own. Champion Park is 4.6 miles from the start point at Twin Lakes, so this might well be the point where you decide to turn back.

From Champion Park, the trail continues toward Olsen Meadows along Brushy Creek Road, with the creek and Brushy Creek greenbelt, a narrow strip of thick woods, immediately to your right. This section, some 0.8 mile, is a slow descent into a long valley to the confluence of South Brushy and Brushy Creeks, right at Olsen Meadows. As the name implies, this is a large, open meadow area, which you cross on 0.5 mile of unshaded track. Egrets hide behind the trees along the creek. Leave Olsen Meadows, and it's a third of a mile to Great Oaks Drive, 6.5 miles from Twin Lakes Park. You will pass a swimming pool under the lee of some cliffs. This portion of the hike feels most like a walk in a city park, but keep going—a prize awaits you.

Use the pedestrian crossing signal to cross Great Oaks Drive and its wide median, staying on the south side of the street, and continue on to the delightfully named Hairy Man Road. Suddenly you are on a country lane. Thick brush covers every inch of the ground below tall trees. It's a sharp contrast. Look for the sign that tells the legend of the Hairy Man. After 0.4 mile along this road, you will come to Fern Bluff, where water seeping down the cliff sustains maidenhair ferns and has carved out a grotto at its base. It's a surprising piece of wild Texas in the midst of suburban neighborhoods and worth a visit. This is the turnaround point. If you wish, you can continue along Hairy Man Road and scramble up a rough path into Fern Bluff Park. Brushy Creek flows through some undeveloped land across I-35 and into Round Rock, broadening as it approaches the dam at Veterans Park. The Round Rock for which that city is named lies in the creek at Chisholm Trail Road, just west of the freeway.

## Nearby Activities

Brushy Creek Lake Park has kayak rentals, a ramp for hand-propelled boats only, picnic facilities, and a labyrinth. Champion Park has shaded picnic facilities, its own trails, and playgrounds. Creekside Park has a swimming pool, open May–September.

### GPS TRAILHEAD COORDINATES
**N30° 29' 43.5"  W97° 48' 33.1"**

From Austin, take US 183 North, and eventually join the TX 183A toll road. Take the US 183 N exit to Avery Ranch Boulevard, and turn left. Immediately turn right onto South Bell Boulevard, US 183. One mile north of Avery Ranch Boulevard, turn right onto East Little Elm Trail. Park on the right after the entrance to the YMCA.

# 19 Comanche Bluff Trail

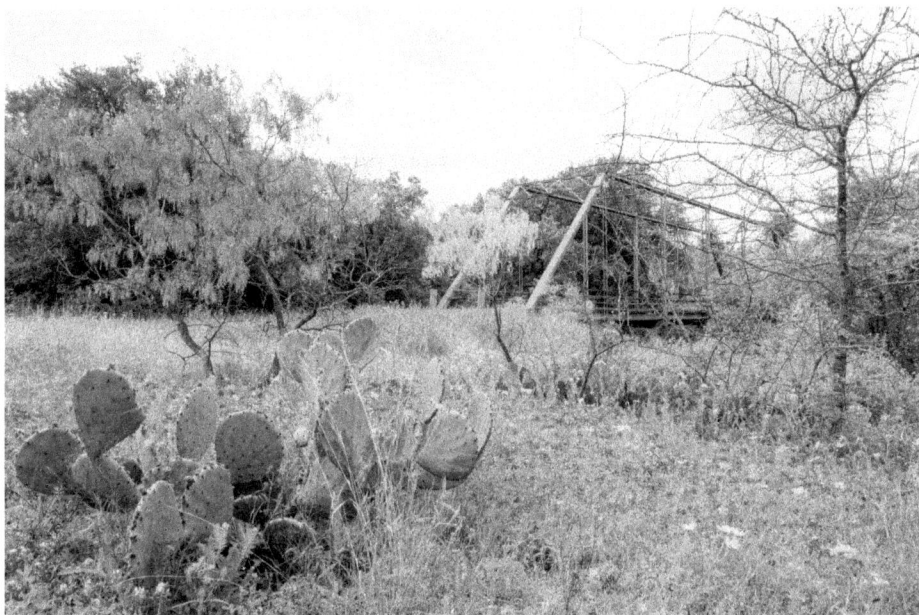

*A meadow along the Comanche Bluff Trail*

## In Brief

This gorgeous hike travels along the shoreline of Granger Lake, a low-key fishing haven on the blackland prairie north of Taylor. You'll walk through thick deciduous forest and across open meadows. Two historical bridges, which spanned the now-flooded waters of the San Gabriel River, have been moved to the path.

## Description

This trail might surprise Central Texas hikers used to the limestone and cedar of the Hill Country. You will pass through dense hardwood savanna and traverse open areas overlooking sleepy inlets to reach a fishing camp in a green glade that feels a long way from the demands of civilization. The combination of moist surroundings and rich bottomland is reminiscent of eastern forests. Granger Lake, formed by a dam on the San Gabriel River, is rimmed with willow, not cypress, and the bottomland is covered with oak, elm, cottonwood, hackberry, and pecan trees. There are some lovely views of the leafy San Gabriel Valley from Farm to Market Road 1331 as you approach the park.

| | |
|---|---|
| **LENGTH:** 7.8 miles (with an option for a shorter hike) | **HIKING TIME:** 3 hours |
| **CONFIGURATION:** Out-and-back | **DRIVING DISTANCE:** 47 miles from the state capitol |
| **DIFFICULTY:** Moderate | **ACCESS:** Daily, 6 a.m.–sunset; $4 day-use fee |
| **SCENERY:** Wooded lakeshore and open meadow | |
| **EXPOSURE:** Mixed | **WHEELCHAIR ACCESS:** No |
| **TRAFFIC:** Moderate in summer, very light in colder months | **MAPS:** At entrance booth |
| | **FACILITIES:** Restroom at trailhead |
| **TRAIL SURFACE:** Dirt singletrack | **CONTACT INFORMATION:** 512-859-2668; tinyurl.com/comanchebluffstrail |

Leave the east trailhead, immediately descending on the Comanche Bluff Trail. You quickly reach an iron trestle bridge that far exceeds the dimensions of any normal trail bridge. This is a special bridge, for it is both historic and haunted. The Hoxie Bridge was erected 3.5 miles east of Circleville around 1900, spanning the San Gabriel River where Granger Lake lies today. During the devastating 1921 flood, the Hoxie Bridge was washed 300 yards downstream. In November of that year, a firm was awarded the contract to restore the bridge. A team of convict laborers was sent from Huntsville to aid in the reconstruction. One of the prisoners was labeled a troublemaker. A guard made an example of him, shooting him in the head and hanging him in a nearby tree at the worksite as a grisly reminder. After the bridge was finished, residents and passersby began to report that the bottomland around the bridge was patrolled by a headless ghost on Friday nights during a full moon. A priest was brought in to pray for the convict's soul, allegedly ending the haunting. In 1979 the bridge was removed from the river before flooding of the lake and was repositioned here by the U.S. Army Corps of Engineers. Moving the bridge may have stirred the wrath of the convict ghost, so keep an eye out on Friday nights during a full moon.

Ahead, uphill, is the recreation area campground. The Comanche Bluff Trail veers right and circles the campground. Granger Lake is to your right. You pass several cross-trails connecting the lake to the campground, while keeping west in tall hardwoods growing out of impenetrable brush. The singletrack path works up little hills and down wet-weather drainages. Watch out for spiderwebs that span the trail. Climb away from the lake at nearly 1 mile, out to mesquite-dotted grass and cacti, where a last path from the campground merges with the main trail. Shortly you'll reach the Friendship Bridge. It once spanned Willis Creek, a feeder branch of the San Gabriel River, which now flows into the north arm of Granger Lake.

Bridges like this were important to the development of Williamson County. The rich soil of the blackland prairie grows fertile crops, but getting them to market was another matter. The deep stream channels and muddy banks made permanent bridge building difficult, and the structures were often swept away by periodic floods. In the 1880s new, stronger iron bridges with higher abutments made the crossings more reliable. The same

## Comanche Bluff Trail

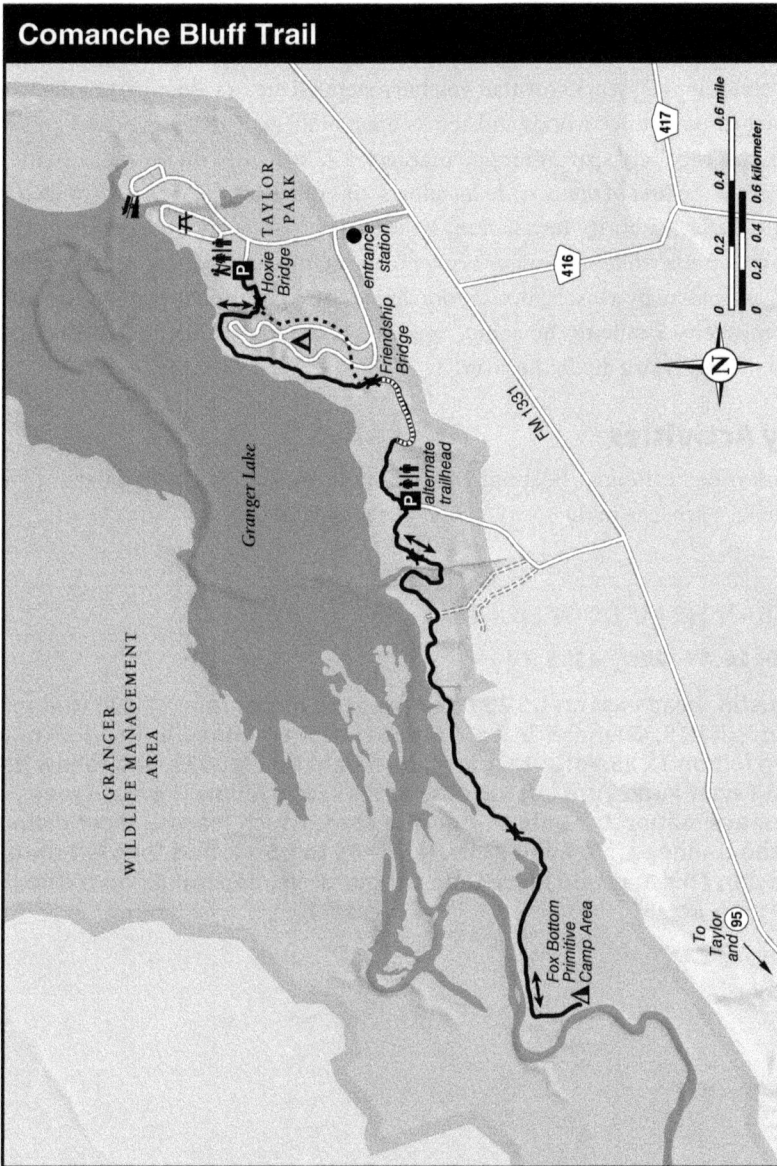

flood of 1921 that ruined the Hoxie Bridge also devastated the Friendship Bridge. Today prairie wildflowers grow extensively in this former farmland during the spring months.

Leave to the right, away from the Friendship Bridge, shortly spanning a stream on a long boardwalk. Briefly pick up an old roadbed before climbing away from the lake to reach the west trailhead of the Comanche Bluff Trail at 1.2 miles. Here are a parking area and restrooms. If you want a shorter hike, turn back here. Otherwise, pick up the trail again through a gate at the western end of the parking lot. It continues nearly 3 more miles to the Fox Bottom Primitive Camp Area, accessible only by foot or boat. (You must call the park beforehand to register if you intend to camp overnight.) Louder birdsong and stronger aromas let you know that you have stepped into a wilder part of the world.

Wander through thick woods and across open prairies. Though the track gets indistinct at places, regularly spaced orange markers will keep you on the right route. At 2 miles you cross the first of many wide meadows, this one bisected by a jeep track leading to a Brazos Water Authority installation. Boardwalks span many of the streams leading into the lake. After a while the trail goes over a bayou, dips into a thick coppice to cross a fence line, and passes by a lost lagoon before diving back into the hardwoods. Keep going: it is only another 0.5 mile to the camp. You'll want to tarry awhile in that shady green clearing and likely take a dip in the river.

## Nearby Activities

Taylor Park offers camping, boating, and fishing in season. For meat eaters, a visit to Louie Mueller Barbecue in the town of Taylor is mandatory.

### GPS TRAILHEAD COORDINATES

**N30° 40' 16.4"  W97° 22' 3.7"**

From Austin, head east on US 290 (toll road) 10 miles. Take TX 130 (toll road) north to Exit 419, Chandler Road. Continue east on Chandler Road 10 miles, and turn left on TX 95. After 1.6 miles, turn right on FM 1331, and follow it 4.7 miles to Taylor Park. Turn left into Taylor Park, and follow the main road past the entrance station 0.3 mile to the side road, which leads a short distance left to the trailhead. (To avoid tolls, take I-35 to US 79, and turn left onto TX 95 in Taylor. This may add more time to your drive, depending on traffic.)

# 20 Crockett Gardens and Falls at Cedar Breaks Park

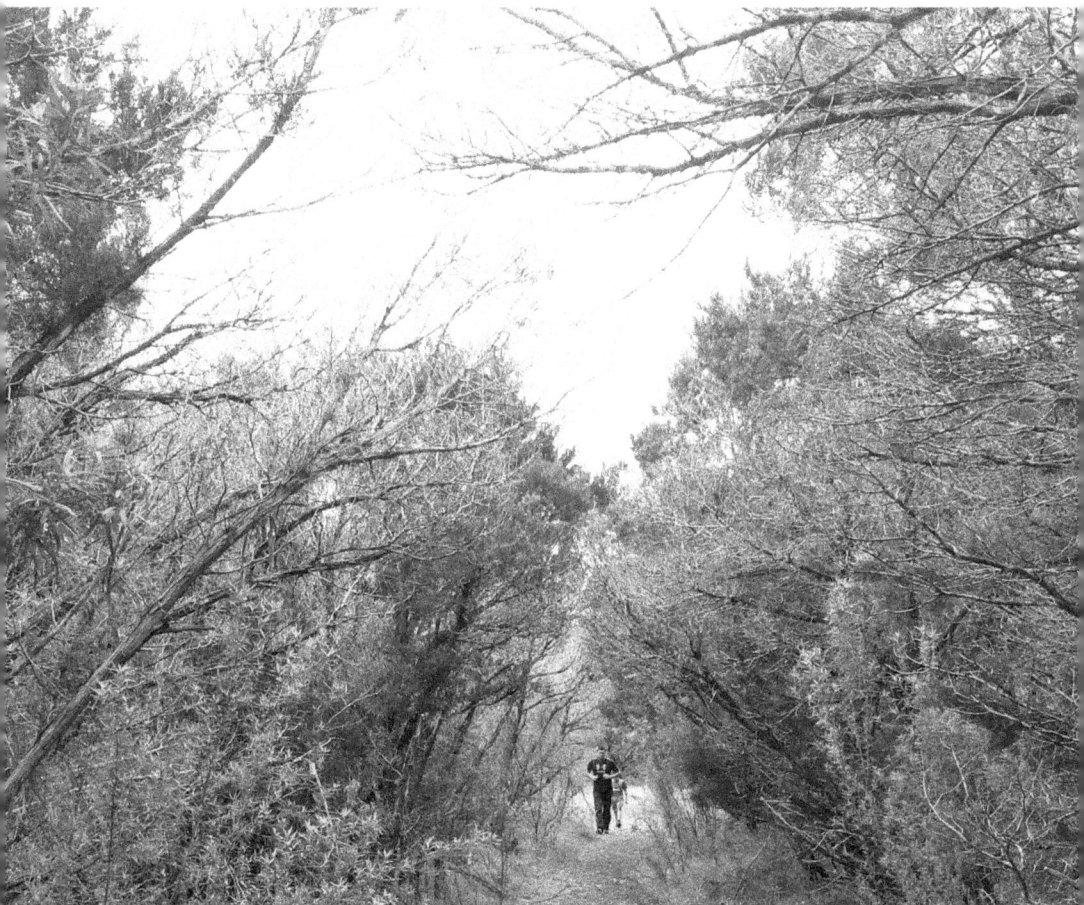

*Cedar breaks above Lake Georgetown on the Crockett Gardens Trail*

## In Brief

Justifiably gaining in popularity, this section of the Good Water Loop is one of the best hikes in the area. After tunneling through the cedar breaks that give the park its name, the route opens onto tall bluffs with grand views over Lake Georgetown. The destination is Crockett Falls, where a spring rains down an overhanging rock.

| | |
|---|---|
| **LENGTH:** 5 miles | **DRIVING DISTANCE:** 33 miles from the state capitol |
| **CONFIGURATION:** Out-and-back | |
| **DIFFICULTY:** Moderate | **ACCESS:** Daily, 6 a.m.–10 p.m.; $4 day-use fee per vehicle with up to 6 people |
| **SCENERY:** Cedar woods, lake bluffs, springs | |
| **EXPOSURE:** Mostly shady | **WHEELCHAIR ACCESS:** No |
| | **MAPS:** tinyurl.com/goodwaterloop |
| **TRAFFIC:** Moderate, busy on weekends | **FACILITIES:** Restrooms, water at park picnic area |
| **TRAIL SURFACE:** Rock, dirt | |
| **HIKING TIME:** 3.5 hours, including lunch at springs | **CONTACT INFORMATION:** 512-930-5253; tinyurl.com/cedarbreakspark |

## Description

There's a lot to enjoy at every stage of this delightful hike. It takes you along part of the Good Water (or Goodwater) Loop, itself part of the San Gabriel River Trail network, which has grown to link the circuit around the lake to the city of Georgetown (see the entry for the Randy Morrow Trail, page 107). This section takes you through cedar woods made for shady summer hiking and along sheer 100-foot bluffs where the vistas extend the length of Lake Georgetown. Beyond that point, the trail crosses a stream to reach an old homestead and Crockett Falls. The spring, surrounded by rich vegetation, flows a few feet to tumble over a rock overhang, bright green with moss and ferns. This unexpected oasis makes a great picnic locale.

Leave the large trailhead on a gravel path that leads into the cedar woods and soon gives way to rocks and dirt. After almost 0.3 mile of level terrain, stone steps begin the descent into a sudden steep ravine. Cross the creek, and the trail turns right along the side of the ravine and doglegs back on itself to avoid the almost technical climb on the other side, though it's obvious that some hikers enjoy the challenge of the direct ascent. Ahead, a stone marker denotes the site of Russell, or Second Booty's, Crossing, which in pre-dam days was the second ford on the North Fork San Gabriel River above Georgetown. The trail descends slowly under cedar arches toward the bluffline. You might hear a boat engine and will certainly glimpse water through the trees, until suddenly you reach the edge and can see across the lake to Russell Park. The gnarly limestone underfoot follows the bluffline west, passing an inviting bench by the 1-mile post. Views open up across the expanse of the lake. Step to the bluff's edge, but tread carefully—some of the drops are sheer and 100 feet or more down to the blue-gray water.

Slightly before the 2-mile point, pass through an old wire fence, and open onto a clearing with cacti, rock, and grass. Begin to circle around an unnamed cove, passing the mile-marker post. Dip down into a green valley and across a sycamore-lined stream, quickly climbing out into a clearing where stone relics of an old homestead stand near a cedar-post corral in various stages of decay. Enter the corral, and reach a trail sign at 2.4 miles. Crockett Spring is straight ahead, but turn right here toward the base of the falls.

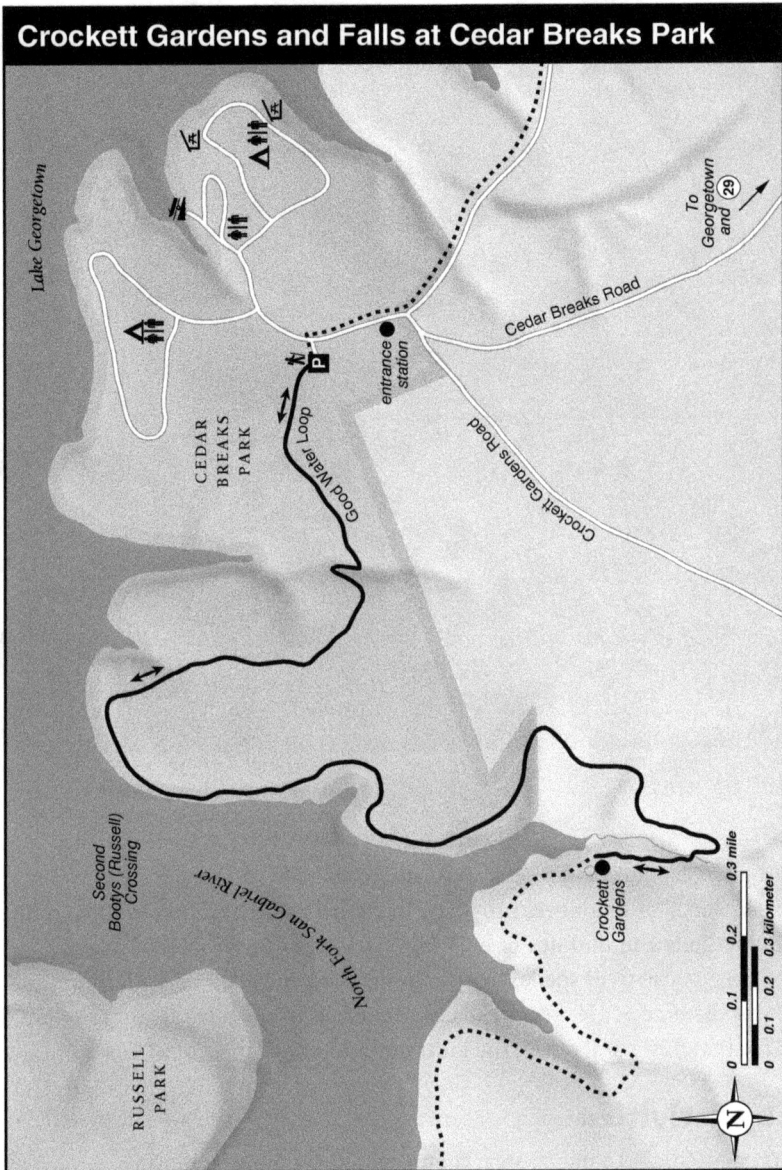

Crockett Gardens and Falls at Cedar Breaks Park

Work your way down the streambed as it stair-steps to the lake, and you come to a little grotto—the overhang mentioned earlier—where you might decide to refresh yourself under the natural shower the spring provides.

Return to the main trail, and reach the spring run and upper falls. Many a settler has coveted this area. It went through several hands until James Knight operated a flour mill and grew fruits and vegetables in the area, including the first strawberries in Williamson County. Later, R. M. Crockett, who gave the area its name, operated a truck garden.

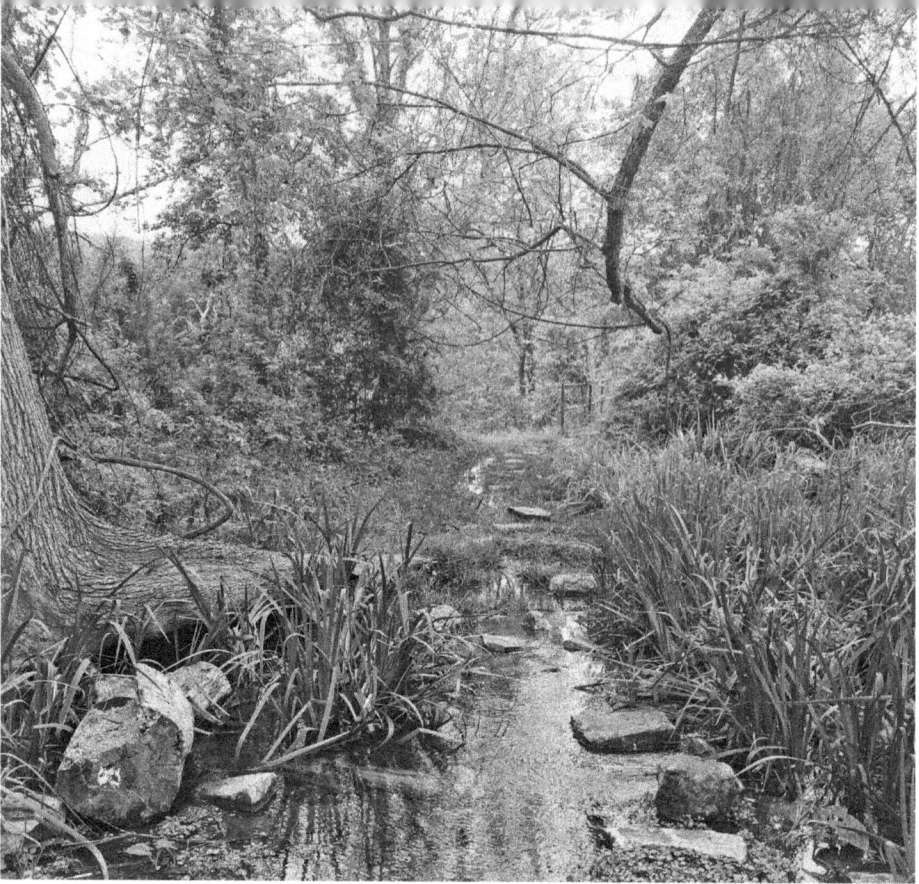

*Crockett Gardens*

Crockett grew produce and took it to Austin to sell. On the far side of the fence, outside U.S. Army Corps of Engineers property, longhorn cattle and horses stand among concrete foundations and outlines of buildings, as well as the stone house and ranch relics nearby. Large pecan trees shade the spring run and benches. The outflow of the spring is visible near the base of a low rock ridge, and the falls from above are quite a sight too. It is easy to see that this is still one of the most desirable spots in Central Texas.

## Nearby Activities

Cedar Breaks Park has a picnic area, campground, and boat landing.

---

**GPS TRAILHEAD COORDINATES**

**N30° 40' 12.5" W97° 44' 19.6"**

From Exit 261 on I-35, take TX 29 west. Travel west 1.1 miles, and then turn right onto D. B. Wood Road. Follow D. B. Wood Road north 1.8 miles, and turn right onto Cedar Breaks Road into the park. Take the first left beyond the entrance station to reach the trailhead.

---

# 21 Dana Peak Park at Stillhouse Hollow Lake

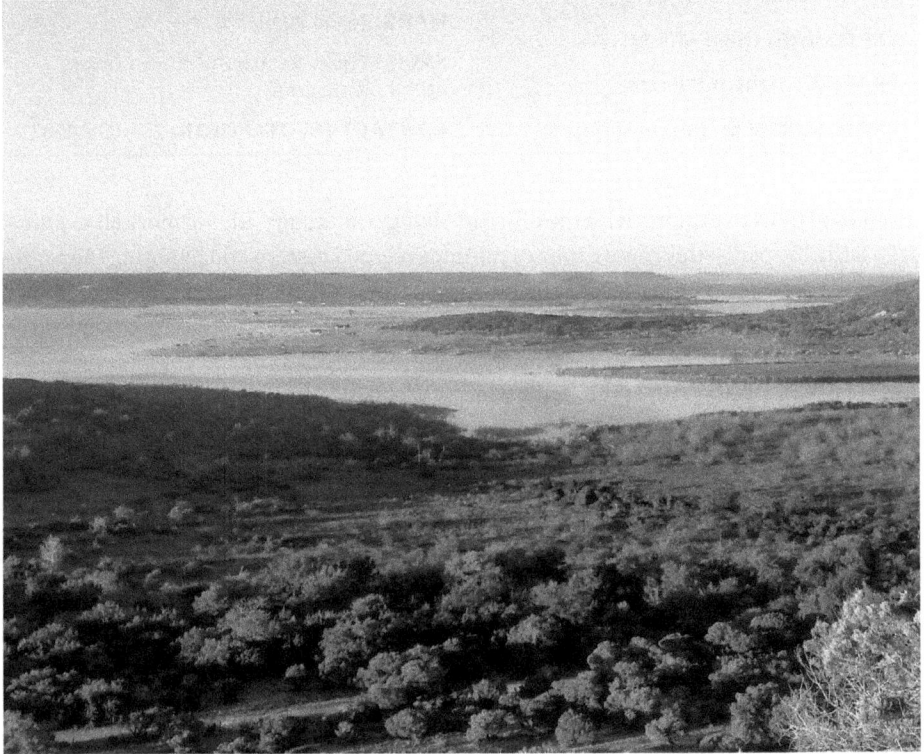

*View of Stillhouse Hollow Lake at Dana Peak*

## In Brief

Explore rocky coves and headlands along the lake, walk through dense woodland, and enjoy the view from limestone peaks at this uncrowded park on the shore of Stillhouse Hollow Lake, part of the Lampasas River.

## Description

Stillhouse Hollow is one of the many U.S. Army Corps of Engineers facilities in the area that not only cater to fishermen, recreational boaters, and the RVers who pack the campsites on weekends but also provide opportunities for hiking and biking. At Dana Peak Park, on the north side of the lake at the edge of Harker Heights, there are perhaps

| | |
|---|---|
| **LENGTH:** 4 miles | **HIKING TIME:** 2.5 hours |
| **CONFIGURATION:** Balloon loop | **DRIVING DISTANCE:** 60 miles from north Austin, 66 miles from the capitol |
| **DIFFICULTY:** Moderate–difficult | **ACCESS:** Daily, 6 a.m.–10 p.m.; free |
| **SCENERY:** Overgrown creek bottoms, cedar breaks | **WHEELCHAIR ACCESS:** No |
| **EXPOSURE:** Open–shady | **MAPS:** None available |
| **TRAFFIC:** Light–moderate | **FACILITIES:** Restrooms and showers at the picnic area |
| **TRAIL SURFACE:** Natural surfaces | **CONTACT INFORMATION:** 254-698-4282 |

20 miles of trails to explore, with the off-road biking community adding more all the time. It's a fairly big park—this route explores the undeveloped eastern end, ignoring the campsites and picnic areas on the large main peninsula. The trails are mostly unmarked, though the strips of colored tape wound round the occasional wooden marker post may mean something to the bikers.

The park's main trail, at this end a wide, washed-out sandy road, runs from the trailhead for a mile to the east, straight as a Roman road except for one diversion around one of the lake's many coves. This route takes you along this track to the next promontory, where you will climb the tallest of the twin peaks. First, however, you will detour around the contours of Dana Peak itself. Take the path diagonally across from the parking area that heads up the cedar-covered hillside, ignoring any forks that would divert you from the ascent. The surface is covered with small limestone rocks, so watch your footing. It's a sharp 120-foot climb to where the path levels out to follow the contour around the top, but there are some good views from this part of the trail. After 0.4 mile you begin to descend, and after 0.1 mile more, you arrive at the junction with the main trail. Turn right.

You can see the track stretching out in front of you across a wide basin at the head of a bay, split by a small peninsula that sticks out between the mouths of two of the three streams that flow into the bay. To your left, a metal rail fence marks the boundary, and at the end of the fence, a path goes up into the northern reaches of the park. Keep forward, passing side trails that lead back to the boat dock and camping areas. By this point, you are well into the most exposed section of the trail, crossing a grassy valley dotted with dead juniper and clumps of salt cedar. Roughly 0.5 mile north are bluffs that ring the northern side of the valley from Dana Peak to a similar peak in front of you. Ahead of you and to the right are the twin peaks that occupy the promontory at the eastern side of the bay and that you will explore.

After another 0.1 mile you cross the first creek and then soon come to a T junction. Turn left up the indistinct muddy (or dusty) track that curls around the head of the second cove in this bay. In a little while, you will cross the second creek, and the path starts to maneuver itself back into a straight line. Bushes and trees start to crowd in on the narrowing track. At 1.3 miles, turn right along a short, deep trench that disappears

## Dana Peak Park at Stillhouse Hollow Lake

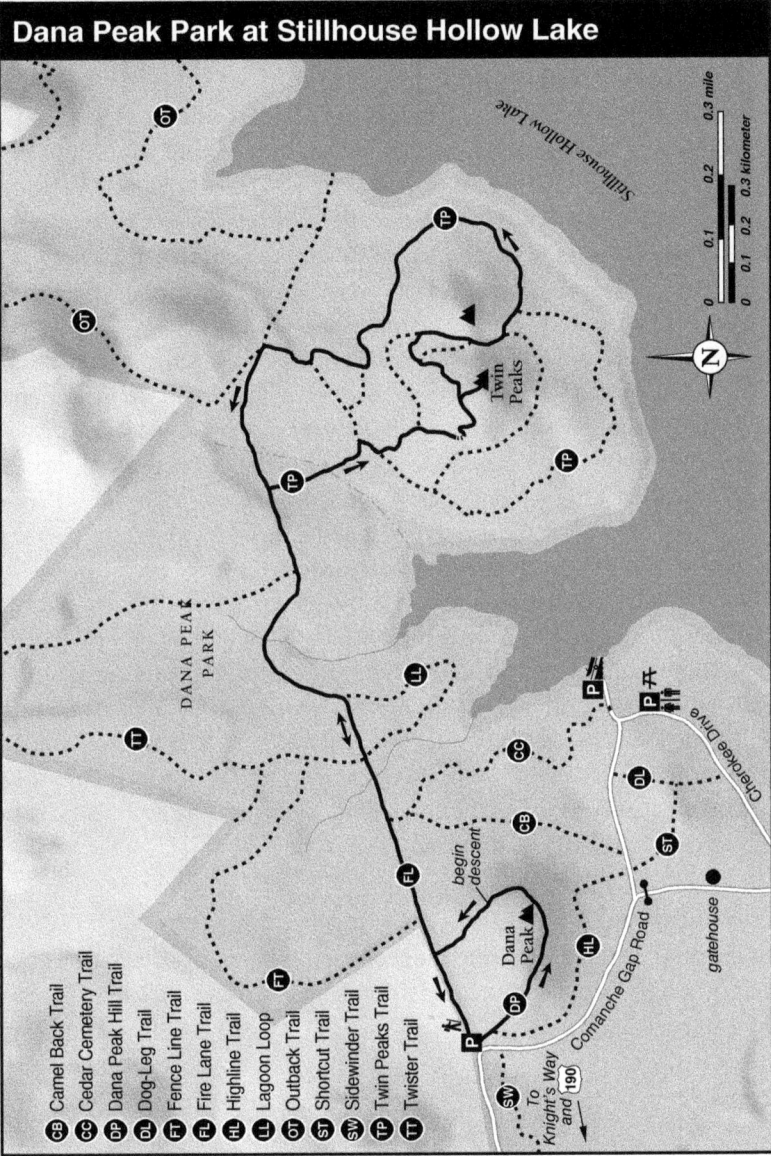

CB  Camel Back Trail
CC  Cedar Cemetery Trail
DP  Dana Peaks Hill Trail
DL  Dog-Leg Trail
FT  Fence Line Trail
FL  Fire Lane Trail
HL  Highline Trail
LL  Lagoon Loop
OT  Outback Trail
ST  Shortcut Trail
SW  Sidewinder Trail
TP  Twin Peaks Trail
TT  Twister Trail

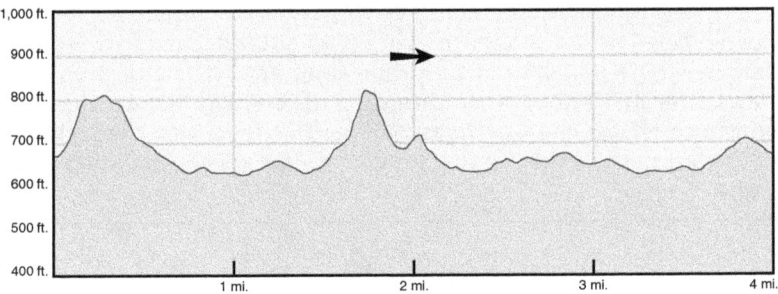

through the hedgerow toward the right of the twin peaks, and continue across the open valley made by the third stream. Once across the muddy stream, take the left fork and start to climb a washed-out channel toward the thick cedar on the hillside. Gnarled trunks and many dead trees give the woods a slightly sinister look. At the next fork, 1.7 miles in, head right. The way gets steeper as it zigzags toward the top, and you will go up some short sections of wooden steps. The trees are thicker and taller here. At 1.8 miles, take a sharp right and scramble up some tall rock steps into a small grove. You have reached the top of the hill. Walk across the flat summit to an inviting lookout area, where someone has built a fire pit. Rest here, eat your energy bar, and enjoy the view through the trees across the lake to the Bell County Expo Center off in the distance.

When you are ready, retrace your steps across the peak, and scramble back down to the trail, where you will turn right. The trail dives back down the hill. After a couple of hundred feet, there's a fork where you turn left (look for the checkered tape), then shortly after that a second fork, where you turn right. Cross a creek bed at the bottom of a small ravine, and you will start to loop back across the saddle between the two peaks. Come down the other side, take a left at the next two junctions, and go straight at the third one, continuing down toward the lake. The path goes through the untidy scrub on the shallow slope between the hill and the water. After a while, the path turns away from the shore. For a while, dense undergrowth crowds your passage along this fertile valley before the earth (and possibly mud) underfoot gives way to sand and the lush foliage is replaced by cedar. At 2.7 and 2.8 miles, turn right at each of two junctions. Continue another 0.1 mile, and you will come to a wooden post striped with colored tape. This is where you turn left to rejoin the main trail, though for a while the narrow trail is hemmed in by trees and bushes covered with creeper. It soon straightens out and takes you back across the floodplain and past Dana Peak to the parking lot.

## Nearby Activities

Camp, fish, swim, and bike at the park. The shops and artist galleries of Salado are a short drive away. So Natural Organic Restaurant in Harker Heights has delicious, healthy food for when you tire of energy bars.

---

### GPS TRAILHEAD COORDINATES

**N31° 1' 54.5" W97° 36' 30.3"**

From Austin, head north on I-35 to Exit 286 in Salado. Take Farm to Market Road 2484 west 7.7 miles; then turn right onto FM 3481. After 3 miles turn right onto Cedar Knob Road; then turn right onto Knight's Way. After 1 mile, turn right onto Comanche Gap Road. Follow this road into the facility, and park on the left in the little parking lot where Comanche Gap Road makes a sharp right.

# 22 Overlook Trail at Lake Georgetown

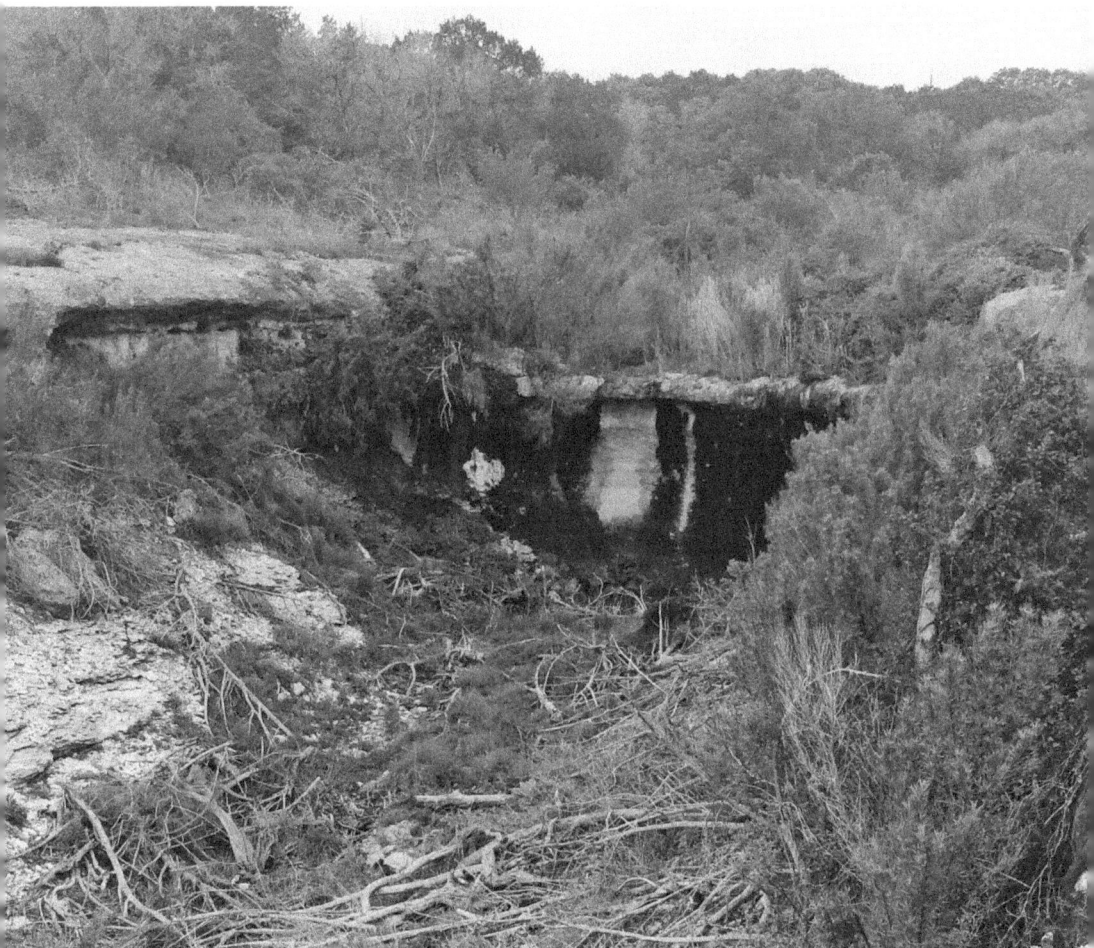

*A dry creek bed along the Overlook Trail*

## In Brief

The hike uses the San Gabriel River Trail at Lake Georgetown to connect two developed recreation areas, passing numerous watery vistas, an old ranch site, and an aboriginal Texan village along the way.

**LENGTH:** 7.2 miles

**CONFIGURATION:** Out-and-back

**DIFFICULTY:** Moderate

**SCENERY:** Lakeside woods and meadows

**EXPOSURE:** Partly sunny

**TRAFFIC:** Heavy on weekends

**TRAIL SURFACE:** Gravel, natural surfaces

**HIKING TIME:** 3 hours

**DRIVING DISTANCE:** 31 miles from the state capitol

**ACCESS:** (Overlook Park) Daily, 7:30 a.m.–sunset; no fees required

**WHEELCHAIR ACCESS:** From beginning of trail to nearby fishing platform

**MAPS:** tinyurl.com/goodwaterloop

**FACILITIES:** Overlook Park and Jim Hogg Park have restrooms, water, picnicking, and shelter. Jim Hogg Park also has camping.

**CONTACT INFORMATION:** 512-930-5253

## Description

The San Gabriel River Trail, also known as the Good Water (or Goodwater) Loop, is one of the region's best trails. It makes a 28-mile circuit around Lake Georgetown within U.S. Army Corps of Engineers property that envelops the reservoir. Civilization is springing up all around this lake, situated just west of the pretty city of Georgetown, but the lakeshore has retained its natural beauty. This particular hike starts near the reservoir dam, which backs up the North Fork San Gabriel River and then travels the scenic shoreline, wandering through groves of live oak and cedar separated by grassy clearings, where you can enjoy views of the large main lake as well as intimate coves. Highlights of the hike include these watery vistas, an aboriginal Texan village site, and the stone foundations of a forgotten ranch. Recreation areas on both ends of the trail expand your outdoor opportunities. This path is popular with mountain bikers, so listen for their comings and goings.

Leave the parking area, passing the restrooms, and come to a concrete junction. The path in front of you leads to a fishing platform. Turn right here, joining a gravel track, with the trailhead uphill to your right and the lake to your left. Initially there is some confusion because multiple paths lead from the parking area, but as long as you're heading away from the dam, you'll be fine. Cedar Breaks Park and stone bluffs are clearly visible across the water. Travel an open area, and another gravel path splits left toward the lake, but stay right, circling around an embayment and staying in the open on the wide foreshore between the trees and the water. The trail narrows and becomes quite rocky as you pass an old concrete water cistern. Note the sloped rock walls bordering the lake.

Cross the normally dry head of the embayment, passing mile marker 23 at 0.7 mile. The entire San Gabriel River Trail is marked at 1-mile increments. Just ahead you will see a sign indicating the T. H. Godwin aboriginal site, near the water's edge. A rock shelter, midden, and quarry site reveal that aboriginal Texans once lived here. The shelter, ample wood, a spring, and chert made the locale appealing. The aboriginals chipped the chert for tools in the shade of the rock shelter. A trail leads down toward the site, but it is now submerged. Continue on through a vegetational mosaic of cedar, grass, cacti, brush, and

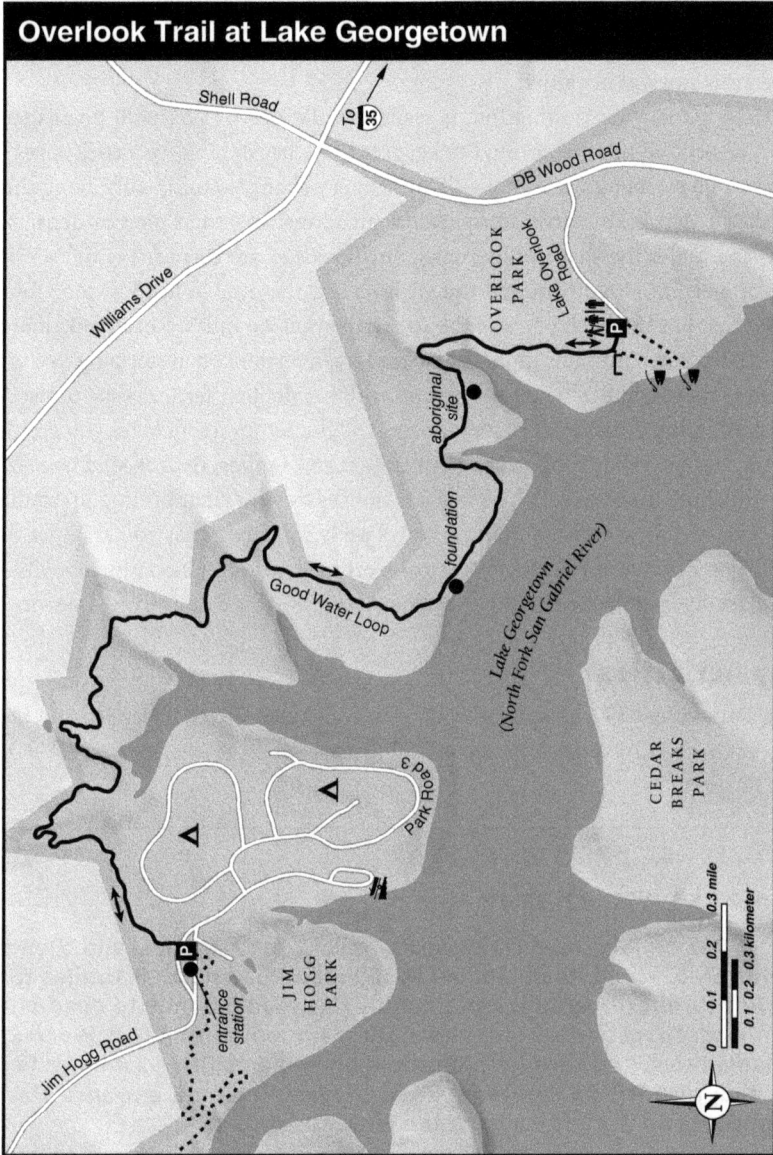

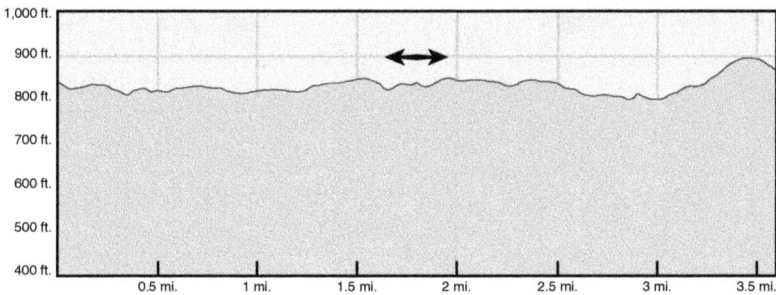

lacey and live oaks along a rocky track. At 1.2 miles look left for the stone foundation of a ranch house or corral. A long stone fence runs parallel to the lake, still the San Gabriel River when this site was occupied.

Jim Hogg Park, your destination, is visible to the north. The path begins to wind around a long second inlet, entering thicker trees, the brush pink with rock roses in the spring. Pass mile marker 22 at 1.7 miles. The scenery changes continually along the trail, which makes a thin gash across stony cactus meadows and then pierces dense woods before passing under the shade of live oaks. Small washes are carpeted with their leaves. Another view of Jim Hogg Park and the wide valley, the double head of the aforementioned inlet that lies between you and the park, opens at 2.6 miles. Reach mile marker 21 at 2.7 miles. Dip down into this mullein-covered open terrain, soon stepping over a trickling branch to meet a line of wet bluffs, green with maidenhair fern, that lie between you and your destination. Distant lake views open. A slight detour north takes you around the bluffs and across the valley. Hop over a clear stream at 3.1 miles; then ascend from the wet meadow and climb a stone bluff. You will see houses to your right butting up against the Corps boundary. Join a well-maintained gravel path indicating that you are near the Jim Hogg trailhead. Emerge at Jim Hogg Park at 3.6 miles. The entrance station is visible from here, and parking is available should you choose to make this a one-way endeavor.

## Nearby Activities

Jim Hogg Park offers 142 campsites with water and electricity. It is also the western trailhead for this hike. Overlook Park has fishing accesses.

### GPS TRAILHEAD COORDINATES
**N30° 40' 27.5"  W97° 43' 26.1"**

From Exit 261 on I-35, take TX 29 west. Travel west 1.1 miles, and then turn right onto D. B. Wood Road. Follow D. B. Wood Road north 3.1 miles to the signed left turn for Overlook Park. Follow this road 0.2 mile to dead-end at the trailhead. To reach the other end of the trail, continue on D. B. Wood Road to Williams Drive, and turn left. Continue on Williams Drive 2.4 miles to Jim Hogg Road; turn left on Jim Hogg Road to reach the park entrance station. The trail starts on the left just past the entrance station.

# 23 Randy Morrow Trail

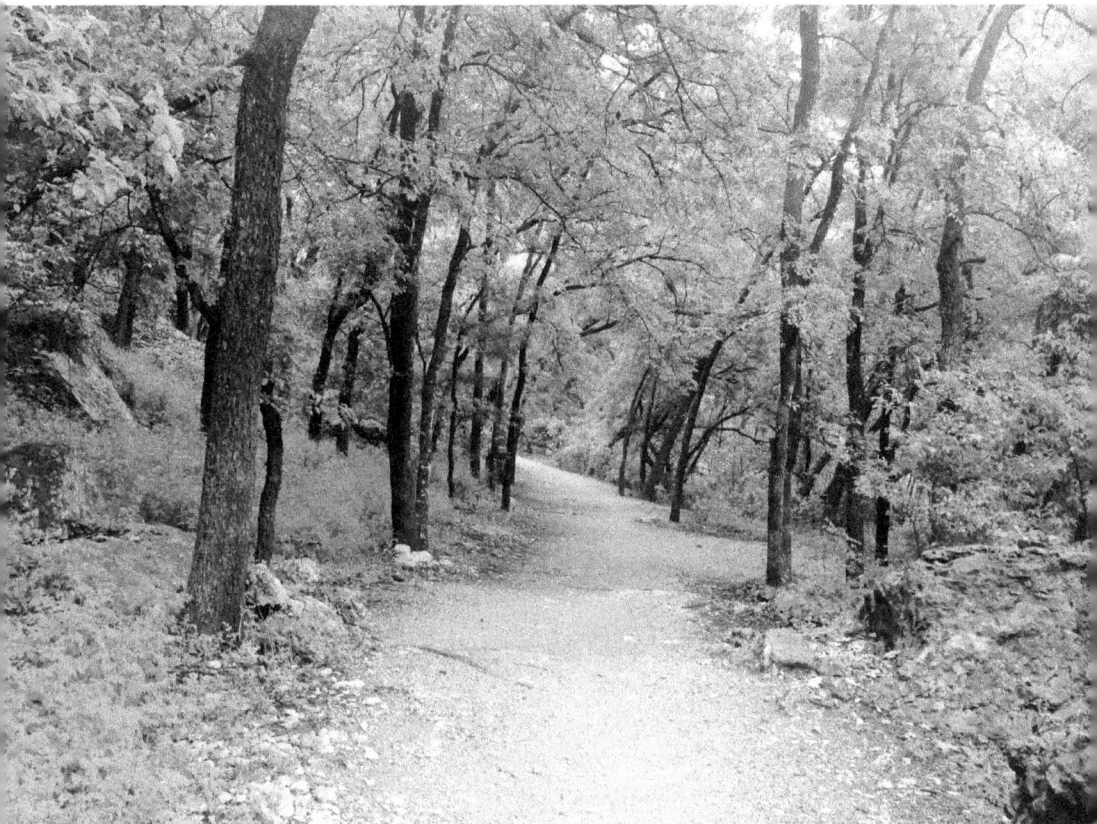

*A tree canopy shades the Randy Morrow Trail.*

## In Brief

Formerly the North San Gabriel River Trail, and renamed in 2013 in honor of a city employee, this trail is a serious rival to Austin's Barton Creek Greenbelt for best urban trail of the region. It connects the city of Georgetown to the Good Water Loop around Lake Georgetown, via the North Fork San Gabriel River.

## Description

This well-maintained trail is an important piece of Georgetown's appeal as a place to live and visit. It winds along the lush North San Gabriel River Valley to the Lake Georgetown dam and then climbs a cedar-covered slope to reach Overlook Park on the lakeshore. The

| | |
|---|---|
| **LENGTH:** 11.2 miles | **ACCESS:** (Overlook Park) Daily, 7:30 a.m.–sunset; (hike-and-bike trail) daily, 5 a.m.–11 p.m.; no fees required |
| **CONFIGURATION:** Out-and-back | |
| **DIFFICULTY:** Moderate | |
| **SCENERY:** River bottom, neighborhood | **WHEELCHAIR ACCESS:** All but one short section is accessible. |
| **EXPOSURE:** Mostly shady | **MAPS:** tinyurl.com/randymorrow |
| **TRAFFIC:** Moderate; busy on weekends | **FACILITIES:** Restrooms at Booty's Road Park, Rivery Park, and San Gabriel Park, which has sports and picnic facilities |
| **TRAIL SURFACE:** Concrete, gravel, asphalt | |
| **HIKING TIME:** 3–4 hours | **CONTACT INFORMATION:** 512-930-3595, parks.georgetown.org |
| **DRIVING DISTANCE:** 29 miles from the state capitol | |

mostly smooth surfaces make for easy hiking, and the scenery is a constant delight. In 2006 Secretary of the Interior Dirk Kempthorne designated it as a National Recreation Trail, a well-deserved honor. A hike-and-bike trail, it is very popular with off-road bikers as well as walkers, so keep your eyes open.

From the parking lot in urban San Gabriel Park, walk toward the water, and turn right on the gravel path that runs along the bank. This is the trail. The river is a lagoon at this point because of the dam at the eastern end of the park. Trees line the south bank. In front of you is a low bridge, a favorite of fishermen, situated at the confluence of the North and South Forks of the San Gabriel. Follow the concrete trail past the bridge and into a little meadow where trees line both sides of the river. At the 0.5-mile mark you will go under Austin Avenue. Bluffs rise from the opposite bank. The apartments perched at the top of these cliffs are a striking juxtaposition of the man-made and the natural.

At 0.9 mile the North Fork turns north, passing under the four bridges that make up I-35 and its frontage roads. The huge concrete blocks of the roadways and their piers are an impressive sight, and once again there is a nice contrast between the infrastructure and the lush greenery of the shrubs and aquatic grasses growing in and around the stream. The sound of traffic flying across the valley way above you seems to belong to a different world.

A low concrete bridge takes you across the river, under the eastern frontage road, and the trail continues up a long slope under the highway. Watch for cyclists on this section in particular, as the narrow path has solid handrails that prevent escape. You emerge into an open meadow, where a few cedars grow. This is Rivery Park, with restrooms and parking. The trail skirts the thick woods of the riverbank, heading north. Keep right at the end of the park. Trees crowd the trail as it descends through a disc golf course. The river bends left and passes under some striking bluffs and then under Rivery Boulevard, as does the path. At 1.8 miles another concrete bridge takes you back to the north side of the river, avoiding Georgetown Country Club and the Middle Fork of the San Gabriel, which flows through the club's property. You will notice the large sluice gate of a dam

## Randy Morrow Trail

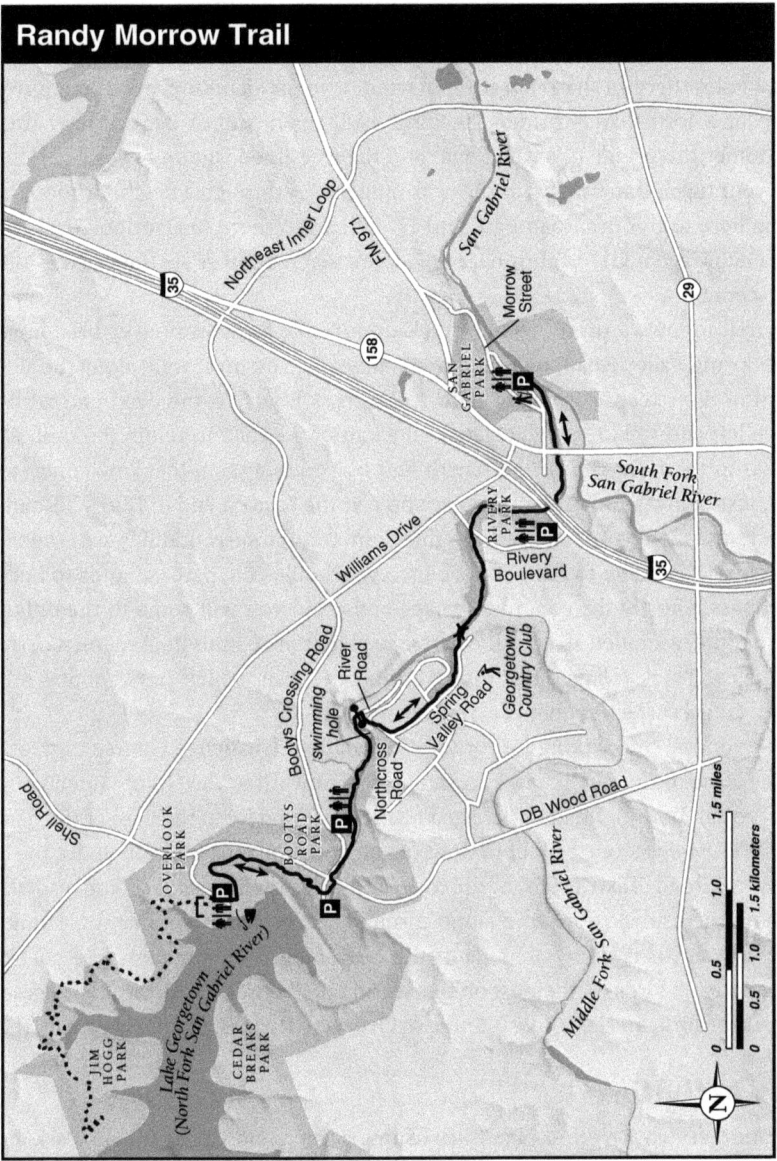

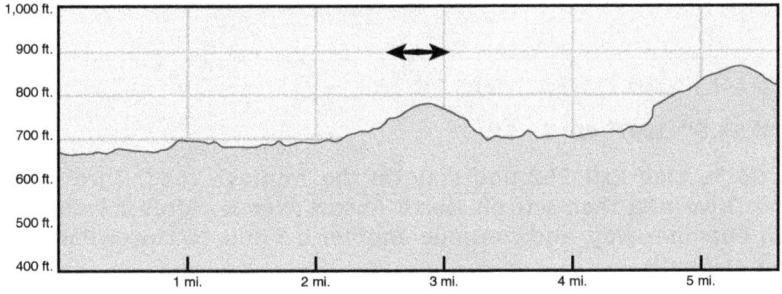

where that fork meets the river. The parks department has put up some Victorian-looking streetlights along this more open section of the trail.

At 2.2 miles there's a sharp left turn. In front of you is an unimproved concrete crossing, more of a ford than a bridge, heading back to the south bank. Enjoy the view up-river, under the bridge to a small dam and the tree-lined lagoon beyond it. This spot might be your turnaround point, as the next mile passes through a neighborhood. It is 2.2 miles from here to Booty's Road Park and 1.1 mile from there to Overlook Park. Should you need encouragement to continue, remind yourself that those sections of the route are the most scenic.

The trail follows a pretty feeder creek up a valley as it flows over bare limestone alongside Spring Valley Road. It ends after 0.5 mile and you must walk along the sidewalk to the end of the street. Turn right onto Northcross Road. At the dead end with River Road, turn left and walk through a gate at the end of the road to rejoin the trail. A ramp leads down to the river and to the fourth and last crossing, another low concrete construction, just below another dam. You are now at the eastern end of Booty's Road Park. There are houses to the north, but from this point on, the surroundings are wilder. Continue past a track leading to the water's edge. At 3.5 miles the path expands to become a stone compass. Shortly the concrete surface ends, and you will come to the only rough part of the route, a sudden steep hill where a feeder creek comes in. Around a corner are three benches. Thick foliage lines the river and the trail, which passes along a line of bluffs. The gravel surface soon gives way to concrete.

When you see the parking lot for the Georgetown Challenge Course to your right, you will be close to the 4-mile mark. A sign points onward to the Good Water Loop. It is half a mile to the Booty's Road Park restrooms and parking lot at the base of the dam. You will see this imposing stone barrier in front of you once you emerge from under the bridge at D. B. Wood Road. Take a right at the fork, and cross the access road and a small open area. Follow the asphalt trail up a slope through sparse cedar woodland 0.7 mile. The steepest part, and it is quite steep, is at the beginning. Bird-watchers can check both lake and woodland birds off their list on this section of the trail. Cross the dam access road, take a left at the fork, and continue 0.3 mile to Overlook Park. Enjoy the view over the lake.

## Nearby Activities

At Lake Georgetown, Overlook Park has fishing access, and Cedar Breaks Park and Jim Hogg Park have camping and picnic areas.

---

### GPS TRAILHEAD COORDINATES

**N30° 38' 54.5"  W97° 40' 15.1"**

From I-35 N, take Exit 262 and stay on the frontage road. Turn right at Williams Drive and then left on North Austin Avenue. After 0.3 mile, turn right on Chamber Way, and continue another 0.3 mile to Lower Park Road. Turn left and park.

# 24 Rimrock, Shin Oak, and Creek Trails at Doeskin Ranch

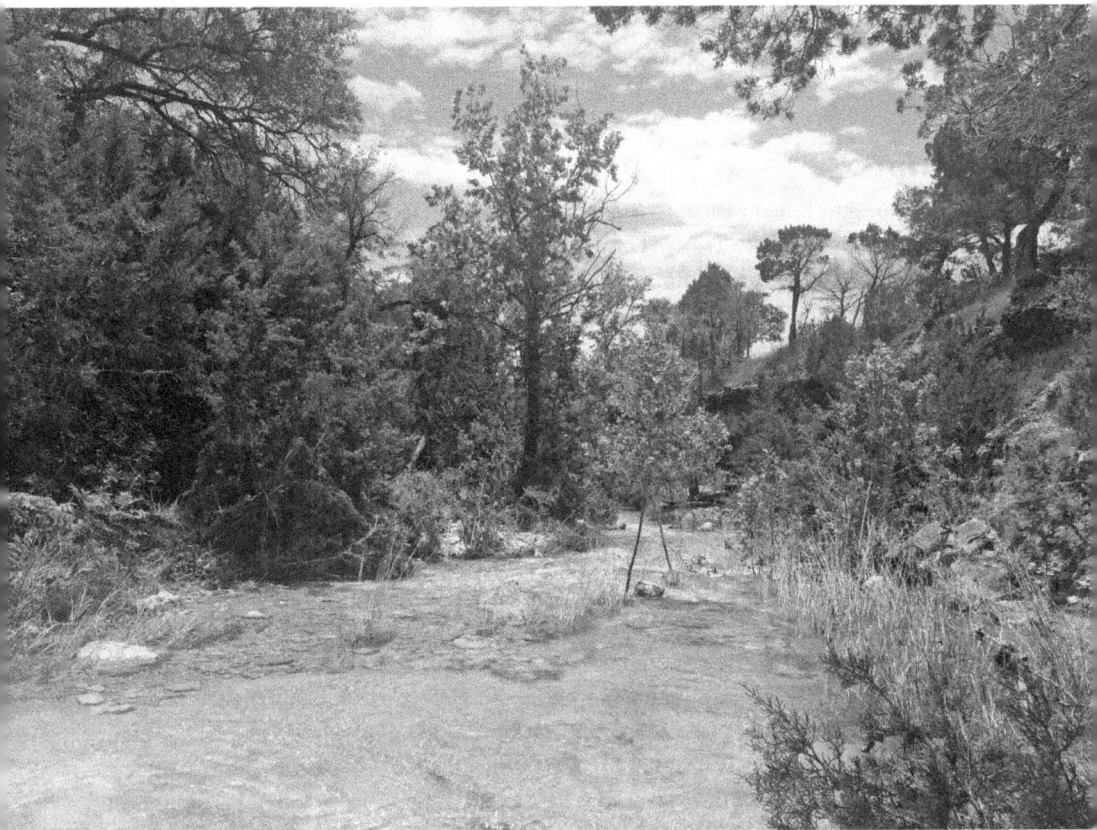

*A creek flows through Doeskin Ranch.*

## In Brief

This set of trails, a lesser-known gem of Austin-area hiking, allows access to a small but varied section of the Balcones Canyonlands National Wildlife Refuge, 24,000 acres of Hill Country between Lake Travis and Liberty Hill. Climb from a creek to a plateau dotted with thickets of shin oak, and enjoy wide-ranging views.

| | |
|---|---|
| **LENGTH:** 2.3 miles | **DRIVING DISTANCE:** 47 miles from the state capitol |
| **CONFIGURATION:** Figure eight | |
| **DIFFICULTY:** Moderate | **ACCESS:** Daily, sunrise–sunset; no fees or permits required |
| **SCENERY:** Riparian creek, prairie, open plateau | **WHEELCHAIR ACCESS:** No |
| **EXPOSURE:** Mostly exposed | **MAPS:** fws.gov/refuge/balcones_canyonlands |
| **TRAFFIC:** Moderate | **FACILITIES:** Restroom at trailhead |
| **TRAIL SURFACE:** Dirt, grass, rocks | **CONTACT INFORMATION:** 512-339-9432; fws.gov/refuge/balcones_canyonlands |
| **HIKING TIME:** 1.5 hours | |

## Description

South of Doeskin Ranch, Farm to Market Road 1174 makes a dramatic descent through Hickory Pass toward Lake Travis. This pass and Tater Hill and Chalk Knob, the hills to its west and east, are the main points of reference in the jumble of hills and ravines visible from the unnamed plateau to which you will ascend on this hike. On the way up, you will explore a Cow Creek tributary and cross ecologically diverse grassland before the steep climb through Ashe juniper to the open cap. These particular and fast-disappearing habitats are home to the black-capped vireo and to the golden-cheeked warbler, the sole avian species that breeds only in Texas. Protecting these and other flora and fauna is the reason for the Balcones Canyonlands National Wildlife Refuge (not to be confused with Austin's Balcones Canyonlands Preserve), one of more than 500 refuges nationwide that together comprise more than 150 million acres. Please remember that pets are not allowed here. The refuge is in the Colorado River watershed, and water flowing to the river has carved these ravines from the hills. Go north, and by the time you get to Liberty Hill, you have crossed into the Brazos River watershed.

At the trailhead, take a moment to peruse the information boards; then head left, north, toward the Creek Trail, which will make the first and shorter part of the figure eight. An asphalt path leads to the trail proper. Shortly you will pass an information sign that names possible past stewards of the land and then a small wooden barn with a tin roof—the first and most noticeable relic of the unknown ranchers' activities. Cross a meadow, walk through a shady stand of cedar, and at 0.1 mile come to the creek. This unnamed branch of Cow Creek carved out the valley through which FM 1174 descends from the upland savanna. At 0.2 mile a side trail leads to a bench by the water's edge. The singletrack Creek Trail continues along the stream's eastern bank, skirting the divide between riparian woodland and grassy meadow. After a rain, little waterfalls might add a soothing background sound to your hike. Tall oaks and cottonwoods add a touch of shade to the idyllic surroundings.

Half a mile into the hike, you will come to a jeep track. This is the Rimrock Trail, and you will return down this path. For now, cross the jeep track and bear left to pick up the

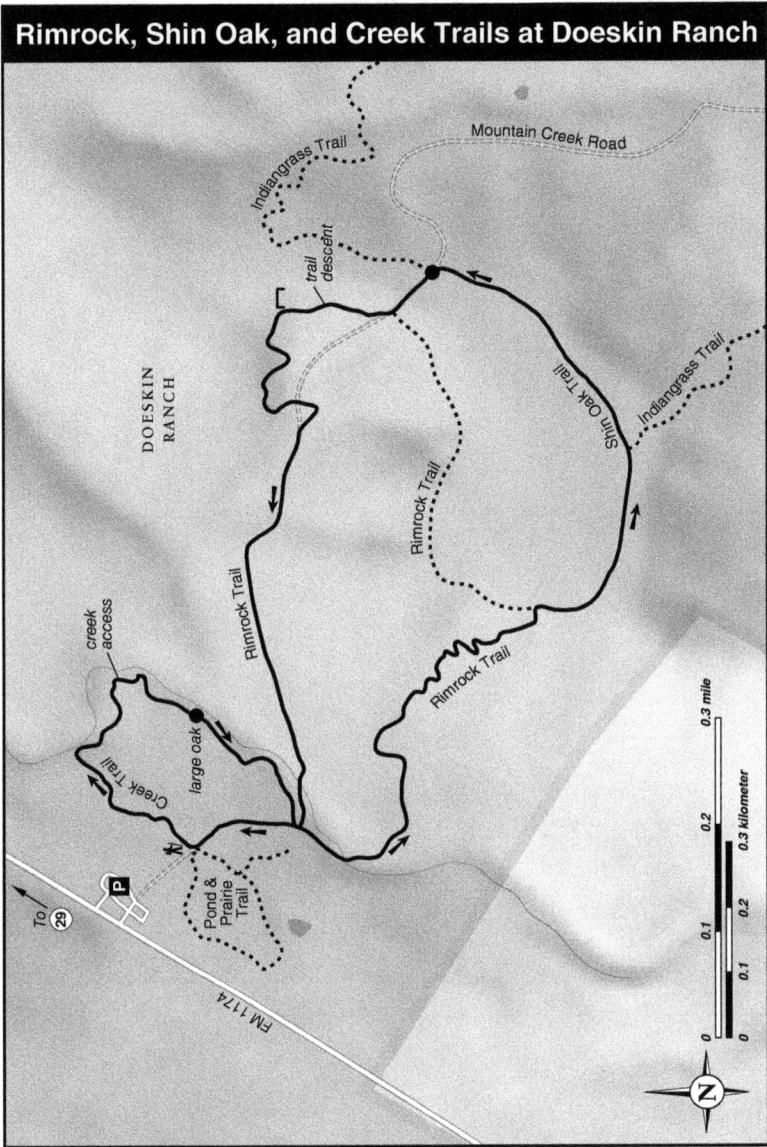

**Rimrock, Shin Oak, and Creek Trails at Doeskin Ranch**

Indiangrass Trail

Mountain Creek Road

trail descent

Shin Oak Trail

Indiangrass Trail

DOESKIN RANCH

Rimrock Trail

Rimrock Trail

Rimrock Trail

creek access

large oak

Creek Trail

P

Pond & Prairie Trail

To 29

FM 1174

0.3 mile
0.3 kilometer
0.2
0.2
0.1
0.1
0

N

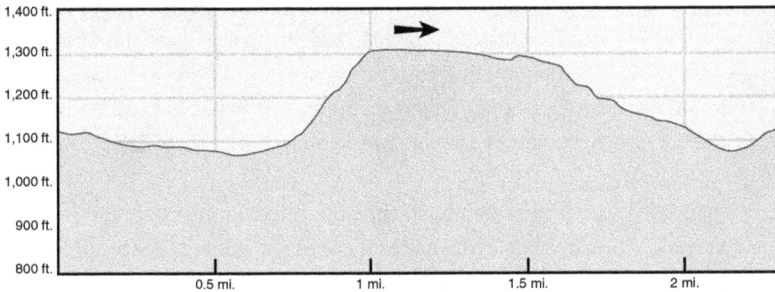

1,400 ft.
1,300 ft.
1,200 ft.
1,100 ft.
1,000 ft.
900 ft.
800 ft.

0.5 mi.          1 mi.          1.5 mi.          2 mi.

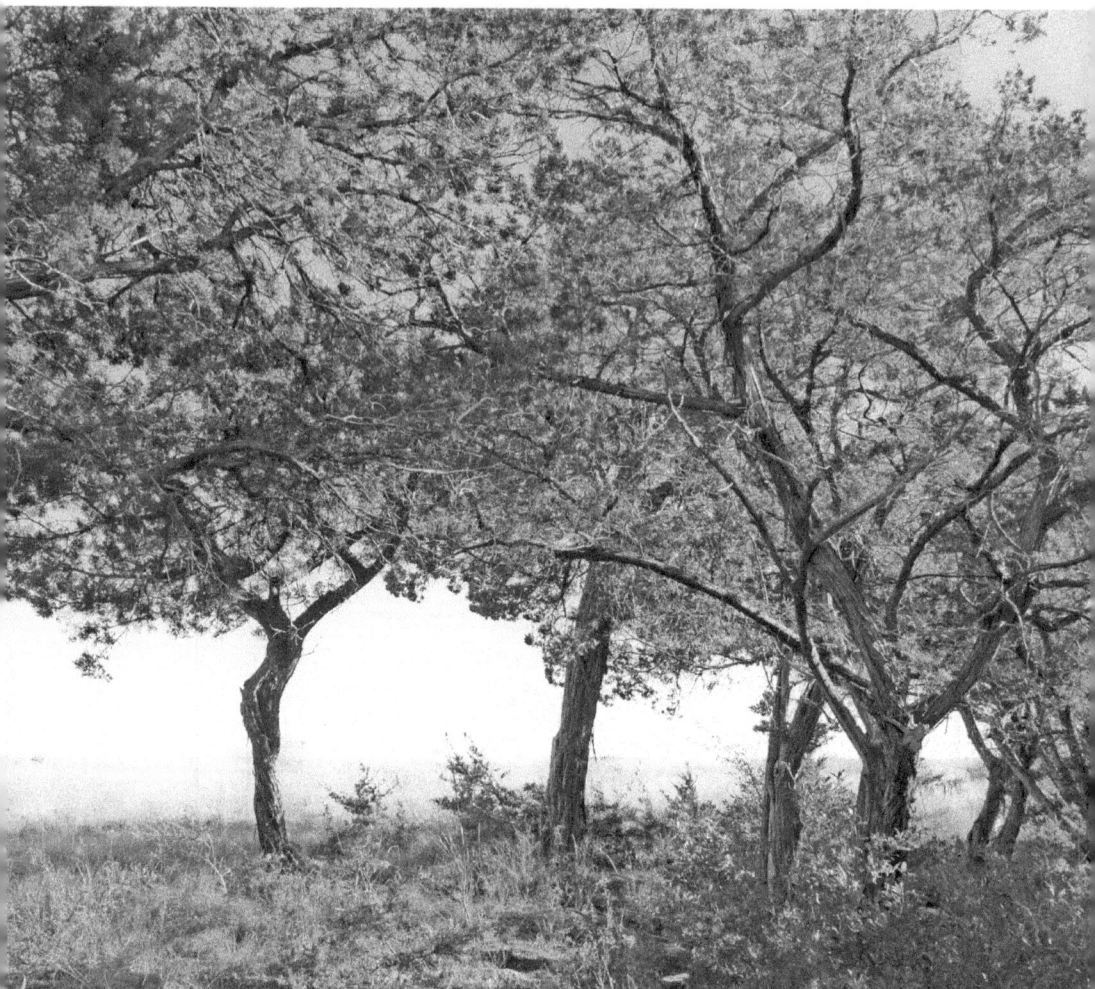

*Oak trees line the ridge at Doeskin Ranch.*

Rimrock Trail going counterclockwise. It descends into a pretty canyon and crosses the creek a few yards farther on.

Clamber out of this canyon and through the woods to head across a meadow toward the lines of exposed rock on the hillside. A shady oak motte stands at the bottom of the slope, but take your time reaching it while you notice the riot of different grasses, flowers, and shrubs that make up the grassland. This is prime butterfly habitat—in early October, the refuge is one of the best places to observe monarchs as they make their annual migration.

Underbrush crowds the trail as you push through the oaks and start the steep zigzag climb to the rim rock. The juniper forest shades most of the hillside. A chasm lies to your left. At 1 mile you clamber over the last *balcón* of harder rock and emerge onto the savanna at the top. Thickets of cedar, mesquite, and oak dot the open ground. The thickets of scrubby oak, called shinneries, are home to the black-capped vireo—the golden-cheeked warbler prefers the juniper. Turn right onto the wide Shin Oak Trail, which follows the 1,300-foot contour around the southern brow of the spur, allowing views over the Cow Creek valley. At 1.4 miles you come to the junction with the Indiangrass Trail, a backcountry trail that would add 1.5 miles to the hike, should you wish to take it. Otherwise turn left; the Shin Oak Trail crosses the cap to join the Rimrock Trail.

Turn right, and the scenery shifts again as the track scrambles over the edge of the plateau, diving back into the juniper forest. The trail stays just below the line of rock for a few yards, coming to a bench with a nice view of the valley. The trailhead is out of sight behind a north-facing flank. From here you will go down another steep ravine and pass through a thickly vegetated valley. Pick up a jeep track that angles around the flank and leads back to the creek. Look for the bat houses set on poles just before the trail crosses the creek at 2.1 miles; stepping-stones will help you avoid wet feet. A rock ledge at the ford might be a waterfall. From here, the gravel trail takes you to the junction with the Creek Trail. Go straight to return to the trailhead.

## Nearby Activities

The half-mile Pond and Prairie Trail at Doeskin Ranch is also worth your time. The Friends of Balcones Canyonlands organize bird-watching events in the refuge. Find out more at friendsofbalcones.org/calendar. And visit the Shin Oak Observation Deck, on FM 1869 toward Liberty Hill.

---

**GPS TRAILHEAD COORDINATES**

**N30° 37' 12.7"  W98° 4' 24.7"**

From Austin, take US 183 north to TX 29. Follow TX 29 west 2.6 miles to Liberty Hill. Turn left onto FM 1869. Follow this road 10.2 miles to the junction of FM 1174. Turn left, and continue 2.4 miles to the Doeskin Ranch access, on the left. A short paved path leads from the parking lot to the trailhead.

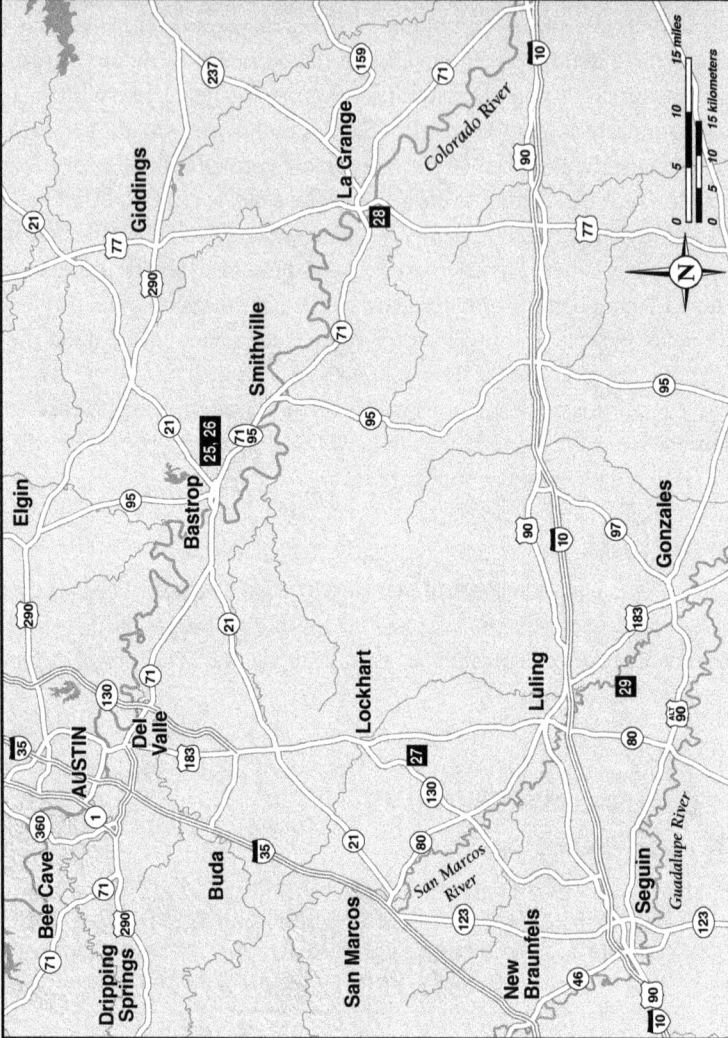

Southeast of Austin *(Hikes 25–29)*

# SOUTHEAST OF AUSTIN

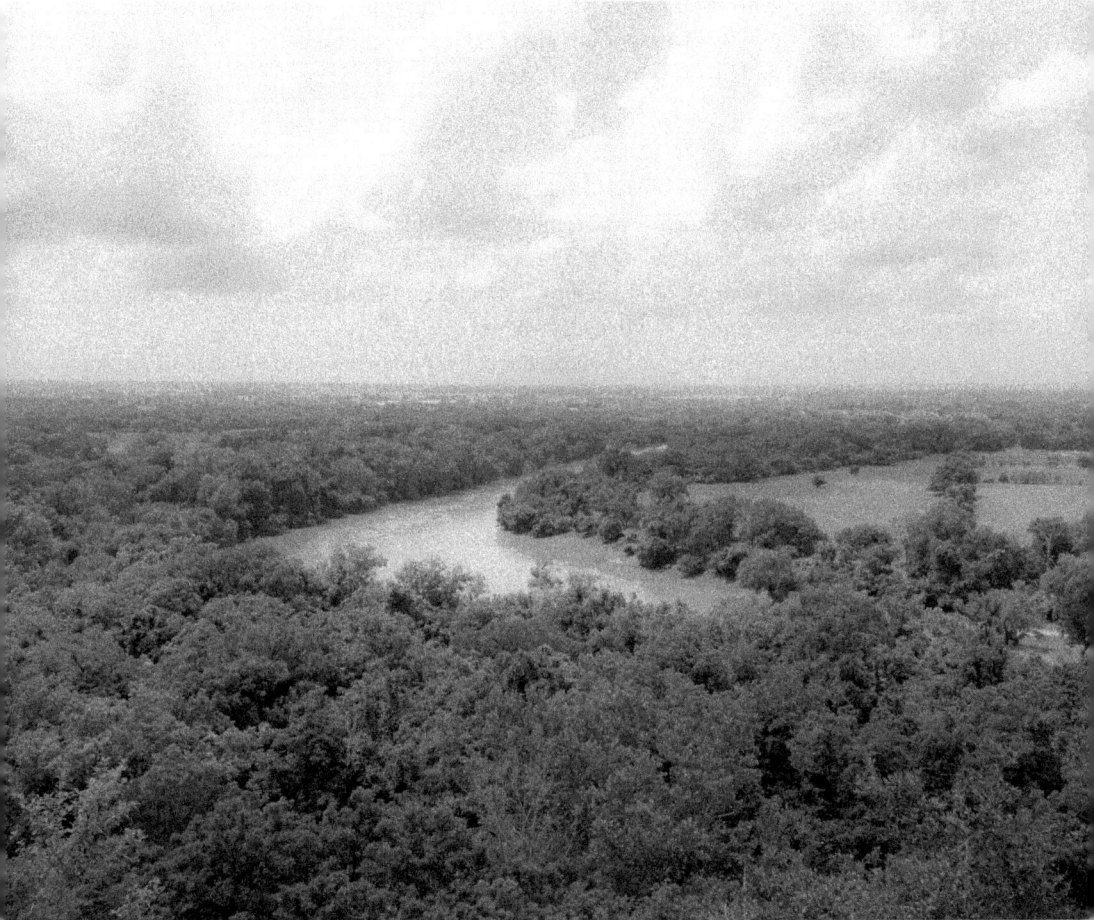

*View of the Colorado River from Monument Hill (see page 129)*

# 25 Bastrop State Park Loop

## In Brief

This hike makes a loop over the sandy hills and dales of Bastrop State Park, now bursting with fresh life after the devastating fire of 2011. From the stone gazebo at the lookout on Park Road 1A, the Red Trail winds south along Copperas Creek before breaking off to join the Orange Trail and heading back to the start point.

## Description

Charred trunks cover the sandy hills and valleys around the parking lot on Park Road 1A. If you visited the park before the fire and remember the sight of the pine trees surrounding you, the current vista is heartbreaking. But beneath the dead trunks, the forest is regenerating. Though your hike won't be shaded by loblollies and the sand underfoot is bare of pine needles, you will see new growth everywhere.

Join the Red Trail from the northwest corner of the parking lot, and immediately make a steep descent on a gravel trail into the unsettling landscape. You are making your way down a canyon that descends into the Copperas Creek valley. The charred trunks provide no shade, so remember sunscreen and a hat. Take the time to look around you, as the sandy soil supports a unique array of flora. To learn more about the plants in the park, sign up at headquarters for a walk with a Master Naturalist, who will instruct you in its botanic delights.

Step over a little drainage at 0.2 mile. At 0.4 mile you make the first of several quick crossings of a deep, overgrown gully full of fallen timber. A little climb and some steps precede the dip into the Copperas Creek watercourse, verdant with cottonwoods and salt cedar. The Blue Trail comes in from the right, as does the creek. Walk over a wooden bridge, the first of many stream crossings you will make as the trail winds down the lush valley. Immediately after this, the Gold Trail leaves to the right. Shortly after, the Black Trail leads again to the right, and then the Gray Trail goes left.

At 1.1 miles a very short spur leads to an old, out-of-service water fountain. It's a lovely example of the fairy-tale architecture scattered through the park by the Civilian Conservation Corps (CCC) in the 1930s. If you've never seen the stone cabins, go take a look.

The folds of the creek valley are visible behind the fountain, and a narrow tuck leads the eye back up to a ridge and a campground. Returning to the trail, you must immediately turn left at the junction with the Yellow Trail, crossing Copperas Creek for the last time. (If you find yourself going up some steep steps, turn back, as you have taken the Yellow Trail.) This bridge is the lowest point of the hike. From it, you head east toward a surviving grove of pines up on the hillside.

Some energy is required to get you up the spur onto a flat ridge. Cross the hill, and come down an equally steep red dirt path on the other side to a parking lot and the park

## Bastrop State Park Loop

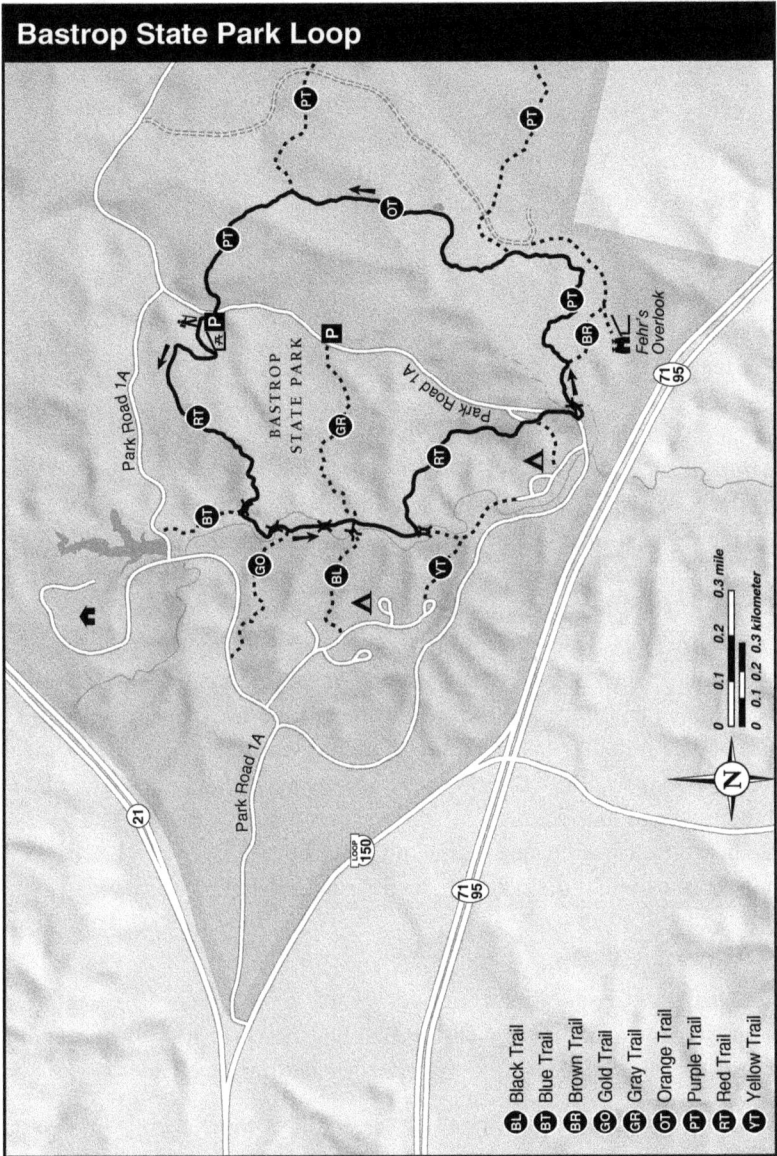

Map legend:
- BL Black Trail
- BT Blue Trail
- BR Brown Trail
- GO Gold Trail
- GR Gray Trail
- OT Orange Trail
- PT Purple Trail
- RT Red Trail
- YT Yellow Trail

BASTROP STATE PARK

Park Road 1A

Fehr's Overlook

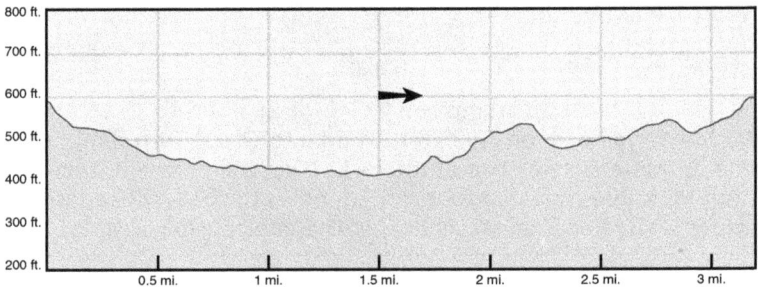

| | |
|---|---|
| **LENGTH:** 3.2 miles | **DRIVING DISTANCE:** 36 miles from the state capitol |
| **CONFIGURATION:** Loop | |
| **DIFFICULTY:** Moderate | **ACCESS:** Daily, 8 a.m.–10 p.m.; $5 entrance fee per person over age 13 |
| **SCENERY:** Sandy hills, creek bottoms | |
| **EXPOSURE:** Exposed | **MAPS:** At park or at tinyurl.com/bastropparkmap |
| **TRAFFIC:** Moderate | **FACILITIES:** Water, picnic table, restrooms in day-use area near park pool |
| **TRAIL SURFACE:** Dirt, sand | |
| **HIKING TIME:** 2 hours | **CONTACT INFORMATION:** 512-321-2101; tpwd.texas.gov/state-parks/bastrop |

road. Turn right. Walk down the road a few yards; at 1.7 miles turn off the road to the left, picking up the Purple Trail.

This path crosses a little feeder creek and then clambers up a long set of steps on the other side of the valley. Fehr's Overlook, another CCC landmark, is visible on the hilltop to the right. At the top of the steps, at 2.3 miles, is the junction with the Orange Trail. Turn left onto this trail. The landscape stays the same in general, but a closer look at any plant reveals a world of detail. Every flower attracts a battalion of hardworking harvester insects.

At the 2.5-mile mark, you walk over a narrow dam next to a pond. This is home for the Houston toad, an endangered species native to these pine forests. The little toad is the most famous of the resident fauna, but there are others worth noting. Birders should look for the pileated woodpecker and the pine warbler. The park is also the western boundary for the southern flying squirrel.

At 2.8 miles turn left at the junction with the Purple Trail, cross the feeder drainage one last time, and then make the steep climb up the hillside back to the parking lot.

## Nearby Activities

Bastrop State Park has two good campgrounds, cabins, a pool, picnic areas, and a fishing lake. The historic town of Bastrop has a charming downtown with restaurants and boutiques. Drive or bike the scenic road that connects Bastrop State Park to Buescher State Park to the east.

## GPS TRAILHEAD COORDINATES
**N30° 6' 40.9" W97° 16' 8.1"**

From the Austin airport, head east on TX 71 for 25 miles to TX 95 in Bastrop. Turn left, and drive north on TX 95 for 0.4 mile to TX 21. Turn right, and head east on TX 21 to reach Bastrop State Park. Pass the park entrance station, turn left on Park Road 1A, and follow it 1.5 miles to the trailhead (look for a stone gazebo). The Red Trail starts behind the information sign.

# 26 Bastrop State Park: Purple Trail

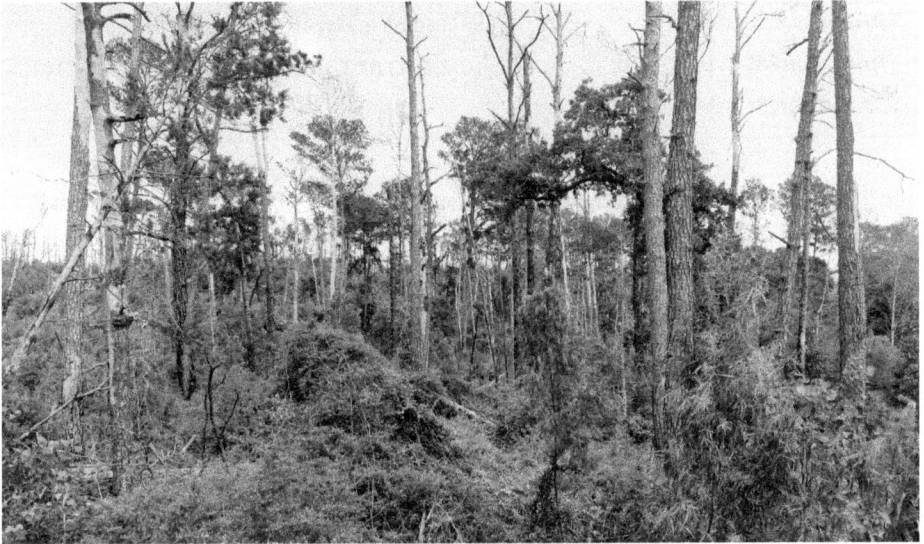

*New growth under burnt trunks at Bastrop State Park*

## In Brief

The Lost Pines were indeed nearly lost in the great fire of 2011, Texas's worst wildfire, but replanting efforts have reinvigorated the forest, and fresh growth is everywhere. Much of the park remains closed, however, and with it half of the celebrated Lost Pines Trail. This shortened version, now called the Purple Trail, takes you to Harmon Road and back. Efforts are under way to reopen the rest of the trail, but no date has been made public.

## Description

The view from the parking lot on Park Road 1A is one of both devastation and regeneration. Before the 2011 fire, the stone gazebo here was hidden in a sea of tall trees; now only their burnt trunks cover the surrounding sandy hills and valleys. But in the shadows of these stark remains, the forest is coming back with vigor. Young pine, red oak, and cottonwood trees are flourishing wherever you look, and the forest floor is alive with bushes, berries, ferns, fungi, and flowers. It is obvious that staff and volunteers have made a herculean effort to clear and replant the park. The Lost Pines Forest Recovery Campaign, a program run by the Arbor Day Foundation in conjunction with Texas Parks and Wildlife

| | |
|---|---|
| **LENGTH:** 4.3 miles | **DRIVING DISTANCE:** 36 miles from the state capitol |
| **CONFIGURATION:** Balloon loop | |
| **DIFFICULTY:** Moderate | **ACCESS:** Daily, 8 a.m.–10 p.m.; $5 entrance fee per person over age 13 |
| **SCENERY:** Sandy hills, creek bottoms | |
| **EXPOSURE:** Mostly exposed | **MAPS:** tinyurl.com/bastropparkmap |
| **TRAFFIC:** Moderate | **FACILITIES:** Water, picnic table, restrooms in day-use area near park pool |
| **TRAIL SURFACE:** Dirt, sand | **CONTACT INFORMATION:** 512-321-2101; tpwd.texas.gov/state-parks/bastrop |
| **HIKING TIME:** 2–3 hours | |

and Texas A&M, has enabled the planting of more than 10,000 seedlings as part of a five-year program that aims to restore this unique loblolly pine forest to its former glory.

Cross the road, and look for a metal post marked with a purple square. The trail immediately makes a sharp descent into the wide bowl of dead trees and green shoots spread out before you. Without the pine foliage, it becomes much easier to understand the terrain through which you are hiking. Bastrop State Park has some higher points—the stone gazebo is on one—but mostly the paths traverse a jumble of washes and banks, always going up or down, sometimes quite steeply, but never for too long. When I was there, recent heavy rains had cut deep channels into many sections of the trail, turning sandy paths into tannin-laced pools, and making some stretches quite challenging.

At 0.2 mile you cross a draw. Climb out of the valley to find a fork at 0.4 mile. Veer left to stay on the Purple Trail. The right-hand track is the Orange Trail (previously known as Roosevelt's Cutoff), by which you will return. The trail bed narrows to a singletrack footpath winding through a prehistoric-looking landscape. Birds flit from bush to tree. The path sticks to the contour line to follow a spur where you will see a grove of trees that somehow survived the fire.

At 0.7 mile cross the Old Road Bed, a sandy jeep track now only for hikers, that bisects the park. Shortly there's a climb up the side of a ridge. Flourishing young pine trees dot the slope. Look to the right for a view over the odd landscape, blighted stakes standing as memento mori over a riot of green. The trail continues, passing through an area where a band of loblollies survived the fire and then a hilltop covered by an oak motte. Drop down from this ridge, and at 1.3 miles cross a wash on a tiny wooden bridge. Listen for the wind through a larger stand of pines, a sound that's been missing from the hike so far.

Reach Harmon Road at just over 1.5 miles. Turn right on the wide, sandy roadbed, and continue 0.8 mile until you come to the next trail junction, where you turn right again, picking up the narrow hiking path. Ferns, salt cedar, and young cottonwoods add to the varied flora of the nascent forest. Enjoy the shade of another oak glade, and at 2.8 miles cross a drainage. In less than half a mile, you will be back at the Old Road, and then at 3.4 miles you reach the junction with the Orange Trail. The Purple Trail

## Bastrop State Park: Purple Trail

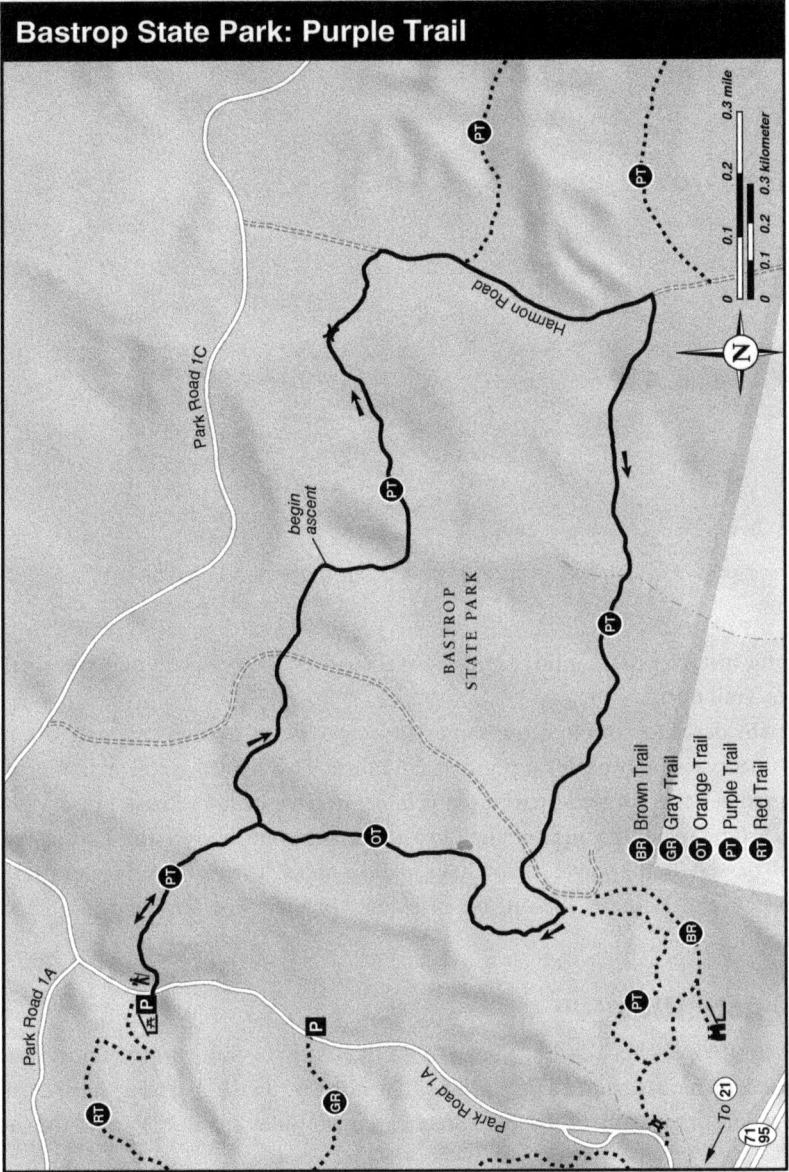

Park Road 1C

Harmon Road

begin ascent

BASTROP
STATE PARK

0.3 mile
0.1    0.2
0    0.3 kilometer
0    0.1    0.2

BR Brown Trail
GR Gray Trail
OT Orange Trail
PT Purple Trail
RT Red Trail

Park Road 1A

Park Road 1A

To 21

71
95

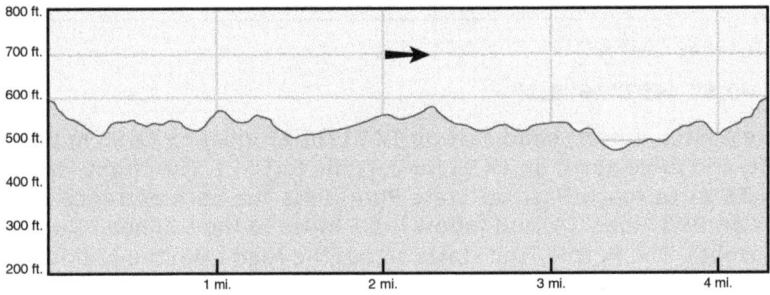

800 ft.
700 ft.
600 ft.
500 ft.
400 ft.
300 ft.
200 ft.

1 mi.        2 mi.        3 mi.        4 mi.

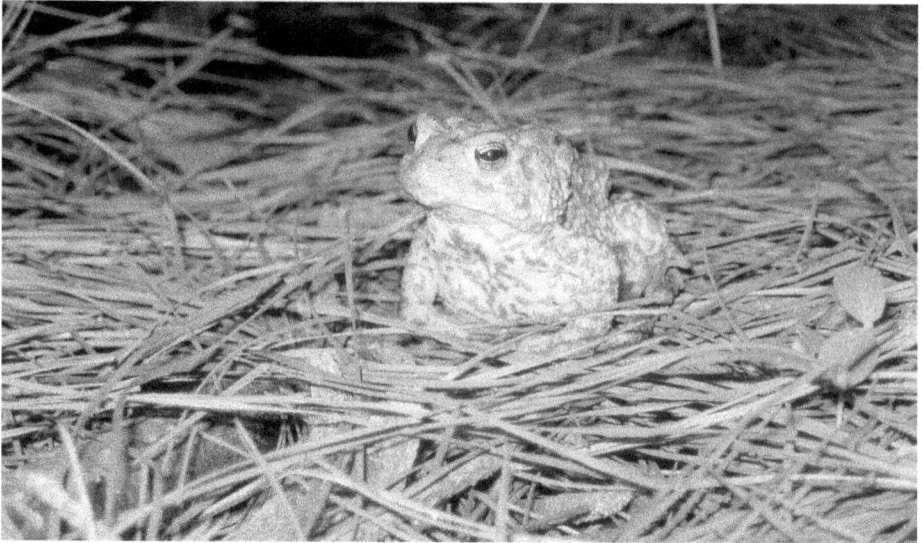

*The endangered Houston toad might be seen near a pond toward the trail's end.*

PHOTO: PAIGE NAJVAR/U.S. FISH & WILDLIFE SERVICE

continues for just over half a mile to end at Park Road 1A, but you will turn right, taking the Orange Trail north.

The path descends through the same landscape we've seen throughout the hike, then loops back east and passes a pond at 3.6 miles. This brown water is home to the Houston toad, a native of these parts that is lucky to have its home base preserved in a state park. From the pond, you climb up onto a spur and come back to the Purple Trail at the fork we passed on the way out. You have hiked 4 miles. Turn left, and make your way 0.3 mile back to the trailhead, looking for a last burst of energy on the steep climb back to the parking lot.

## Nearby Activities

Bastrop State Park is chock-full of things to do. It has two good campgrounds, historic cabins, a pool, picnic areas, and a fishing lake. The historic town of Bastrop is also close by. A 13-mile scenic drive connects Bastrop State Park with Buescher State Park to the east.

---

### GPS TRAILHEAD COORDINATES

**N30° 6' 40.9"  W97° 16' 8.1"**

From the Austin airport, head east on TX 71 for 25 miles to TX 95 in Bastrop. Turn left, and drive north on TX 95 for 0.4 mile to TX 21. Turn right, and head east on TX 21 to reach Bastrop State Park. Pass the park entrance station, turn left on Park Road 1A, and follow it 1.5 miles to the trailhead (look for a stone gazebo). The Purple Trail starts across the road from the parking area.

# 27 Lockhart State Park Loop

## In Brief

This is a short but rewarding hike around the park's southern hills and along Plum Creek, through undisturbed forest. The swimming pool and golf course are the popular attractions at this park, so you will likely have the trail to yourself.

## Description

President Franklin D. Roosevelt founded the Civilian Conservation Corps (CCC) to give young men a living and some purpose during the Great Depression. Of the more than 1,400 work camps in the nation, 15 were located in Texas, and they were responsible for a great number of the state park and forest facilities still in use today. At Lockhart, they built the spring-fed swimming pool, as well as dams, bridges, and picnic tables. These features, historically interesting in themselves, blend in nicely with the park's geography. The CCC also constructed the refectory building (now the Recreation Hall) at the trailhead, which recently reopened after renovations.

The loop takes in eight short named trails, starting with the Caddy Trail. This trail leaves the parking lot down a short series of steps to the right of the refectory and plunges through the woods to meet Park Road 10. This is your first encounter with the terrific variety of flora growing in the park—look for live oak, black walnut, ash, elm, and pecan. Yaupon, kidneywood, and other shrubs cover the ground. Much of this forest has been undisturbed for centuries. Keep an eye out for spider webs. Many of the trails might not have been hiked for a few days, and the resident arachnids—some of which grow to a remarkable size—seem to relish the challenge of bridging the trail. Yawning while hiking can have unpleasant consequences.

It's less than 0.1 mile to Park Road 10, where you turn left and then shortly right, coming to the Chisholm Trail, which starts by skirting the golf course. Make your way around a metal gate onto a wide, grassy path leading into the woods. To your right, there is a small ravine. At 0.2 mile you cross a seasonal drainage where Rattlesnake Run Trail leaves to your right. Keep straight, and shortly make a right turn, following the signage, by a bench. The grassy path winds away from the golf course, bends to the left, and then starts to climb, all the while in dense vegetation.

At 0.4 mile come to the junction with the Comanche Loop, and turn left to follow this short trail around the top of this little rise, where cactus and, in season, wildflowers grow in a little open area. A little farther on, a bench allows for contemplation of a modest but leafy vista. Foxes, deer, and rabbits, as well as numerous species of songbirds, hide in the tangled undergrowth.

Returning to the junction, go straight, continuing on the Chisholm Trail. Oak branches shade the path. At 0.7 mile you come to a fence, the park border, where you turn

**LENGTH:** 1.9 miles

**CONFIGURATION:** Loop

**DIFFICULTY:** Easy–moderate

**SCENERY:** Hardwoods, creek

**EXPOSURE:** Shady

**TRAFFIC:** Very light

**TRAIL SURFACE:** Dirt, some tarmac

**HIKING TIME:** 1 hour

**DRIVING DISTANCE:** 40 miles from the state capitol

**ACCESS:** Daily, 8 a.m.–10 p.m.; $3 entrance fee per person over age 13

**WHEELCHAIR ACCESS:** No

**MAPS:** tinyurl.com/lockhartmap

**FACILITIES:** Restrooms, vending machines, swimming pool, 9-hole golf course

**CONTACT INFORMATION:** 512-398-3479; tpwd.texas.gov/state-parks/lockhart

left by a meadow of bluestem grass and mesquite. You can be sure this is bluestem grass, as there is a sign saying so; it's the first of several that usefully identify various trees, shrubs, and flowering plants along the trail. You will notice a windmill and then wooden corrals and ranch buildings to your right, looking somewhat abandoned. The ranchland across the fence, sparsely covered with mesquite, is quite a contrast to the rampant and impenetrable growth in the park.

At 0.8 mile the Hilltop Trail leaves to the left, a shortcut to the beginning of the Clear Fork Trail. Keep straight on what is now the Fence Line Trail. Be aware that the thick ground growth serves as inviting habitat to scorpions, snakes, and tarantulas. In another 0.1 mile, turn left onto the Persimmon Trail. This short trail pushes through a lovely grove of these trees, which you will recognize from their small, plump leaves and peeling gray trunks.

At 1.1 miles you reach the end of the Persimmon Trail. Turn left onto the Creekview Trail, which meets the Clear Fork of Plum Creek, the park's main watercourse. Soon turn right at a junction to make a little loop to the Old Fishing Hole, a deep, wide pool that almost always has water. Continue on. More signs identify Virginia creeper and inland sea oats. At 1.2 miles you exit the forest at an open picnic area. Follow the edge of the woods around to the right, coming to the Clear Fork Trail. This begins by crossing the creek at a stone dam, possibly quite a challenge after heavy rains.

Once across the creek, walk along the flat path back to Park Road 10, crossing some feeder creeks along the way. At the beginning—really its end—the Clear Fork Trail is narrow and quite overgrown but soon widens. The drainages can be very slippery if they are wet. The creek bottomland is a touch more open than the dense vegetation by the fence line, and light darting through the treetops makes shadows dance across the forest floor. You may see nutrias swimming in the creek. At 1.5 miles you pass another dam and a little wooded island that you may want to explore. The Wild Rose Loop leaves to the right, just before you cross a larger feeder creek. Walk through a glade of red oaks opposite the RV camping area.

At 1.7 miles you emerge from the woods onto the road opposite a pretty dam, a feature of the park and another CCC construction. Turn left onto the road, passing fairways

## Lockhart State Park Loop

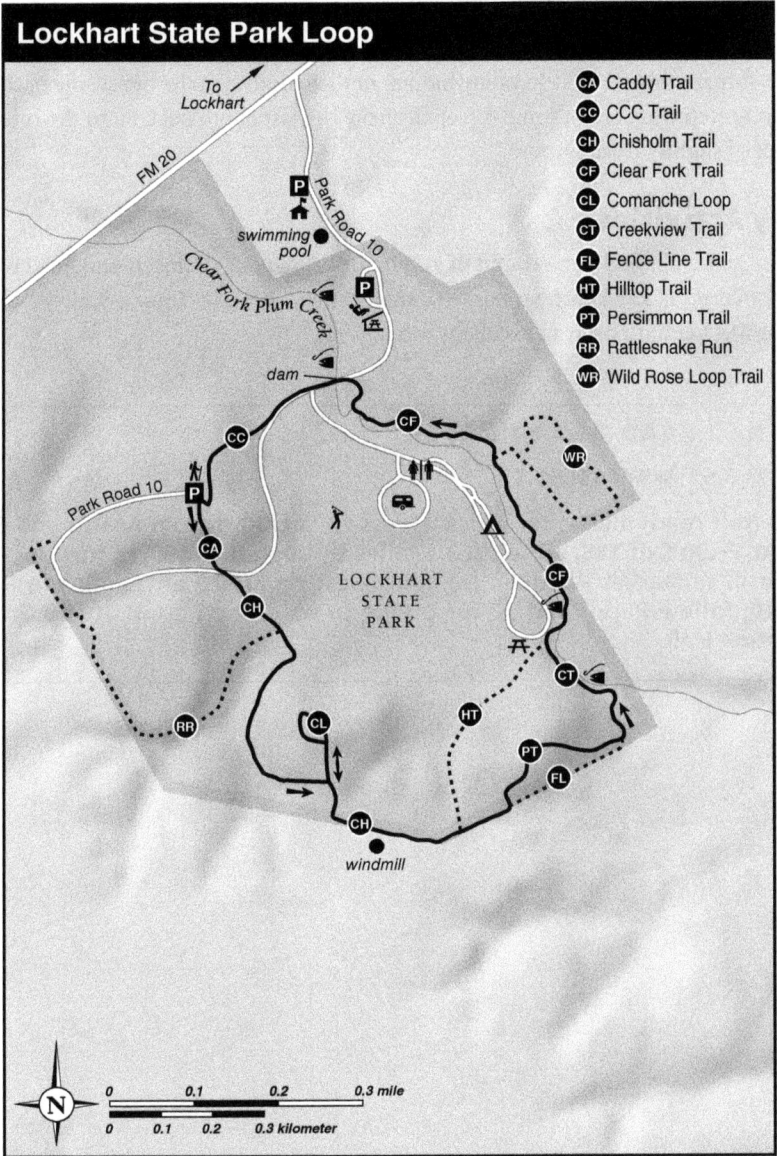

Trail legend:
- CA Caddy Trail
- CC CCC Trail
- CH Chisholm Trail
- CF Clear Fork Trail
- CL Comanche Loop
- CT Creekview Trail
- FL Fence Line Trail
- HT Hilltop Trail
- PT Persimmon Trail
- RR Rattlesnake Run
- WR Wild Rose Loop Trail

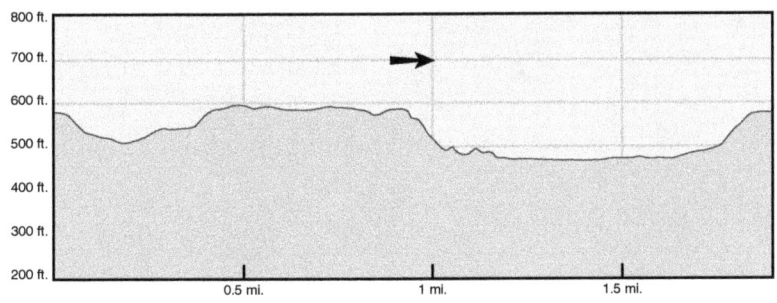

on either side. After 0.1 mile look for the beginning of the CCC Trail at the corner of the woods. Turn right onto this trail, and immediately ascend a steep slope, which leads you through a surprisingly wide little valley hidden in the woods. On the other side of the valley, concrete steps that are in some disrepair make the last climb back up to the refectory and trailhead slightly treacherous.

## Nearby Activities

Bring your golf clubs and get a round of golf in, or bring your swimsuit and head over to the spring-fed pool. Lockhart has some of the best barbecue in Texas—Smitty's Market and Kreuz Market both have an excellent reputation.

---

### GPS TRAILHEAD COORDINATES

**N29° 51' 2.5"  W97° 41' 58.7"**

TX 130 (toll road) allows for quick access to Lockhart from Austin and San Antonio. From Exit 183, go south 3.1 miles through the town to the junction with Farm to Market Road 20. Go southwest on FM 20 for 2 miles to Park Road 10; follow Park Road 10 for 1 mile to its end on a hill at the Group Recreation Hall.

---

# 28 Monument Hill History and Nature Walk

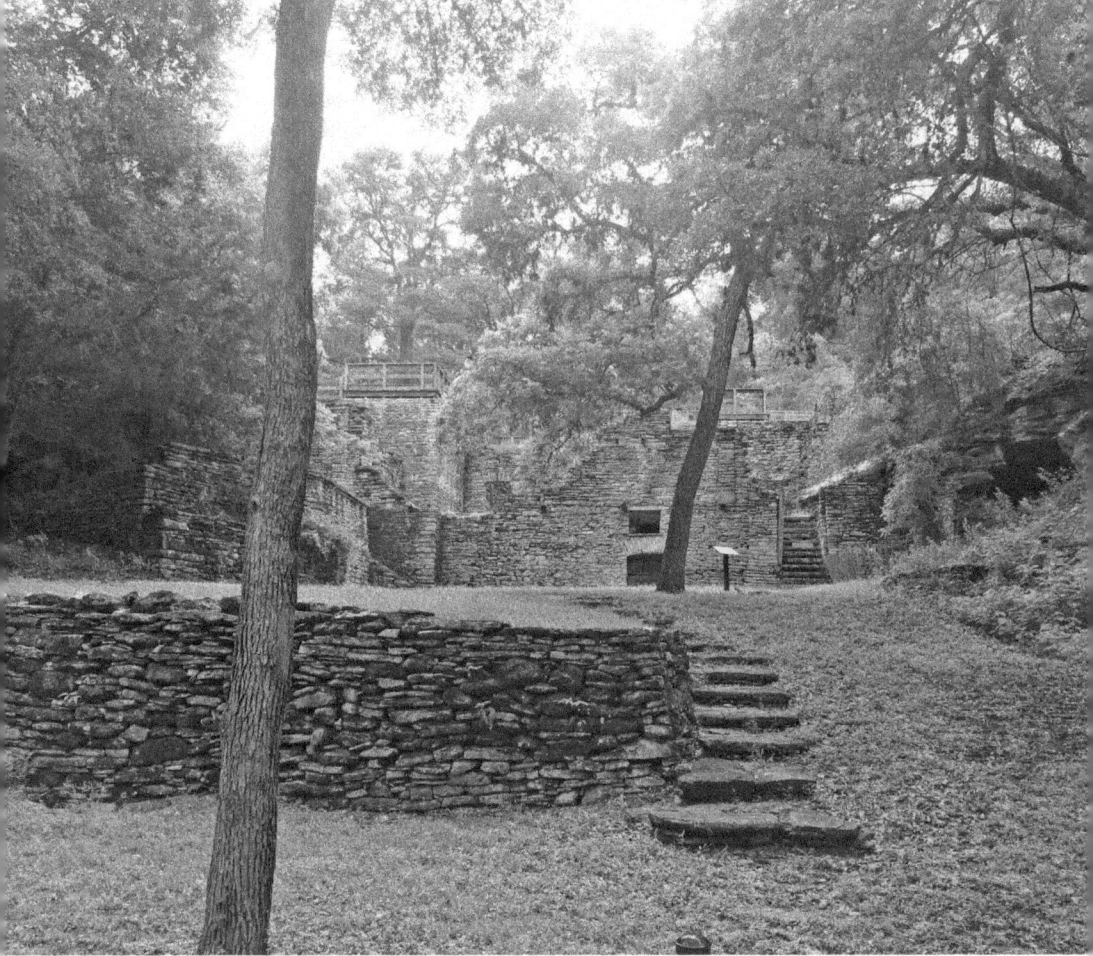

*Brewery ruins at Monument Hill*

## In Brief

This hike visits the tomb of the fallen heroes of the Dawson Massacre and Mier Expedition, along with a pioneer's house and brewery. From a bluff offering extensive views into the Colorado River Valley, you will hike down into a secluded ravine.

| | |
|---|---|
| **LENGTH:** 1 mile | **DRIVING DISTANCE:** 67 miles from the state capitol |
| **CONFIGURATION:** Loop | |
| **DIFFICULTY:** Easy–moderate | **ACCESS:** Daily, 8 a.m.–5 p.m.; no entrance fee required |
| **SCENERY:** River bluff, sculpted lawn, oak woods | **WHEELCHAIR ACCESS:** Yes, to monument and overlook |
| **EXPOSURE:** Mostly shady | **MAPS:** tinyurl.com/monumenthillmap |
| **TRAFFIC:** Moderate on weekends | **FACILITIES:** Picnic area, restrooms |
| **TRAIL SURFACE:** Wood, rock, gravel, sidewalk | **CONTACT INFORMATION:** 979-968-5658; tpwd.texas.gov/state-parks/monument-hill-kreische-brewery |
| **HIKING TIME:** 30–45 minutes | |

## Description

Have you heard of the Black Bean Incident? In 1842, Mexico made one last attempt to retake the Republic of Texas. A group of militiamen from La Grange went to battle with the Mexican army, led by Gen. Adrián Woll, who routed the militia at Salado Creek. Some Texans crossed into Mexico in retaliation and were attacked after the militiamen took Ciudad Mier. Most were captured and forced to march toward Mexico City. Some escaped but were soon recaptured, and a furious President Santa Anna ordered every 10th captive executed. One hundred seventy-six beans were put in a pot, and 17 were black. Each Texan was ordered to pull a bean. Those who plucked a black bean met their death by firing squad on March 23, 1844.

In 1847, survivor John Dusenbury led an expedition to retrieve the remains of his companions, which, along with those of the men who had battled Woll in 1842 at Salado Creek, were buried on Monument Hill, though the tomb and monument were built later. The grounds were acquired by the state in 1907 and opened to the public in 1983 as a State Historical Site.

Leave the visitor center and walk across the smooth oak- and pecan-studded lawn to the mausoleum. Signs and plaques tell the story. Beyond the monument, there is an escarpment overlooking the town of La Grange and a majestic bend in the Colorado River. This bluff is an important ecological marker, as it is the boundary between the upland post oak woodlands and the Fayette prairie environments. In addition, pockets of alkaline soil, caused by the erosion of the sandstone cap, support species normally found 70 miles west. These travelers, born down the river, have formed their own little Lost Hill Country.

A few yards farther, you will see the handsome Kreische house, set over the ridgetop on the side of the steep little valley in which Heinrich Kreische built his brewery. Kreische knew a good spot when he saw it. Tours of the home are conducted occasionally—check the events page of the park's website for more details.

## Monument Hill History and Nature Walk

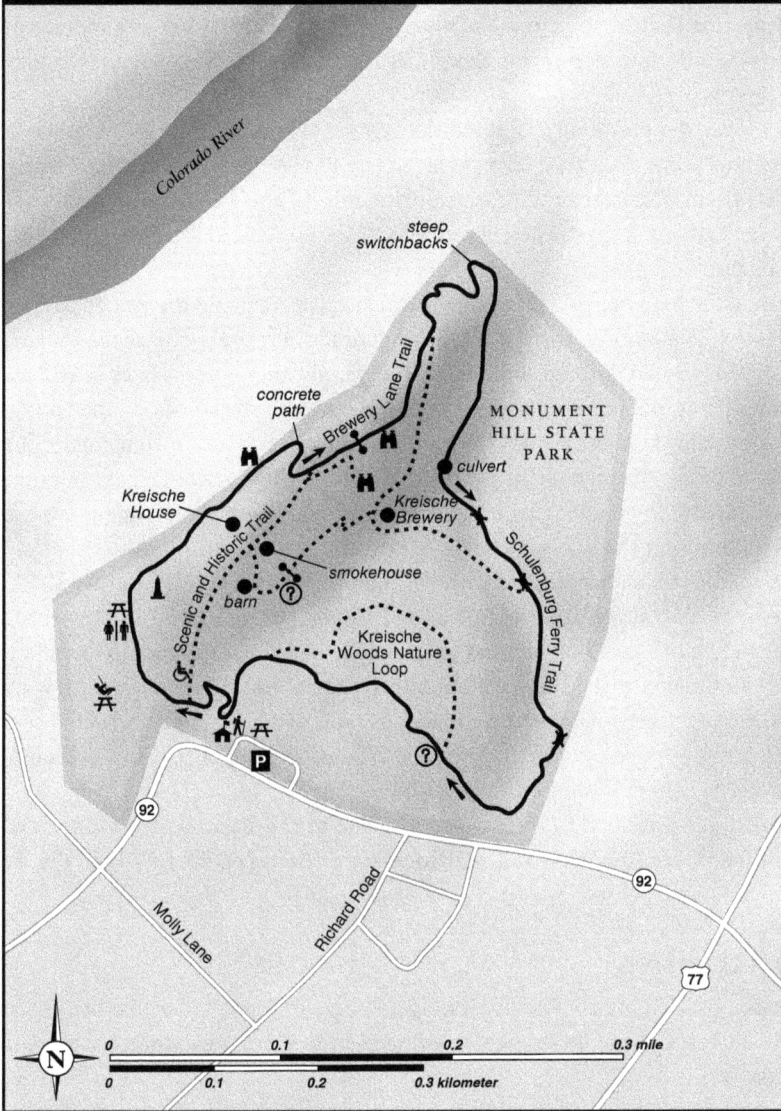

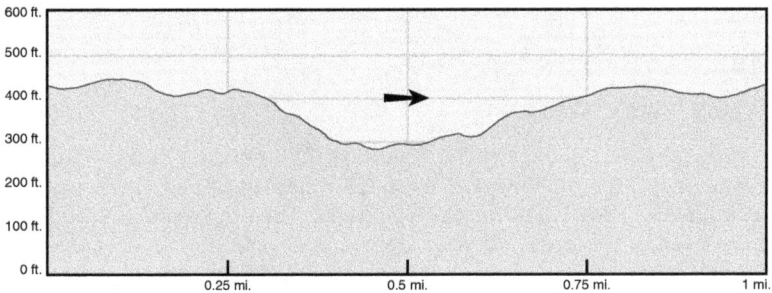

Colorado River

steep
switchbacks

concrete
path

Brewery Lane Trail

MONUMENT
HILL STATE
PARK

culvert

Kreische
House

Kreische
Brewery

Scenic and Historic Trail

smokehouse

barn

Schulenburg Ferry Trail

Kreische
Woods Nature
Loop

92

92

Molly Lane

Pichard Road

77

0        0.1        0.2        0.3 mile

N

0        0.1        0.2        0.3 kilometer

600 ft.

500 ft.

400 ft.

300 ft.

200 ft.

100 ft.

0 ft.

0.25 mi.        0.5 mi.        0.75 mi.        1 mi.

The trail heads along the spur, passing a bench from which you can admire the vista. At 0.3 mile you will come to a concrete path with handrails that leads down the hill. Follow this, scattering lizards, and cross a road to reach a platform. From this vantage point you can look over the wooded ravine that hides the old brewery, the ruins of which are visible below you.

Retrace your steps, and turn right on the tarmac, which is the Brewery Lane Trail. Pass a gate, and come to a bench on your right. This is the Lower Bluff Overlook. Rocky outcrops in open areas on the opposite side of the valley bring to mind the mountains around Fort Davis. The chimneys of the Sam Seymour power plant are visible in the distance.

At 0.4 mile the road makes a sharp right turn; keep straight into the woods past a little barrier, onto the Schulenburg Ferry Trail. The handrails here are useful as the trail makes some steep zigzags down through some shady oak woods. It then turns back south, up the canyon, tunneling through more woods, and follows an old roadbed along the spring-fed stream. Water might be splashing down a cliff from a large culvert on your right. Stop by the grand old brewery. You can see Kreische's elaborate rockwork, which incorporated the slope of the land into the brewing process. Beautifully engineered stone walls support the roadbed as it climbs up the valley. Delicate layers of rock outcrop add to the charm. Following rainfall, the stream babbles delightfully, and water pours over little grottos.

You will pass two stone bridges, Lower and Upper. At the latter, the Brewery Lane Trail comes in from the right. The road gets steeper and the surrounding forest a little denser. At 0.8 mile you reach the park boundary, where you turn right over a wooden bridge onto an earth path. Diving into the woods, you will cross four bridges in succession. Keep left at the junction with the Kreische Woods Nature Loop, which will take you back to the visitor center.

You may want to return to the house and walk to the back, where a fine veranda looks over a barn, smokehouse, and millstone set on terraced lawns above the steep, wooded canyon.

## Nearby Activities

In La Grange, visit the Texas Czech Heritage Center to learn more about the strong Czech influence on Central Texas, which you can taste if you buy some kolaches from Weikel's Bakery.

**GPS TRAILHEAD COORDINATES**

**N29° 53' 16.9"  W96° 52' 34.0"**

From Austin, take TX 71 east to TX Business 71 near La Grange. Turn right onto TX Business 71, and follow it east 2.3 miles to US 77. Turn right, and head south on US 77 for 1.6 miles to TX Spur 92. Turn right on TX Spur 92, and follow it 0.4 mile to the park, on your right.

# 29 Palmetto State Park Loop

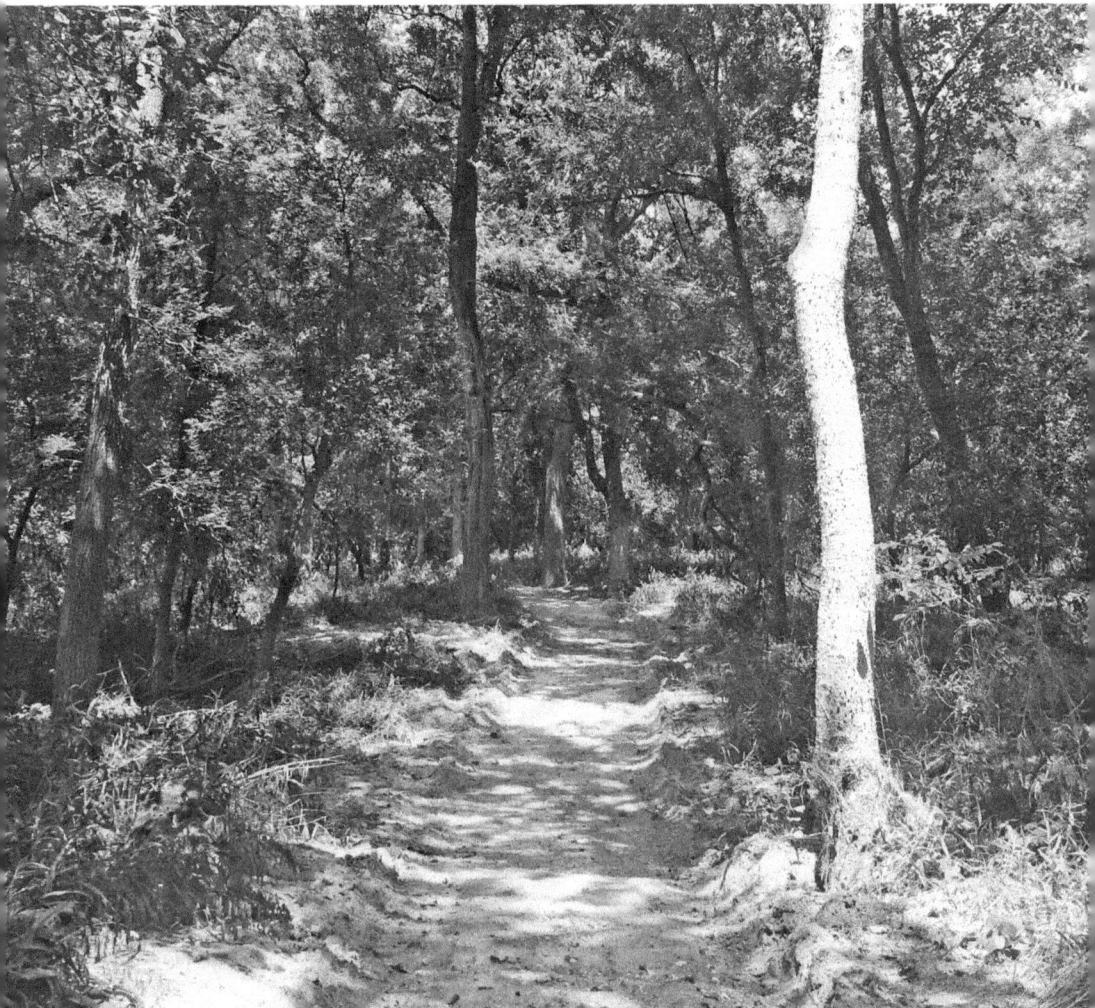

*Look up to find one of hundreds of bird species that visit Palmetto State Park.*

## In Brief

This loop follows the upgraded trail system at this old-time state park. You'll travel bluffs along the San Marcos River on a gravel track and wander through wooded wetlands bridging a jumble of tributaries to come to a swamp forest where palmettos thrive in impressive concentrations.

| | |
|---|---|
| **LENGTH:** 2.8 miles | **DRIVING DISTANCE:** 57 miles from the state capitol |
| **CONFIGURATION:** Loop | **ACCESS:** Daily, 8:15 a.m.–10 p.m.; $3 entrance fee per person over age 13 |
| **DIFFICULTY:** Easy | |
| **SCENERY:** Riverside riparian woods, swamp | **WHEELCHAIR ACCESS:** Yes |
| | **MAPS:** tinyurl.com/palmettomap |
| **EXPOSURE:** Mostly shaded | **FACILITIES:** Restrooms, water, picnicking at trailhead |
| **TRAFFIC:** Busy on weekends | |
| **TRAIL SURFACE:** Gravel | **CONTACT INFORMATION:** 830-672-3266; tpwd.texas.gov/state-parks/palmetto |
| **HIKING TIME:** 1.5 hours | |

## Description

Botanically, east merges with west at the lush, almost tropical Palmetto State Park, which gets its name from the dwarf palmettos that flourish in this preserve's ephemeral swamps. Aside from a relic population in Oklahoma, this is the most northerly and westerly stand of these relatives of the palm tree in the country. They are most numerous on the last portion of this hike, the Ottine Swamp Trail, named after the small village just north of the park. The palmettos are just one of an unusual range of plants found here.

The park is on the Great Texas Coastal Birding Trail, and more than 240 species have been observed within the boundaries. You can download a checklist from the park's website. You'll most likely see more birds and animals on the first section of the hike, the San Marcos River Trail, which follows the river bank for just over a mile through a mix of hardwoods.

Though the park covers only 270 acres, it has a number of distinct environments. In addition to the diversity of the riparian forest and the marshes, there are more western-looking landscapes on the higher ground along the Mesquite Flats Trail, which features drier woods and grassy meadows.

Palmetto State Park is one of Texas's oldest preserves and was developed by the Civilian Conservation Corps in the 1930s. The corps' handiwork can be seen all over the park—a fine example, the refectory building, is next to the parking lot.

Head northeast on the San Marcos River Trail, with the trailer-camping area to your right and the earthen banks of the river to your left. The trail system boasts a wide gravel bed that gently undulates through a shady hardwood forest heavy with hackberry. You may only catch glimpses of the actual stream thanks to the deep trench it has cut in the soil. The San Marcos River flows from a spring in San Marcos, 60 miles northwest; here, it is close to its confluence with the Guadalupe River at Gonzales. Like other rivers that flow across the Texas prairie, the San Marcos is often muddied by its eroding banks. The numerous dead logs, brush piles, and flotsam high above the river itself are evidence of recurrent flash-flooding.

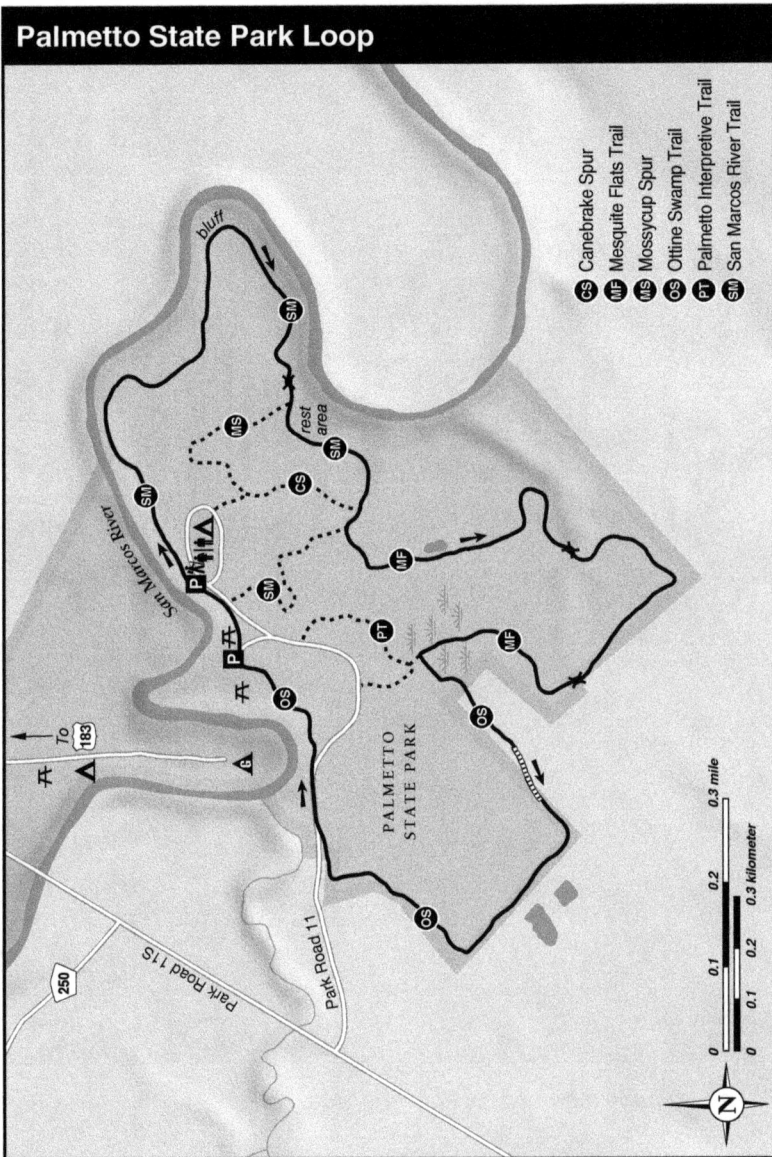

**Palmetto State Park Loop**

CS Canebrake Spur
MF Mesquite Flats Trail
MS Mossycup Spur
OS Ottine Swamp Trail
PT Palmetto Interpretive Trail
SM San Marcos River Trail

Travel rich bottomland through an airy forest of tall deciduous trees. The almost entirely level track makes for an easy hike, allowing you to focus on the scenery and to keep an eye out for wildlife. Deer might spring across the trail in front of you. Look for patches of inland sea oats. The trail follows the river around the bend, with views of crumbling sandy bluffs at the second corner of the roughly rectangular peninsula.

The woods thin subtly and lose some diversity as the trail turns back southwest. At 0.8 mile an iron bridge goes over the first of many intermittent streambeds. Just beyond

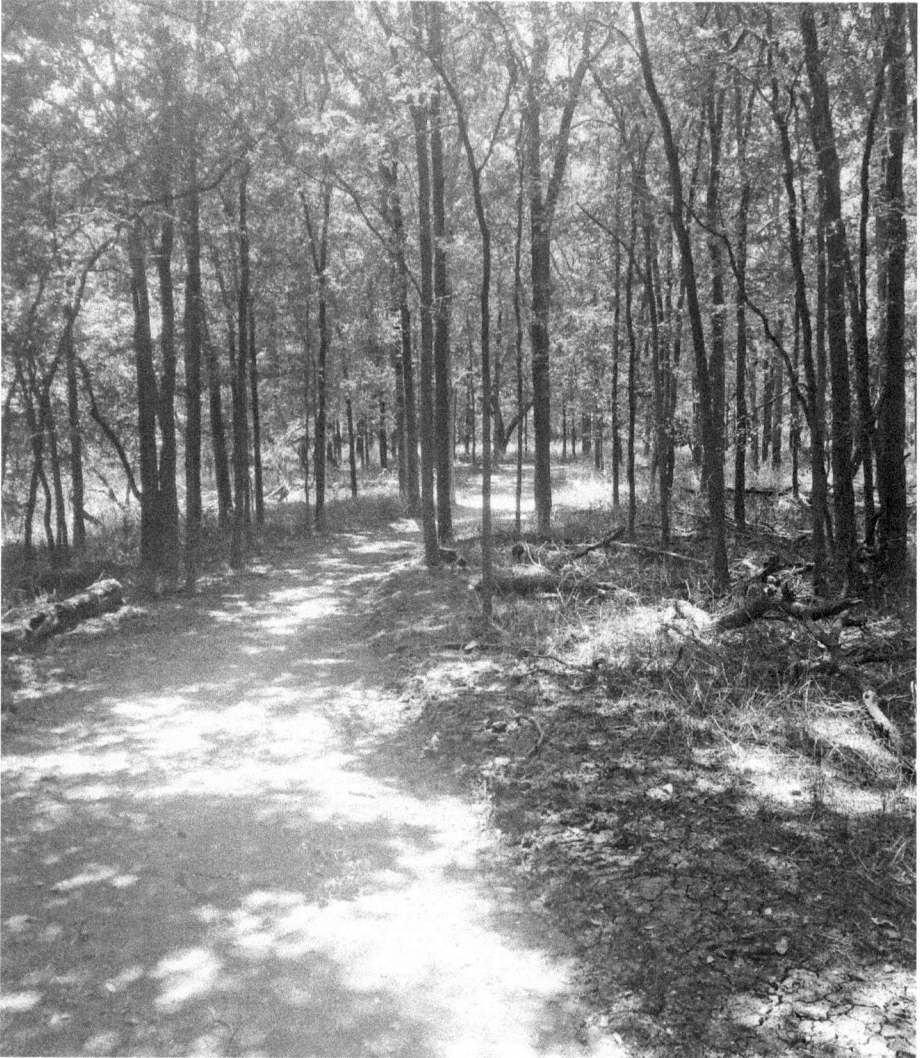

*The trail winds through the woods at Palmetto State Park.*

here, the Mossycup Spur path leads right, looping toward the campground. Pass a bench, and at 0.9 mile the route turns away from the river, crossing a wide wash and following a narrow spur due west. Palmettos thrive in this jumble of drainages. A second shortcut, the Canebreak Spur, leaves right. At 1 mile turn left onto the Mesquite Flats Trail, crossing two wooden bridges. There will be many more bridges and boardwalks as the trail wanders past mesquite-covered meadows and over often-wet sloughs. The transition between these small-scale ecosystems is surprisingly immediate.

At 1.5 miles reach the southern tip of the Mesquite Flats Trail, close to the park boundary. The path turns northwest from here, crossing a larger swath of mesquite savanna and reaching the junction with the Ottine Swamp Trail at 1.9 miles. Turn left here for the last loop of the hike.

At the beginning of this trail, the woods are denser, and there are palmettos all around, looking like a lost alien army. A boardwalk leads to a wildlife-viewing area with a bench. The path makes two right turns as it follows the boundary fence, going over another longer boardwalk before coming to Park Road 11 at 2.5 miles. Turn right, shadowing the park road, passing by sloughs and swampland. Cross the road close to the river, and shortly return to the parking lot.

## Nearby Activities

The park offers camping, fishing, and canoe and pedal boat rental. Paddlers can float the San Marcos River on the Luling Zedler Mill Paddling Trail. The Palmetto Interpretive Trail has more information about the park's ecosystems and visits a CCC water tower.

---

**GPS TRAILHEAD COORDINATES**

**N29° 35' 24" W97° 34' 56.9"**

From Exit 632 on I-10 east of San Antonio and south of Austin, take US 183 south 2.3 miles to Park Road 11. Follow Park Road 11 for 2 miles to a four-way junction. Go straight here. Stop at the park headquarters on your right, and pay the entry fee. Then continue 0.8 mile over three bridges to turn left at the sign for the picnic area. Stay with Park Road 11, and follow it to a fork. Go left to reach a parking area. After parking, walk back to the fork, and then head for the trailer-camping area. Pass one end of the San Marcos River Trail on the way to it and the hike's start at the end of the campsite overflow-parking area.

---

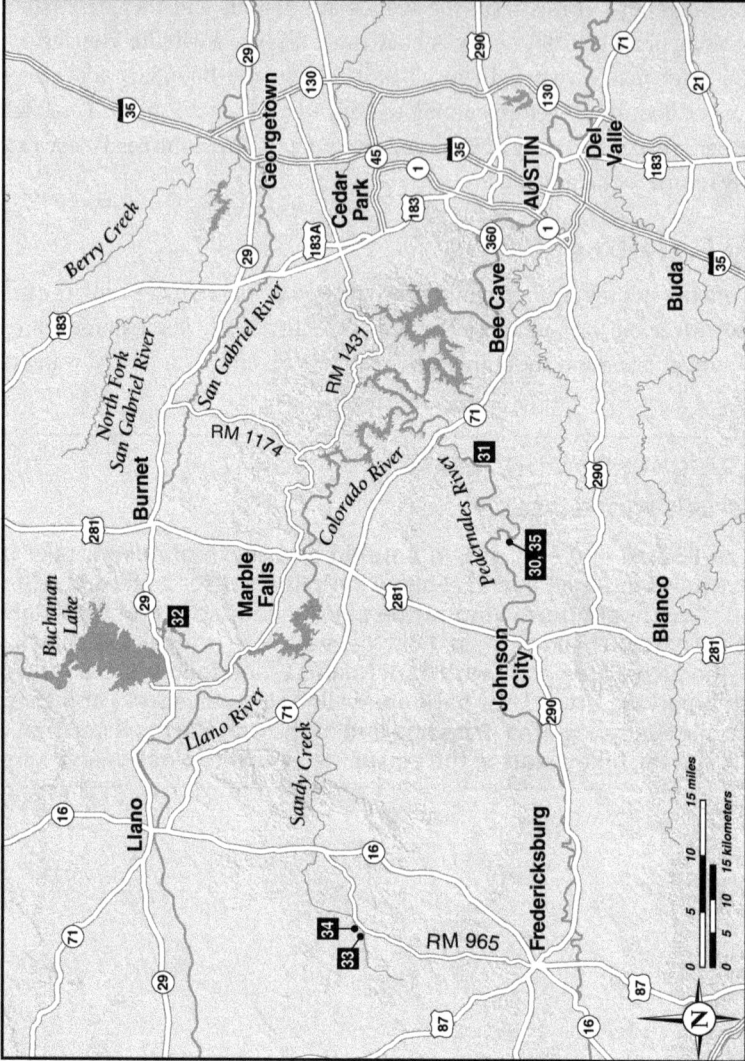

West of Austin (Hikes 30–35)

# WEST OF AUSTIN

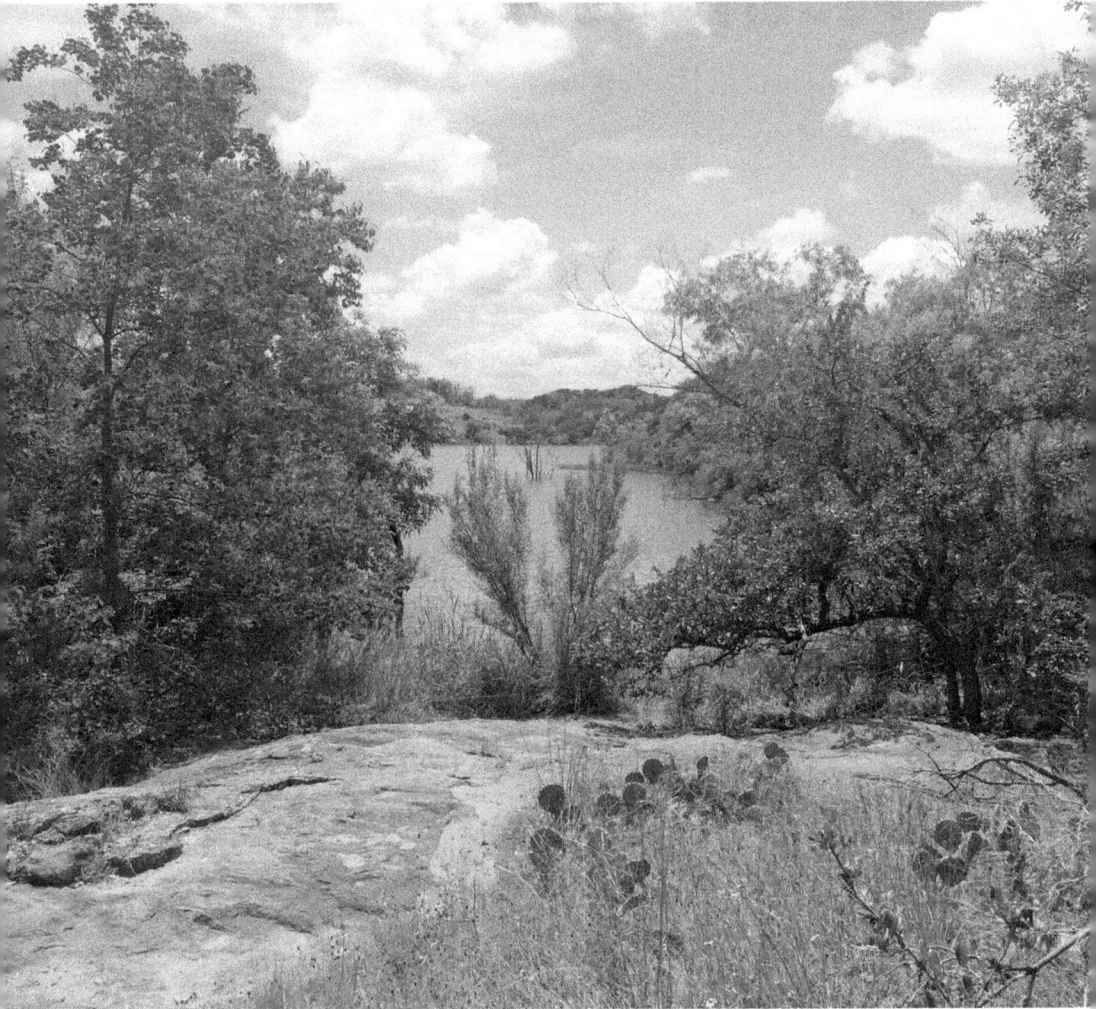

*Hinds Branch at Inks Lake (see page 149)*

# 30 5.5-Mile Loop at Pedernales Falls State Park

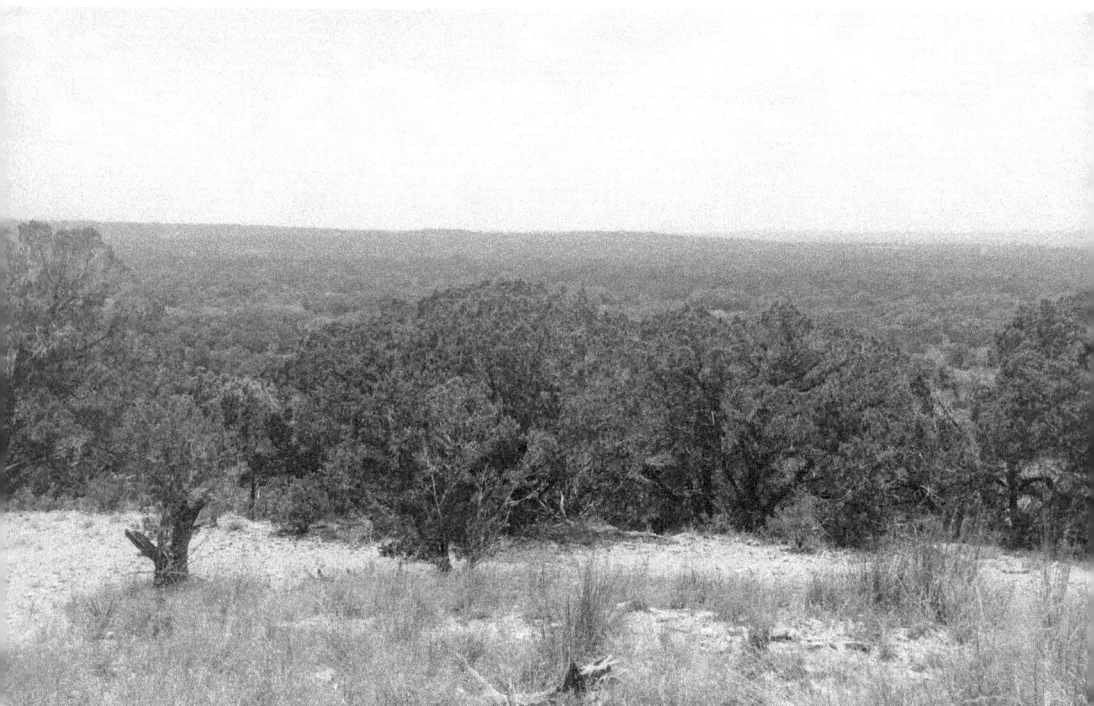

*The view from the overlook on the 5.5-Mile Loop*

## In Brief

The highlight of this long loop around a plateau bordered on three sides by the Pedernales River is a grand view of the park. There are stiff climbs on the farthest section, and you must ford the river to get to the loop, but for the most part this is an easy and underused hike along old ranch roads.

## Description

This hike goes through the northern portion of the park across the Pedernales River and gets much less traffic than the popular Wolf Mountain Trail. The main section is a relaxed ramble around the broad shoulder of the peak at the center of a peninsula created by a winding, southerly bend in the river. The grasslands on this shoulder, a

| | |
|---|---|
| **LENGTH:** 5.8 miles | **ACCESS:** Daily, 8 a.m.–10 p.m.; $6 day-use fee per person over age 13 |
| **CONFIGURATION:** Balloon loop | |
| **DIFFICULTY:** Easy–moderate | **WHEELCHAIR ACCESS:** No |
| **SCENERY:** Wooded plateau | **MAPS:** tinyurl.com/pedernalesfalls trailmap |
| **EXPOSURE:** Mostly exposed | |
| **TRAFFIC:** Moderate to light | **FACILITIES:** Restrooms and water at trailhead and park office |
| **TRAIL SURFACE:** Dirt, rocks | |
| **HIKING TIME:** 3 hours | **CONTACT INFORMATION:** 830-868-7304; tpwd.texas.gov/state-parks/pedernales-falls |
| **DRIVING DISTANCE:** 34 miles from the state capitol | |

riot of flowering plants and shrubs between oak and cedar thickets, should be catnip to naturalists looking to spot plants, birds, and butterflies. The farthest section climbs over two mountain spurs, detours to a scenic overlook, and finally makes a long descent back to the river crossing.

The only possible challenge in this hike is Trammell's Crossing, where you must ford the Pedernales—you'll get wet if the river's flow is particularly untrammeled. From the parking lot, descend through mixed woods past the park amphitheater. The trail drops sharply to the river bottom and makes its way along the sandy bank to a grove of cypresses at the water's edge, where there is a low dam. Cross the river behind the dam on a concrete shelf.

On the other side, the path climbs equally steeply out of the valley on an exposed trail that is surfaced with asphalt to combat erosion. A bend to the left takes you through woods onto the plateau. At 0.8 mile you arrive at the start of the loop. Take the fork on the right, as you will for all five trail junctions. The trail is well signed and not difficult to follow; there is a metal map and wooden bench at this and other junctions, thanks to one Mark Chalberg, who built them as part of a Boy Scout project.

In 0.1 mile you will come to another junction. Turn right to take the Spur Trail, a ranching road now overgrown with grass. This addition to the trail, not marked on the metal maps, has turned what used to be the Four Mile Loop into the 5.5-Mile Loop. The Spur Trail stays closer to the bluffs over the Pedernales River, though the river is not visible from the path. The route wanders through cedar breaks and meadows that see few human visitors. Tall grass on this section means you should wear long pants for this hike to avoid ticks, chiggers, and stickers. Although the vegetation has all but obscured the tracks, the way forward is not difficult to discern. At 1.5 miles there are views of Wolf and Tobacco Mountains across the valley. The path comes close to the edge of the wooded slope to the river and then turns north and rejoins the main trail at the 2-mile mark.

From here, the trail heads north along flat terrain covered with juniper, sometimes sparser, sometimes thicker. The ranch road you are walking along is mostly exposed, though there are woods on either side. A cutoff trail leaves left, offering quick access to the return portion of the loop. At 2.8 miles you pass through a gap in a tumbledown stone

## 5.5-Mile Loop at Pedernales Falls State Park

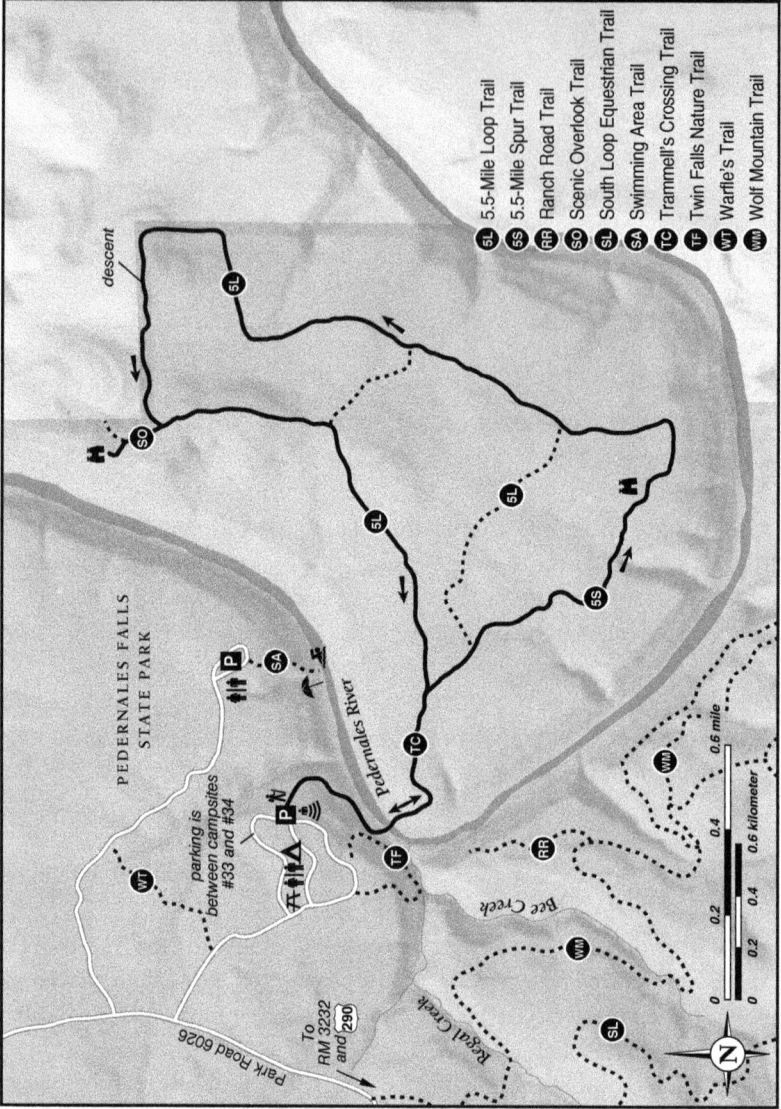

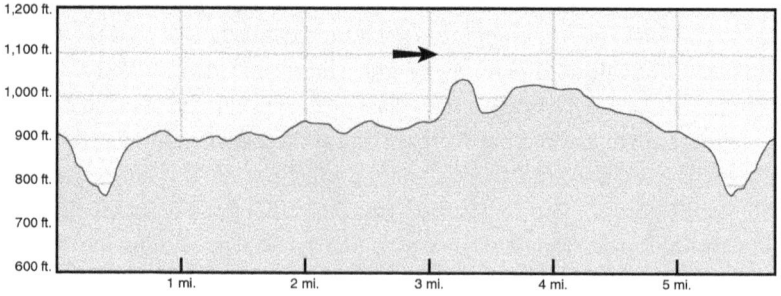

wall and then cross a wide wet-weather drainage in a fold in the hillside. Water has significantly eroded the trail here. The trail veers right, and at the 3-mile mark, you reach the boundary fence and must turn left for the rooty, rocky climb up a spur to the corner of the park. Oak mottes dot the open ranchland beyond the fence—thick oak and cedar forest is a step away to the left. At the top, you turn west with the fence line, crossing the spur on exposed rock outcrops. Look for aoudad (wild sheep) on the ranch to the north.

Big views open to the south as the path descends from the high point to another drainage heavily wooded with live oak and juniper. The basin is wet enough to support a modest wetland where reeds flourish. Watch out for spider webs as you walk through the forest. The trail climbs out of the drainage to level off in a cactus-and-grass flat at 3.7 miles. Leave the rough path, and turn right on a jeep track to find the scenic overlook, only a short walk north at the edge of the drop-off to the river. A bench welcomes you—sit awhile and take in the green Pedernales valley. You might hear the sound of the water rushing below.

Return to the overlook junction, and stay right, heading out along a spur through thin, grassy woodlands. At 4.2 miles the trail starts the long descent to the river down rocky slopes of cedar and oak. Pass the other end of the cutoff trail at 4.4 miles and the start of the loop at the 5-mile point. From there, go back down the hill to the river. Make Trammell's Crossing one more time, and climb back to the trailhead and parking lot.

## **Nearby Activities**

Camp, fish, mountain bike, and swim and tube in the river at Pedernales Falls State Park. Johnson City, 10 miles west, has restaurants, art galleries, and museums. Visit the Lyndon B. Johnson National Historical Park and the Lyndon B. Johnson State Park & Historic Site.

---

### **GPS TRAILHEAD COORDINATES**

#### **N30° 18' 44.2" W98° 14' 43.3"**

This state park is off US 290 at the Hays–Blanco county line, just west of Henly. It can be accessed from Austin via US 290 and from San Antonio via US 281 to US 290. Once at the county line, take Ranch to Market Road 3232 north 6.2 miles to the park entrance. From the park entrance station, drive 0.7 mile and turn right into the camping loop. Follow the loop to the right until you come to the second trailhead parking lot. Look for the Trammell's Crossing River Access and Amphitheater signs.

# 31 Hamilton Pool Preserve Trail

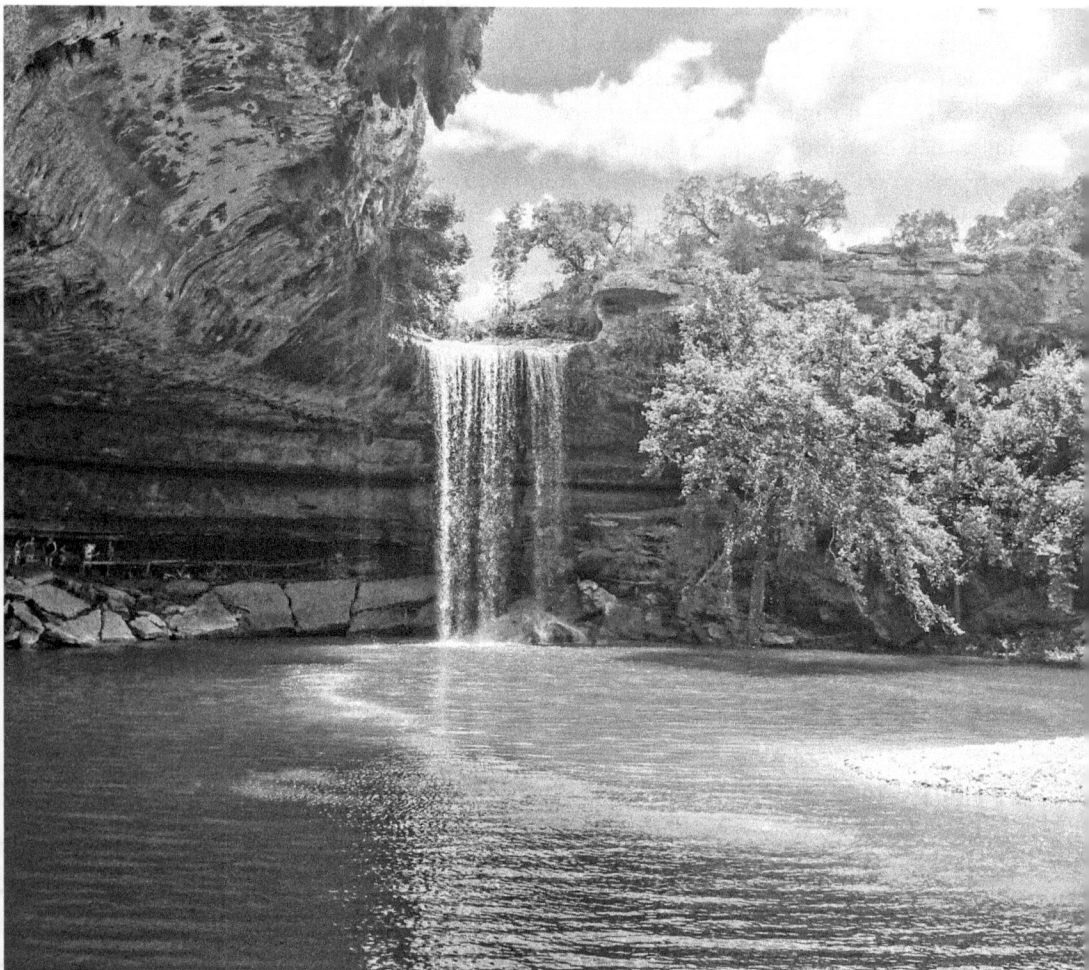

*Hamilton Pool*

## In Brief

This is a wonderful hike through a unique geological area that could be a canyon in Colorado rather than the Texas Hill Country. The magnificent grotto is one of the top natural wonders of the state.

| | |
|---|---|
| **LENGTH:** 2 miles | **HIKING TIME:** 1 hour |
| **CONFIGURATION:** Out-and-back with spur | **DRIVING DISTANCE:** 31 miles from the state capitol |
| **DIFFICULTY:** Easy | **ACCESS:** Daily, 9 a.m.–5:30 p.m.; $15 day-use fee per vehicle, cash or local check only, allows access to all Travis County Parks; reservations required to enter the preserve May 15–Sept. 30 |
| **SCENERY:** Ferns, cypress, and hardwoods along the Hamilton Creek and Pedernales River; pool and collapsed limestone grotto | |
| **EXPOSURE:** Shady | **WHEELCHAIR ACCESS:** No |
| **TRAFFIC:** Light–moderate on trail; busy at pool. Weekends are much busier than weekdays. | **MAPS:** At park |
| | **FACILITIES:** Picnic tables, restrooms |
| **TRAIL SURFACE:** Dirt, rock, roots | **CONTACT INFORMATION:** 512-264-2740; parks.traviscountytx.gov/find-a-park/hamilton-pool |

## Description

Every year, more than 75,000 people visit Hamilton Pool Preserve, which is named after Morgan Hamilton, brother to the 10th governor of Texas, Andrew Hamilton. Morgan acquired the property in the 1860s and then sold the land in the 1880s to the Reimers, German immigrants who wanted to graze sheep and cattle. As the story goes, their son found the collapsed grotto, and the family, not looking a gift horse in the mouth, opened the area for recreational use. For almost a century, the land was trampled by frolickers and livestock and suffered greatly. In 1980 the Texas Parks & Wildlife Department declared Hamilton Pool the "most significant natural area in rural Travis County," and five years later the county purchased 232 acres from the Reimer family and began the restoration process. The park is now part of the Balcones Canyonlands Preserve. Please help preserve this unique environment by staying on the trails, as the land is still recovering from decades of abuse.

Formed by centuries of water erosion, the canyon provides shelter for all kinds of wildlife. The preserve is recognized by the Audubon Society for its value as a bird habitat. The rich plant life found here includes orchids and other plants not found elsewhere in Central Texas.

The trail starts at the end of the parking lot. A bulletin board at the trailhead displays pictures of the wildlife and plants found inside the preserve. Numerous bird species and reptiles, including the Texas coral snake, live here. Although it is poisonous, the coral snake is reclusive and spends its time hidden in dead logs. The preserve is also one of the few places in this part of the state where you might come across a beaver or porcupine. Quiet, early-morning hikers stand the best chance of seeing these creatures.

Walk across the cedar-covered uplands to the steps that lead down into the canyon. A bench lets you sit and watch the traffic coming and going. The trail is steep at times,

## Hamilton Pool Preserve Trail

0.3 mile

0.3 kilometer

0.2

0.2

0.1

0.1

0

0

N

Hamilton Pool

private property

Hamilton Creek

P

HAMILTON POOL PRESERVE

Hamilton Pool Road

Pedernales River

Westcave Preserve

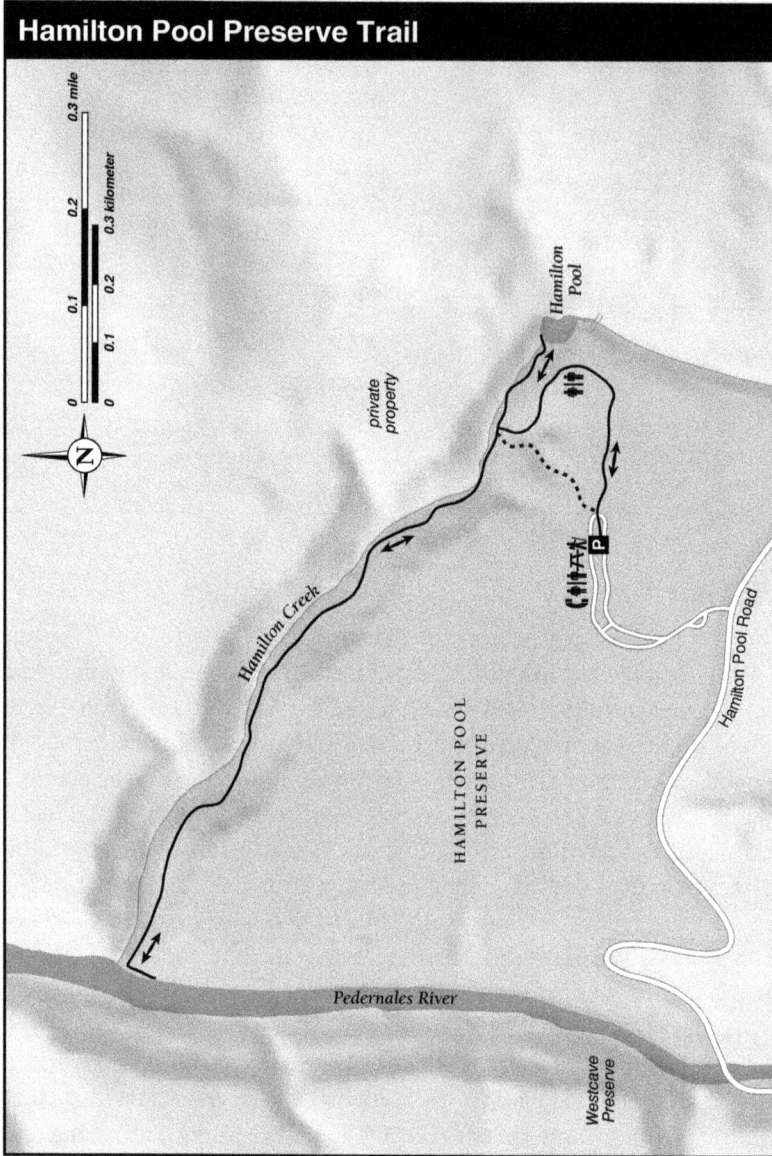

and less-practiced hikers can find it challenging. At the bottom there is a T-junction, where you'll find two portable toilets, garbage and recycling bins, and a directional sign. The pool is to the right, less than 0.1 mile distant, but you'll want to save that until last, so turn left toward the Pedernales River.

Hamilton Creek is to your right, and the clear water flows down the canyon through a series of pools linked by little falls. The steady splashing is the soundtrack for the hike.

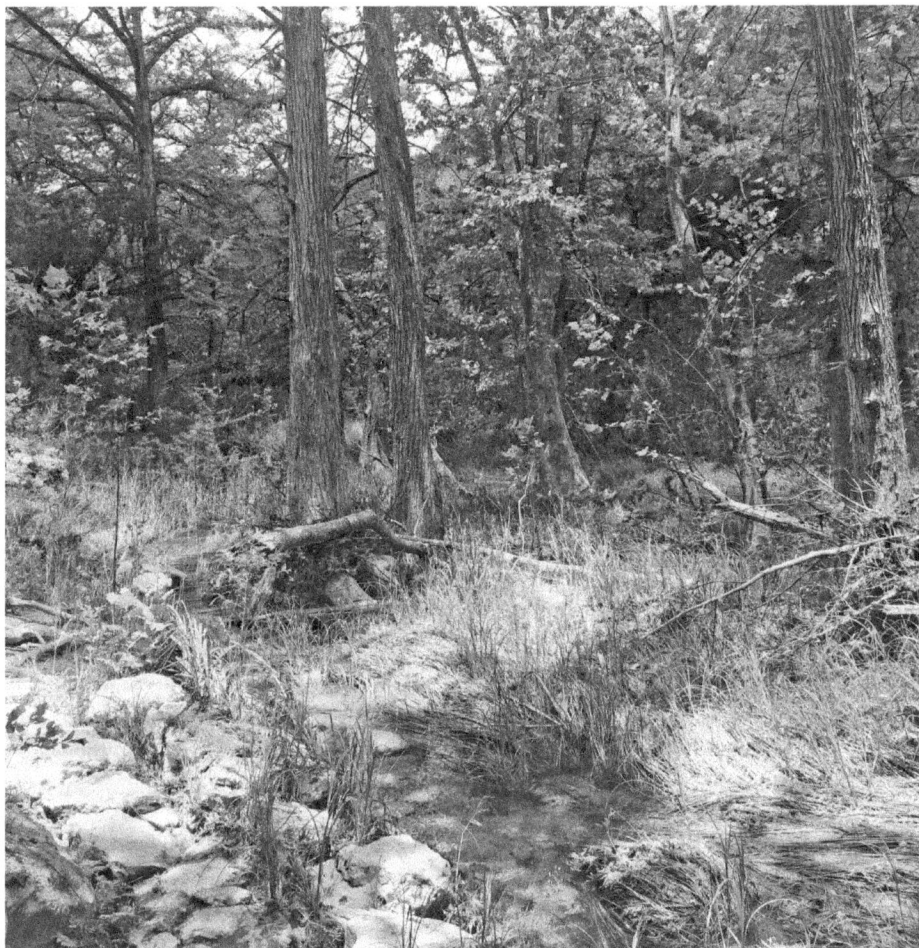

*Hamilton Creek*

Cedar and oak cover the slopes and banks, and very tall cypresses grow everywhere in the creek. Boulders are strewn along the watercourse. It's wild, lush, and beautiful.

The trail has some rough spots as it clambers up and down the banks on the descent to the Pedernales. Quite early on, look for two large boulders that lean on each other. Hikers must duck to pass between them. Take a moment to study the surface of the rocks, and you'll notice they are embedded with shells.

A fork 0.3 mile into the trail leads down to a sandbar in the creek. The trail climbs slowly, ending up about 20–30 feet above the creek. At 0.5 mile a stand of junipers creates a natural tunnel. Keep an eye out for golden-cheeked warblers, which are known to nest in the park. Short spur trails let you look down into the canyon. The water is clear, due in large part to the numerous small rapids in the stream, and you might see fish and snapping turtles. Boulders litter the ever-taller fern-bedecked cliffs to your left.

Come to the junction of the Pedernales and Hamilton Creek, 0.8 mile from the trailhead. Two benches made from cedar posts let hikers rest and enjoy the view of the bucolic valley and wide river. When the water is low, numerous sandbars appear, and you can wade out and bury your toes in the silt and sand of the river. Look for gar, common in this stretch of the Pedernales, and keep an eye out for great blue herons and egrets wading along the banks. If you brought a snack, this is a good place to enjoy it.

Walk back up the trail and go straight at the junction, heading to the pool and grotto. The sounds of people playing in the waters ahead will precede your arrival. You'll pass between two large boulders. To the right, cliffs tower above the trail. At 1.5 miles into the hike, you'll see the clear lagoon, partially shaded by the large outcrop of the collapsed limestone grotto.

It's hard to overstate the magnificence of this formation. Huge limestone stalactites covered with moss and ferns hang from the wide mouth of the grotto. At the southern end, the creek plunges 50 feet from the uplands onto a large rock, sending spray everywhere. Cliff swallows fly around the cave, and their mud nests hang on the rock wall. You would not be disappointed even if you had hiked for days through a tropical jungle to get here.

A large metal staircase leads down about 20 feet, close to the waterfall. Watch your step because the stairs are always very slippery. The trail hugs the inside wall, and you must squeeze behind a large rock. Make your way around to the beach area, which may be very crowded. The water is surprisingly transparent, and you will see catfish and sunfish milling around. If swimming is allowed, take off your shoes and wade into the water. (Quite often, a high bacteria count makes the water unsuitable for swimming, so look for signs, or call ahead to check conditions.)

## Nearby Activities

There are two other parks nearby that are worth visiting. The beautiful Westcave preserve has guided tours on the weekends, and Reimers Ranch offers hiking, climbing, mountain biking, and access to the Pedernales River.

---

### GPS TRAILHEAD COORDINATES

**N30° 20' 30.0"  W98° 7' 49.5"**

From Austin take TX 71 west to Hamilton Pool Road/Farm to Market Road 3238. Turn left, and drive 13 miles west on FM 3238 to the preserve. Note: Entrance is limited to 75 vehicles at a time; once that limit is reached, no one else is let in until someone leaves. Plan to arrive early because no waiting places are nearby. Pets are not allowed. Call 512-264-2740 for updates before you leave.

# 32 Inks Lake State Park

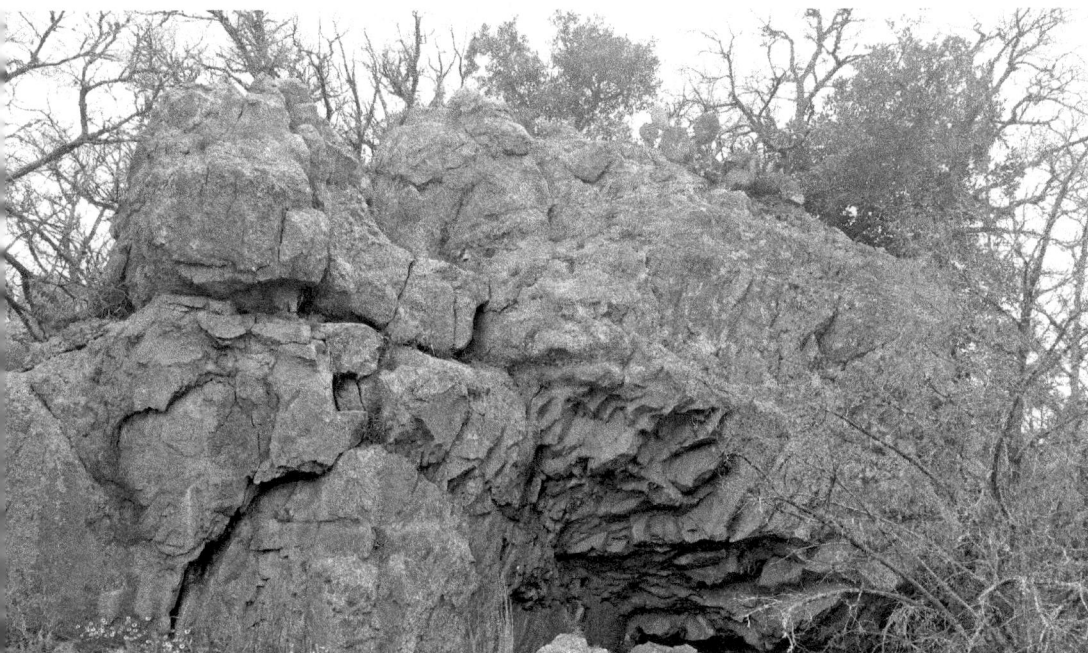

*Rock formation at Inks Lake*

## In Brief

Located in the Highland Lakes chain west of Austin, this moderately challenging hike passes Inks Lake's shoreline and wanders through hills of pink rock and distant woods. Abundant wildlife and few hikers make it a real gem.

## Description

A big chunk of Inks Lake State Park lies south of Park Road 4, and this area is off the beaten track for most visitors, despite the best efforts of the park staff, who have placed encouraging and informative signs at trailheads and major trail junctions. All the more for you and me, then; while the multitudes fish and grill, we can wander the park's more remote peaks and valleys undisturbed.

You will have noticed the pink rock that is exposed everywhere in the park and its surroundings. Inks Lake is on the western end of the Llano Uplift, a dome of Precambrian granite whose main feature is Enchanted Rock, geologically an example of a batholith. The area around Inks Lake is not granite, though; rather, it is Valley Spring gneiss, or rock

| | |
|---|---|
| **LENGTH:** 4.6 miles | **DRIVING DISTANCE:** 69 miles from the state capitol |
| **CONFIGURATION:** Balloon loop | |
| **DIFFICULTY:** Moderately difficult | **ACCESS:** Daily, 8 a.m.–10 p.m.; $6 entrance fee per person over age 13 |
| **SCENERY:** Hills, lake, wildlife, rock formations | **WHEELCHAIR ACCESS:** No |
| **EXPOSURE:** Exposed, with some shady areas | **MAPS:** tinyurl.com/inkslakemap |
| **TRAFFIC:** Light | **FACILITIES:** Restrooms, showers, picnic tables, and camping. Park store sells refreshments and supplies and rents canoes. |
| **TRAIL SURFACE:** Dirt and rock | |
| **HIKING TIME:** 2–3 hours | **CONTACT INFORMATION:** 512-793-2223; tpwd.texas.gov/state-parks/inks-lake |

(mostly granite) that has been metamorphosed by temperature and pressure. The name comes from an old German word for spark, as the minerals in the rock can make it glitter in the sunlight. You'll cross many gneiss "islands" on this hike.

Trails in the park are color-coded, and though there are marker posts, you are more likely to see dots of color painted directly onto the rock. When crossing the "islands," it is very possible to wander off the trail, so keep a lookout for the dots and the more weathered rock at those areas. Occasionally, stone verges and arrows point the way over otherwise trackless expanses of bare hillside.

The route starts on the green Lake Trail, loops around the blue Woodland Trail, and returns via the red Connecting Trail and the yellow Pecan Flats Trail. You will climb more than 1,000 feet three times, making several easy crossings over small streams on the way.

The Lake Trail starts at the information board in the parking lot and heads into some low cedar on a granite trail. Here, as in other parks, a lot of the juniper looks to have suffered from the drought of recent years. Open areas dotted with cactus, grasses, and mesquite, as well as yucca and wildflowers, surround the trail, which nonetheless stays mainly in the shade on this beginning section. Look for examples of the art of rock balancing on an outcrop to the right of the pathway.

At 0.2 mile you meet the water's edge at the end of the narrow cove where Hinds Branch flows into Inks Lake. The view up the inlet demands a picture. The trail continues into a shady grove, where the Pecan Flats Trail joins from the left, marked by a sign that says INTERPRETIVE TRAIL. (You can download the "Hiking Trail Guide for Pecan Flats" from the park's website.) Keep going straight on the Lake Trail, and at 0.4 mile cross Hinds Branch on a wooden bridge.

From here, the path opens up as it heads west past Stumpy Hollow, a popular spot for fishing, and on up to your first peak. This summit is 962 feet above sea level. Keep an eye out for the trail markers on the ascent because there is often no dirt path to follow. Take in the view north over the lake from the bare cap, and then tackle the moderately

## Inks Lake State Park

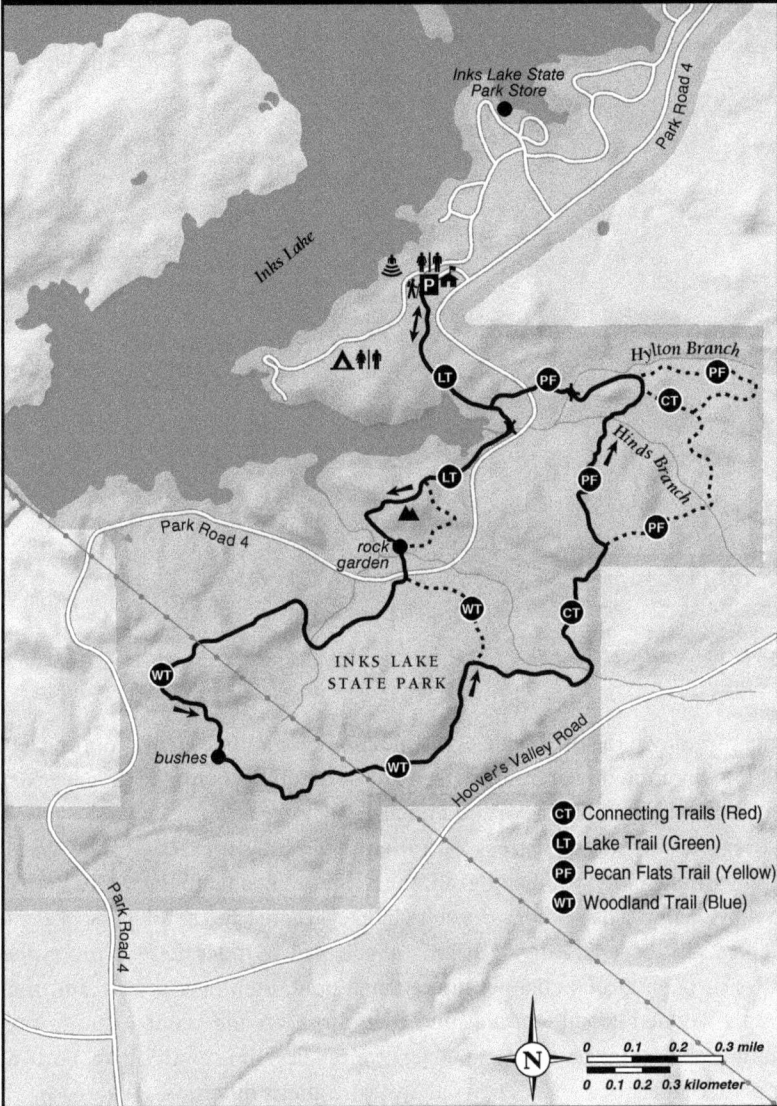

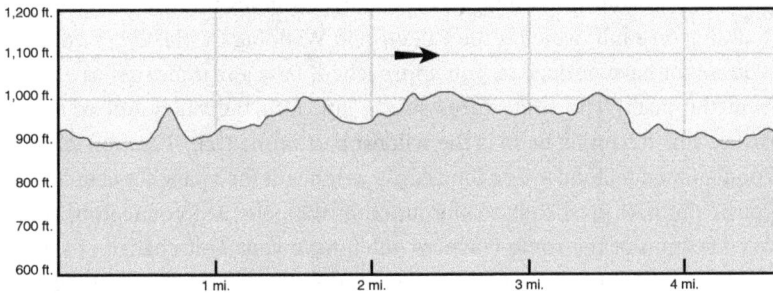

Inks Lake State
Park Store

Park Road 4

Inks Lake

Hylton Branch

PF

CT

LT

PF

Hinds Branch

LT

PF

PF

rock
garden

PF

WT

CT

Park Road 4

INKS LAKE
STATE PARK

WT

WT

bushes

Hoover's Valley Road

CT Connecting Trails (Red)
LT Lake Trail (Green)
PF Pecan Flats Trail (Yellow)
WT Woodland Trail (Blue)

Park Road 4

N

| 0 | 0.1 | 0.2 | 0.3 mile |
| 0 | 0.1 | 0.2 | 0.3 kilometer |

1,200 ft.
1,100 ft.
1,000 ft.
900 ft.
800 ft.
700 ft.
600 ft.

1 mi.   2 mi.   3 mi.   4 mi.

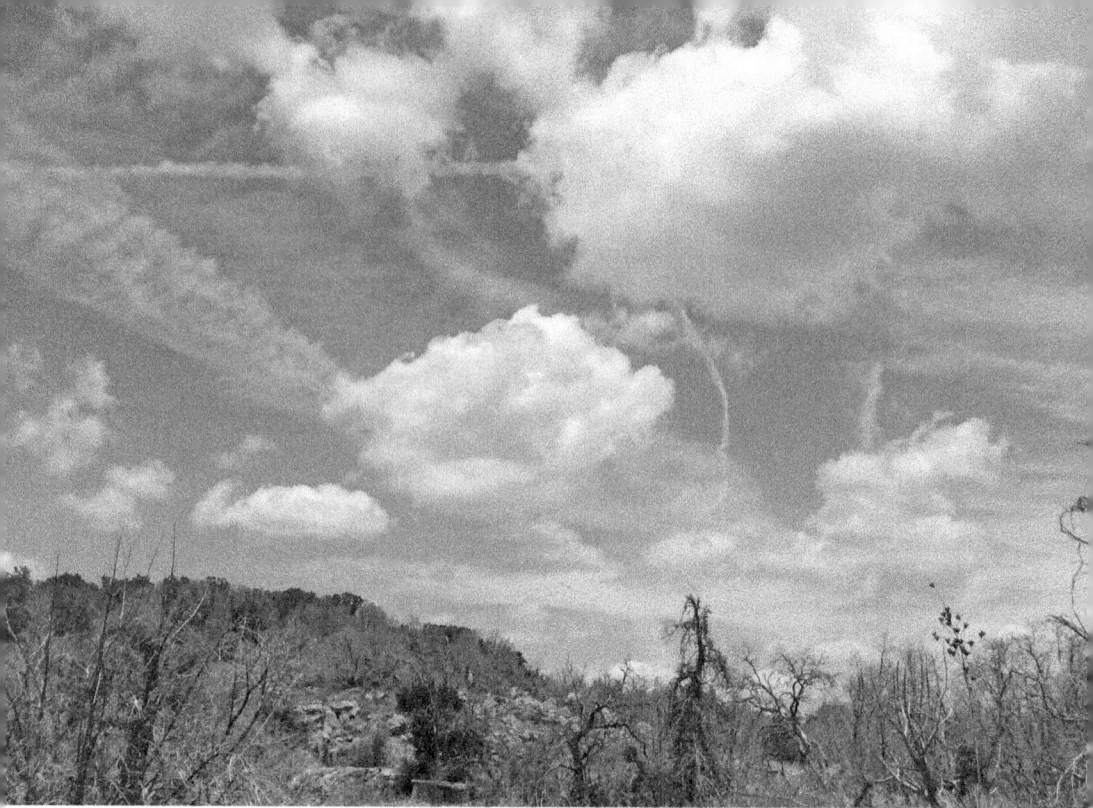

*Clouds over Inks Lake State Park*

challenging track down the other side of the hill. Look for a stone arrow pointing left, and proceed in the direction it is pointing, past a gneiss island decorated with many rock formations constructed by both nature and humans.

Step over a creek, and then cross Park Road 4 carefully at exactly 1 mile, coming to the junction with the blue Woodland Trail. Turn right to head into the park's hinterlands along a shallow valley. The scenery doesn't change—cactus and sotol grow in the sandy pink soil, and stands of cedar offer occasional shade. At 1.25 miles there's a pretty scene: a stream flows through a rock channel into a small pool. Step over the stream; the path clambers up a wooded hillside onto a spur, then turns left and clambers up to the hill's grassy summit, where you are above 1,000 feet for the first time on this hike. Forb, a leafy flowering plant that is not a grass, grows all over the gneiss outcrops.

Enjoy the views from this vantage point, only 1.5 miles into the hike. Look for a castlelike building on a hill, which is the Falkenstein Wedding Castle. Cross under power lines that you might have noticed as you approached. Pass a marker sign as you start to descend from the peak. The route turns south, left, into the valley out of which you climbed earlier. The next mile or so is the wildest part of the trek. The trail starts to live up to its Woodland name, following a long copse as it heads for a pass between two peaks. From the pass, the path descends to the junction with the red connecting trail. This lesser-traveled section of the route is where you'll have your best chance of seeing bird and animal life, and though you might hear the occasional truck rumbling along Hoover's

Valley Road, just south of the park, this area feels remote. The singletrack trail is easy to follow but overgrown, a sure sign that you are off the beaten track.

When you go back under the power lines, you will have hiked 2.4 miles. The trail climbs up the pass, making it to 1,020 feet. The lighter green of deciduous trees gives way to the darker colors of juniper. Rock formations reappear. In springtime, flowers bloom among the cactus.

At 2.8 miles you come to the junction with the red Connecting Trail. Turn right, and make your way cross-country to the left side of the yellow Pecan Flats Trail loop. The sign describes the red trail as "steep and rugged," but it seems no more so than the terrain you have already passed through. The trail crosses three little drainages; then at 3.1 miles it crosses a wider creek in an open area. The water is colored brown like an East Texas stream, presumably from the minerals in the gneiss. The path goes north across a valley floor, crosses a rock outcrop where the path is hard to follow, and makes the last of the three ascents to more than 1,000 feet at a rocky summit. You will come to the yellow trail at the top. Turn left, in the direction of the arrow that points to SCENIC VIEWS.

There are indeed some scenic views from the hill—you can see Buchanan Dam, the largest multiple-arch dam in the country—but the sign that describes the Pecan Flats Trail as "flat but rugged" is wrong. The trail makes quite a rough descent from this spur and is hard to follow at times. At 3.7 miles you cross Hinds Branch again and soon come to a junction with a different section of the red Connecting Trail. Keep left, on a wide gravel track, and go left at the next junction, where the yellow trail splits. The gravel road follows Hylton Branch past the primitive campsites, under the shade of the pecan trees that flourish in the bottomlands. Cross Hylton Branch on a bridge, and at 4.1 miles arrive at Park Road 4. Pick up the trail on the other side of the road. In just under 0.1 mile, you end the loop portion of the hike at the junction with the green trail. Turn right to retrace your steps 0.5 mile to the trailhead.

The unusual scenery, combined with undisturbed nature, makes this hike special. Perhaps once you find out for yourself how "gneiss" it is at Inks Lake, you will want to return again and again.

## Nearby Activities

Rent a kayak or canoe at the park store, and explore Devil's Waterhole, a rocky inlet perfect for swimming and jumping off rocks. The park also offers picnicking, camping, and a nine-hole golf course. Visit the Inks Dam National Fish Hatchery, just below Inks Dam.

---

**GPS TRAILHEAD COORDINATES**

**N30° 44' 12.4"  W98° 22' 12.5"**

**From US 281 north of Marble Falls, turn left on Park Road 4, and follow it 12 miles to the entrance to Inks Lake State Park. The parking lot for the hiking trail is directly across from the headquarters.**

# 33 Loop and Summit Trails at Enchanted Rock State Natural Area

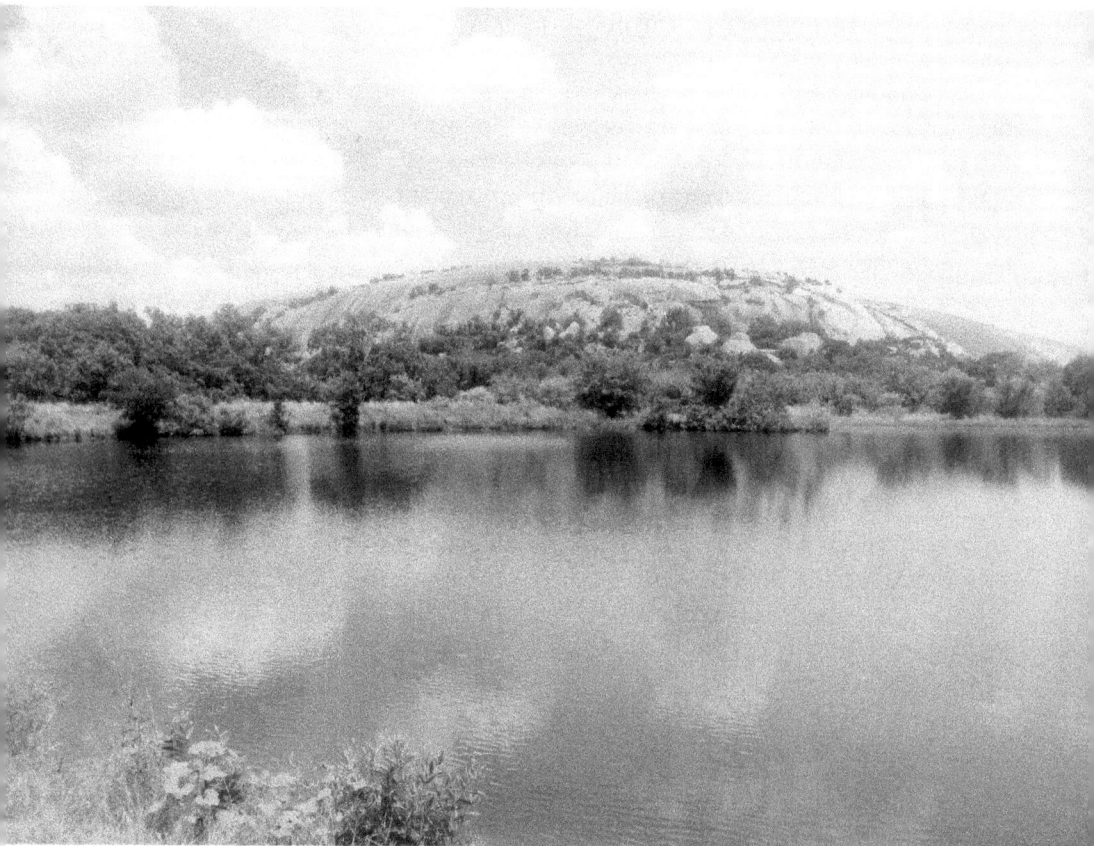

*Moss Lake and Enchanted Rock*

## In Brief

Every Central Texas hiker needs to climb to the top of Enchanted Rock, the most notable landmark in this part of the state. This hike adds the first portion of the park's Loop Trail to the summit ascent for a bracing 4-mile trek. Be prepared to visit during off times, as weekends can be so crowded that park entry is cut off.

| | |
|---|---|
| **LENGTH:** 4 miles | **ACCESS:** Daily, 8 a.m.–10 p.m.; closed during public hunts; $7 day-use fee per person over age 13 |
| **CONFIGURATION:** Loop | |
| **DIFFICULTY:** Difficult | |
| **SCENERY:** Granite mountain, broken woods, canyon walls | **WHEELCHAIR ACCESS:** No |
| | **MAPS:** tinyurl.com/enchantedrock trailmap |
| **EXPOSURE:** Exposed | |
| **TRAFFIC:** Moderate–very heavy on weekends | **FACILITIES:** Restrooms at campground and on trail; water at park headquarters and restrooms |
| **TRAIL SURFACE:** Granite slab, pea gravel, dirt, rocks | **CONTACT INFORMATION:** 830-685-3636; tpwd.texas.gov/state-parks/enchanted-rock |
| **HIKING TIME:** 2–3 hours | |
| **DRIVING DISTANCE:** 95 miles from the state capitol | |

## Description

This is the quintessential Central Texas hike, and as such I have included it despite its being outside this guidebook's distance parameters. Enchanted Rock's pink dome is the most prominent feature of the Llano Uplift block of Precambrian granite, some of which is more than a billion years old. This dome and the others surrounding it were formed when liquid magma, thrust toward Earth's surface, slowly cooled and became granite. Over time, the surface rock eroded, and the domes were left to dominate the surrounding savanna.

The granite soil supports a range of flora very different from the juniper-covered limestone hills elsewhere in the Hill Country. Post, blackjack, and live oaks thrive on the ridges and in the valleys around the dome, with bluestem and grama grasses growing in their shade. Pencil cactus grows alongside the more usual prickly pear. The land is hotter, pricklier, drier, and generally more inhospitable than the green slopes of the Balcones Escarpment. Most of this hike is exposed, including the route to the summit, so bring water and dress accordingly. If you are coming to Enchanted Rock on a weekend, be aware that the park often fills up by 10 a.m.; after that, cars will not be allowed into the park until 4 or 5 p.m., if at all. You might want to call before you come, and it's best to overnight at the campground if you are visiting on a weekend. Better yet, come during the week. Avoid this park completely on holidays and during spring break.

Start the hike on the Loop Trail by passing around a metal gate onto a wide crushed-granite path. The grass- and cactus-strewn terrain is open, broken only by smaller stands of oak, mesquite, and other trees. To your right, Little Rock sprawls westward, bisected by a large fissure. Cabin-size rocks lie around the valley floor. The domes are layered like an onion, and as each layer expands, the layer on top of it cracks and falls away. The scenery is defined by these huge boulders and the pink color of the granite.

At nearly 0.4 mile the trail starts to ascend a steep flank of Little Rock, turning north as it does so. The path leads across an outcrop, and the way is not obvious. At this

Loop and Summit Trails at Enchanted Rock State Natural Area

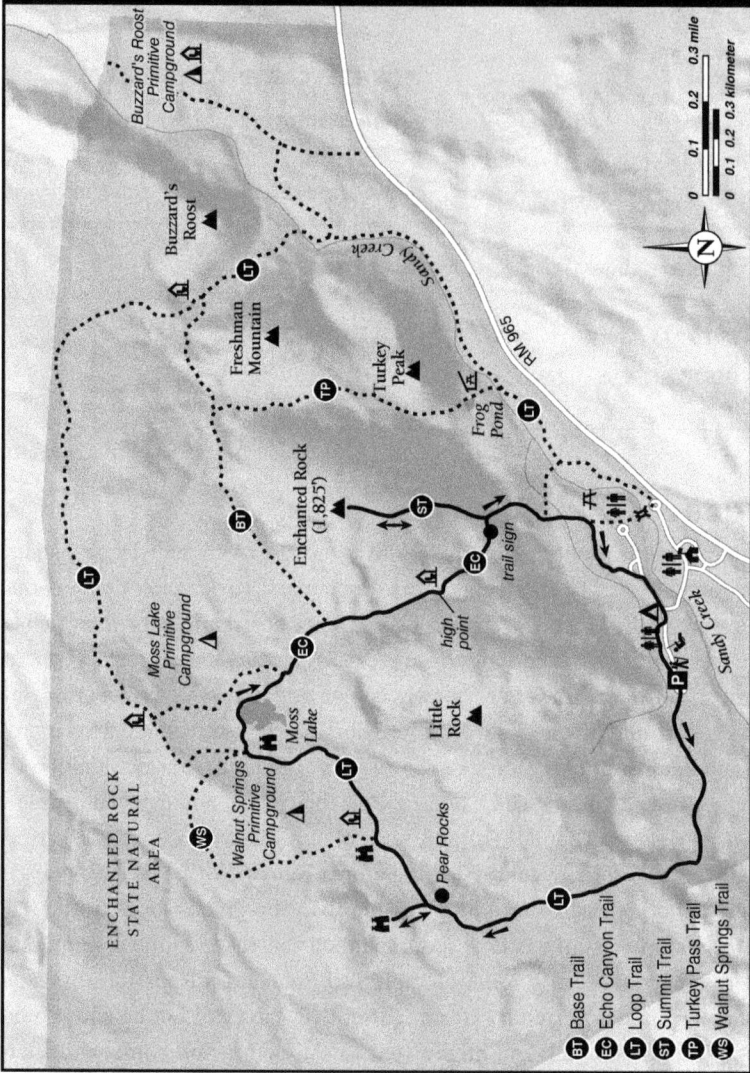

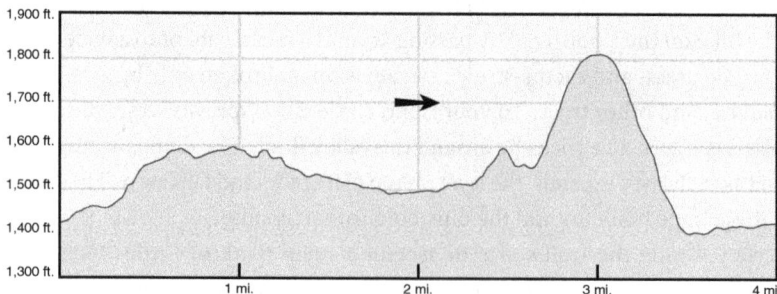

and many other points in this hike, look for the marker at the end of the bare rock to stay on the trail.

The climb levels off at 0.7 mile into the hike, which becomes an undulating walk across the spur. Epiphytes cover stubby oaks, and vistas open up to the left. Two large, pear-shaped boulders ahead of you are a landmark, and the trail passes them at the 1-mile mark. The spur to a scenic overlook comes up on the left shortly. It's worth the extra steps for the wide-ranging vista of dusty, African-looking savanna, though the best views—of the pink domes—are behind you. Other rock formations are visible to the north toward Llano. Lichens growing on the rocks add black, gray, and green to the color palette.

Descend from the spur into the lush, flat savanna. At 1.4 miles a trail leaves left to the Walnut Springs Camping Area. This site is for backpackers, but it does have a restroom. Many large blackjack oaks grow on the flat valley floor.

Leave the Loop Trail at 1.8 miles, and then turn right onto the Echo Canyon Trail, soon passing over the dam of Moss Lake. Live oaks shelter a shady lakeside resting spot for hikers. The perfect curve of Enchanted Rock is reflected in the water of the lake. Come around the eastern side of the lake, keep left at a junction, and come to the information board at the access point for the Moss Lake Primitive Camping Area, another backcountry campsite. You have hiked 2 miles at this point.

Pass another small spur leading to the camping area, and step up onto a rocky outcrop. In this confusing area, aim for the gap between Enchanted Rock and Little Rock, looking for the yellow arrows on wooden posts. Keep straight at the junction with the Base Trail, here unidentified, that leads left around the north side of Enchanted Rock. Vast chunks of the dome that have tumbled to the valley floor now litter the ground ahead of you. After a while, you will find yourself a on rooty path surrounded by vegetation. Trails lead left to climbing routes on Enchanted Rock. Reach a signboard showing these climbing routes. The trail to the right leads to another backcountry toilet. Keep forward up Echo Canyon amid fallen boulders. Climb up rock steps to a high point, and keep left, dipping down to cross a rocky wash. At 2.7 miles come out onto the sheer granite by the Echo Canyon Trail sign. Another sign, straight across the rock face, reads SUMMIT TRAIL, and most likely a steady, antlike procession of humans is filing past it as they scale the dome. Join the line, making your way to the summit while avoiding the vernal pools, where vegetation struggles for life in the places where soil and seeds have been blown into a crack. On a summer evening you might hear the rock groaning as it cools down and contracts.

Reach the top of Enchanted Rock at around 3 miles. Views expand in every direction. The actual highest point is on the rock's northwest side. Look down onto Moss Lake and the main park area below; you'll see what resembles a world of toy cars, buildings, and people. Central Texas stretches off for miles in all directions. A jeep trail leads off to the north into the nearly trackless veldt.

Backtrack on the Summit Trail, descending all the way to a feeder branch of Sandy Creek, heading for a red-roofed gazebo. Before you reach the steps to the gazebo, turn right on a trail that leads along the feeder creek. Keep left at a junction, and cross the

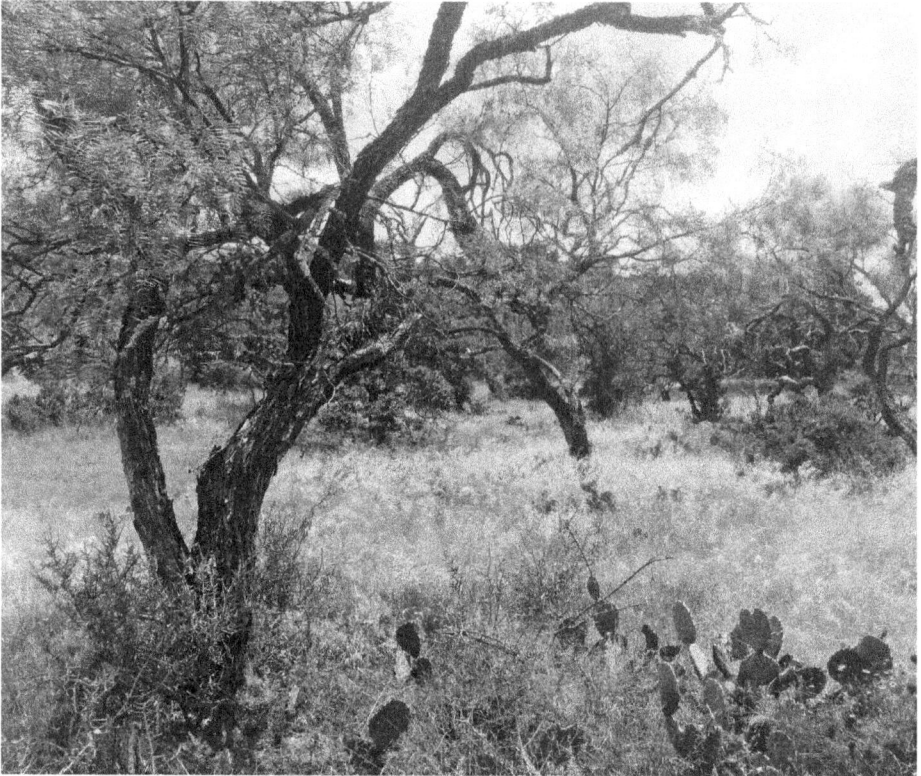

*Mesquite trees at Enchanted Rock*

feeder branch to reach the parking lot at the camping area. Turn right to walk back toward the trailhead and complete the loop.

## Nearby Activities

This State Natural Area offers hiking, picnicking, rock climbing, and walk-in tent camping.

**GPS TRAILHEAD COORDINATES**

**N30° 29' 47.2"  W98° 49' 29.2"**

From the Gillespie County Courthouse in downtown Fredericksburg, take Main Street west 0.4 mile to reach Milam Street/Ranch to Market Road 965. Turn right, and follow the road 17 miles to reach Enchanted Rock State Natural Area. Obtain your entrance permit, and then double-back behind the headquarters, turning right to cross Sandy Creek. Turn left at the T-intersection, drive through the camping areas, and park as close to the end of the road as you can. The Loop Trail begins at the end of the lot.

# 34 Turkey Pass Loop at Enchanted Rock State Natural Area

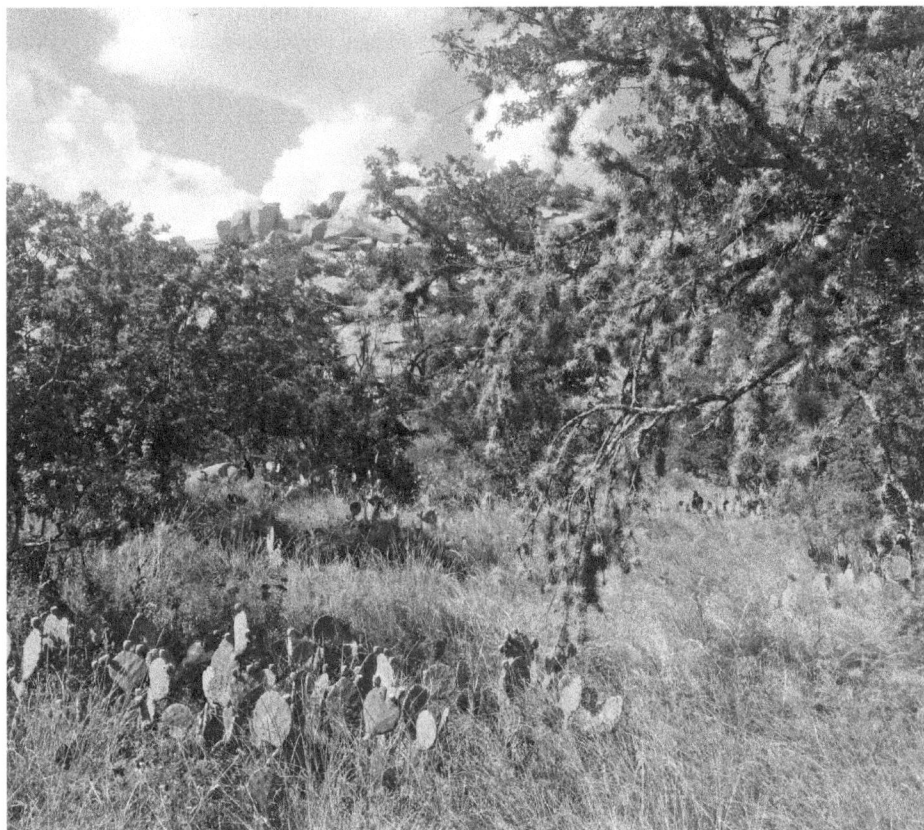

*Grass and cactus under oak trees at Enchanted Rock*

## In Brief

This pretty hike over Turkey Pass at the Enchanted Rock State Natural Area avoids the crowds seeking the summit of Enchanted Rock. It travels along Sandy Creek, passes Frog Pond, and circles around the breathtaking pink-granite mountains that make the area so unique.

| | |
|---|---|
| **LENGTH:** 2.6 miles | **ACCESS:** Daily, 8 a.m.–10 p.m.; closed during public hunts; $7 day-use fee per person over age 13 |
| **CONFIGURATION:** Loop | |
| **DIFFICULTY:** Moderate–difficult | |
| **SCENERY:** Creek bed, granite mountains | **WHEELCHAIR ACCESS:** No |
| **EXPOSURE:** Mostly exposed | **MAPS:** tinyurl.com/enchantedrock trailmap |
| **TRAFFIC:** Moderate–light | **FACILITIES:** Restrooms at headquarters; water at trailhead |
| **TRAIL SURFACE:** Dirt, gravel, rock | |
| **HIKING TIME:** 2 hours | **CONTACT INFORMATION:** 830-685-3636; tpwd.texas.gov/state-parks/ enchanted-rock |
| **DRIVING DISTANCE:** 95 miles from the state capitol | |

## Description

This hike climbs over Turkey Pass and around the less-traveled eastern end of the Loop Trail, taking you close to Turkey Peak, Freshman Mountain, and Buzzard's Roost, the craggier mounds to the east of Enchanted Rock. The scenery takes in all the different ecologies of the park–creek floodplain, mesquite grassland, sparse oak forest, and pink granite. Turkey Pass, which you will come to before you hike a mile, is the high point at 1,536 feet above sea level; from there, your route makes a long descent back to the creek valley.

Heavy use of the park has resulted in many bootleg trails; the official trails, which you should stick to, are marked with low wooden posts inscribed with an arrow and a white plastic diamond. Get used to looking for this sign, as certain sections of the hike are hard to follow. If you are coming to Enchanted Rock on a weekend, be aware that the parking lot often fills up by 10 a.m.; after that, cars will not be allowed into the park until 4 or 5 p.m., if at all. You might want to call before you come, and it's best to overnight at the campground if you are visiting on a weekend. Better yet, come during the week. Avoid this park completely on holidays and during spring break.

From the trailhead, walk through a shady picnic area and down some steps, and then make your way across a feeder branch of Sandy Creek. Abundant grasses grow by the creek, dotted with flowering plants and mesquite and large oak trees. Some parts can be very lush in wetter times. The hike goes up and down along the bank, trail signs indicating the way. Shortly you will join the Loop Trail, keeping right. The walking is easy. Pass a residence, and then at 0.4 mile come to the group picnic shelter. The trail goes to the left of the parking lot and comes to an information sign.

Turn left here, joining the Turkey Pass Trail and rock-hopping the stream, which flows in clear braids over a pink, grainy bed. Frog Pond appears just over the hill from Sandy Creek. Walk over a wooden bridge before reaching a junction. Keep right on the Turkey Pass Trail, heading for the gap between Turkey Peak to the right and Enchanted Rock to the left. Multiple paths spur off toward Turkey Peak, whose crags attract adventurous hikers. The vast face of Enchanted Rock towers to your left.

Turkey Pass Loop at Enchanted Rock State Natural Area

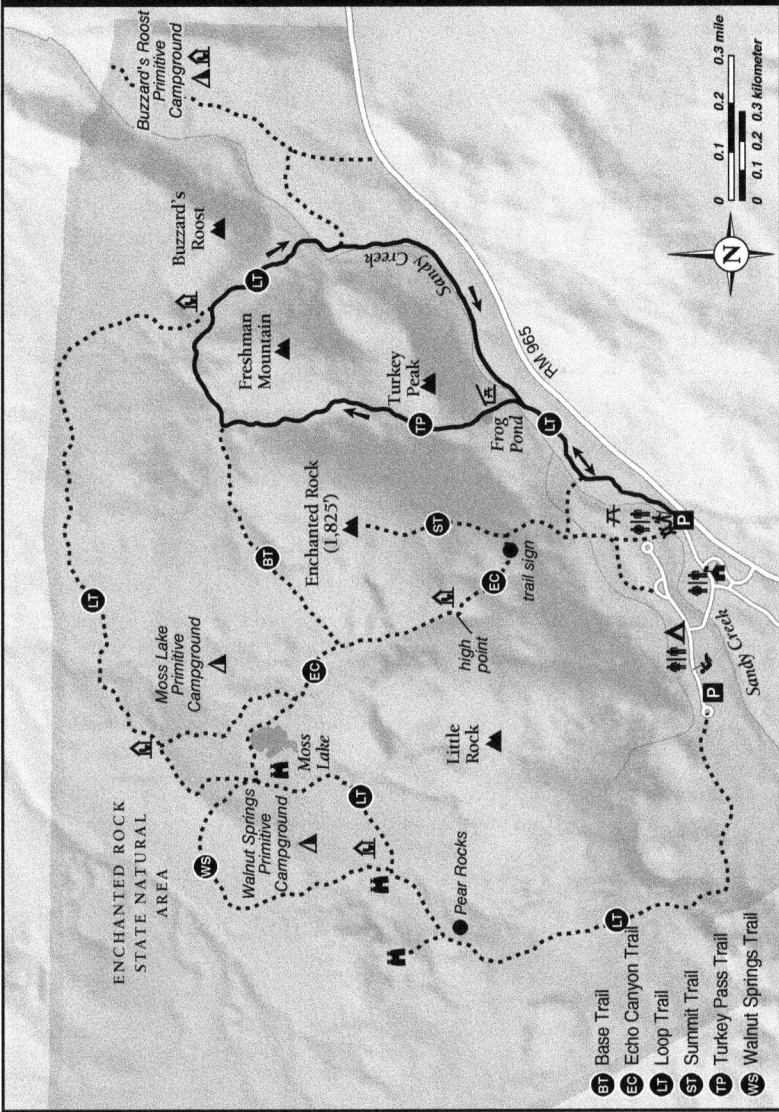

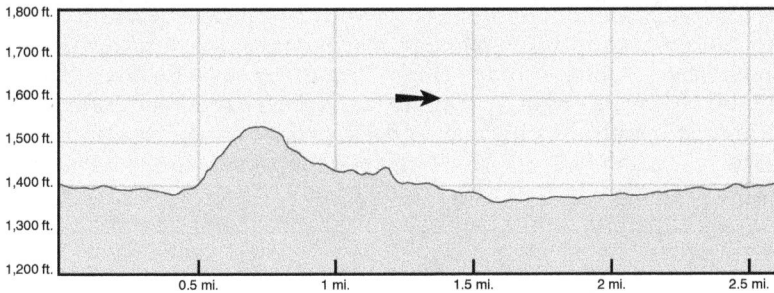

Now comes the steep climb over fallen boulders to the high point between Turkey Peak and Enchanted Rock. There are yellow plastic markers to show the way forward, in addition to the wooden posts. Broken pieces of granite, in all shapes and sizes, lie around the base of Enchanted Rock, which is even odder and more impressive up close. The hill is part of a batholith, which is a vast rock-berg, most of which is hidden underground. Enchanted Rock and the others around it are exfoliation domes, which is to say they are peeling away. The reduction in weight from the loss of the top layer causes the next layer to expand and crack. Enchanted Rock is not even the second largest of these in the United States, as is sometimes claimed, but the smoothness of its surface and the regularity of its curves give it a special magic.

Reach the pass at 0.7 mile, and keep forward over slabs of granite, making for the wide-open panorama in front of you. Freshman Mountain stands ahead to your right. Drift down through oak woods on narrow singletrack to reach a trail junction at just over a mile. Turn right on the Base Trail, immediately crossing a wet-weather drainage. Keep downstream, parallel to the drainage, before climbing over a flank of Freshman Mountain, from which Buzzard's Roost is visible ahead. Dip down into the watershed again, now quite a verdant valley between the two mountains.

At 1.3 miles you come to the Loop Trail. Turn right on an easy-to-follow gravel path. Boulderers and explorers will want to linger in this remote field of stones. Descend into the Sandy Creek watershed, recrossing the feeder branch and then fording the main creek at 1.6 miles. The path to the Buzzard's Roost Primitive Camping Area leaves to the left. Continue upstream along open Sandy Creek, where gravel bars, grassy banks, and many rock formations enhance the scene. Views open of the crags on Turkey Peak and then of Enchanted Rock.

Return to the group picnic shelter at 2.2 miles. This ends the loop portion of your hike. Keep forward along Sandy Creek, and backtrack a little more than half a mile to the trailhead.

## Nearby Activities

Picnic, rock-climb, and tent-camp at this state natural area.

### GPS TRAILHEAD COORDINATES
**N30° 29' 50.5" W98° 49' 4.7"**

From the Gillespie County Courthouse in downtown Fredericksburg, take Main Street west 0.4 mile to reach Milam Street/Ranch to Market Road 965. Turn right, and follow the road 17 miles to reach Enchanted Rock State Natural Area. Obtain your entrance permit, and keep right as you leave the park headquarters. The Sandy Creek Trail begins at the far side of the turnaround/parking area at the end of the road.

# 35 Wolf Mountain Trail at Pedernales Falls State Park

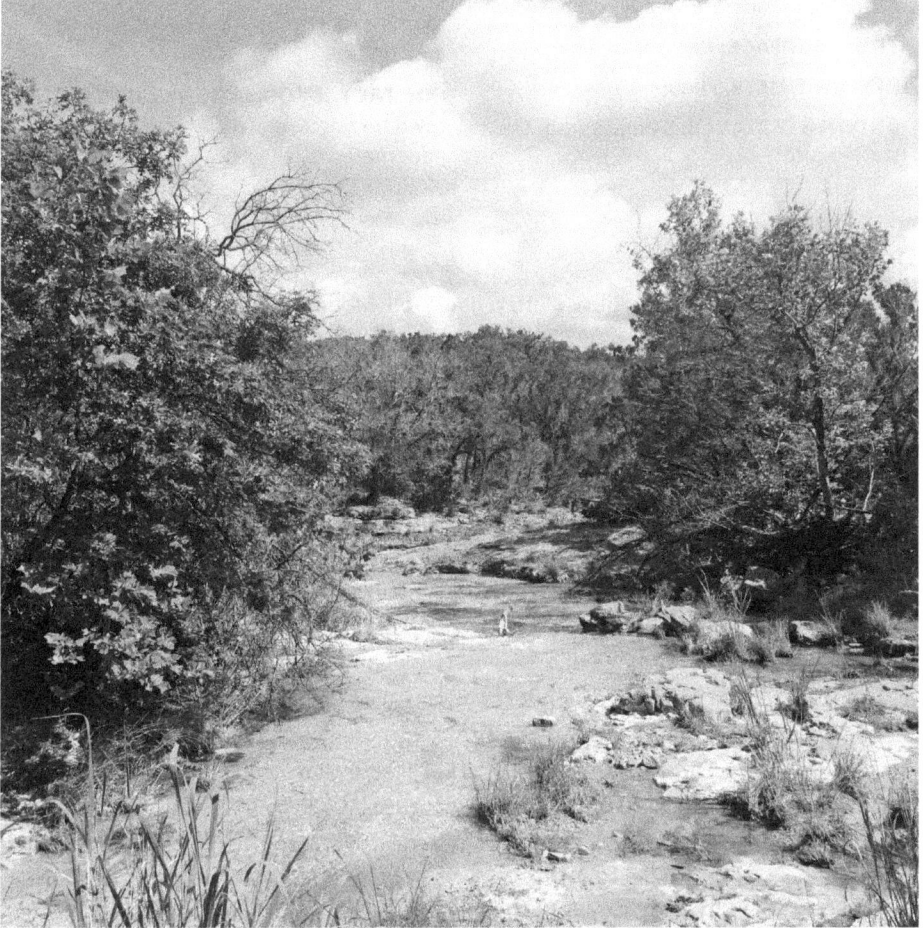

*One of many creeks at Pedernales Falls State Park*

## In Brief

This trail explores the high country of Pedernales Falls State Park, where views, creeks, a spring, and a homesite await the trekker. The park, set in a swath of emerald green Hill Country just west of Dripping Springs, offers the nearest remote wilderness to Austin. The Wolf Mountain Trail also has a popular backcountry campsite.

| | |
|---|---|
| **LENGTH:** 7.4 miles | **ACCESS:** Daily, 8 a.m.–10 p.m.; $6 day-use fee per person over age 13 |
| **CONFIGURATION:** Balloon loop | |
| **DIFFICULTY:** Moderate | **WHEELCHAIR ACCESS:** No |
| **SCENERY:** Juniper woods, creek valleys | **MAPS:** tinyurl.com/pedernalesfalls trailmap |
| **EXPOSURE:** Mostly sunny | |
| **TRAFFIC:** Moderate–heavy | **FACILITIES:** Water at trailhead, restrooms at park office and near camping area on trail |
| **TRAIL SURFACE:** Dirt, rocks | |
| **HIKING TIME:** 4.5 hours | |
| **DRIVING DISTANCE:** 34 miles from the state capitol | **CONTACT INFORMATION:** 830-868-7304; tpwd.texas.gov/state-parks/pedernales-falls |

## Description

A whole day's hike in the Hill Country, the Wolf Mountain Trail is best after a rain-bearing front has blown through, filling the Pedernales River and its tributaries and clearing the skies for far-reaching views. The path traverses several watersheds, the last of which has a spring and homesite nearby. A swimming hole at Bee Creek and the primitive camping area bring people to this trail, which may be heavily trafficked until you pass these attractions. Fewer people will venture to Jones Spring, just over 3 miles in. On the back section of Tobacco Mountain, you'll likely pass only the occasional intrepid hiker or biker.

Leave the parking lot on a shady path through thick juniper that turns out to be an imposter, depositing you in short order on a wide gravel road. Turn left onto this road, which you will follow for much of the route. Though the well-maintained surface makes for easy walking, the path cleared for the roadway leaves the hiker exposed to the elements. Bring a hat, sunscreen, and plenty of water to keep you hydrated on this long hike.

The road descends to cross Regal Creek, where there might be a small cascade. Juniper woodland dominates the landscape, which is broken by rough grasses, rocks, and live oaks. Gray skeletons of dead cedar are scattered through the sparse forest. The trail climbs away from Regal Creek and curves around into the Bee Creek watershed. "Social" trails, as the Texas Parks & Wildlife Department calls them, lead to the bluffs over the creek. Should you wish to make a short detour, at 0.9 mile one such spur makes its way down to a blue pool. Water tumbles down a slippery rock slide into this pool, which is often deep enough for jumping off the bluff. If heat, rainfall, and the weekend have aligned, there will be folks enjoying this picture-perfect spot.

Cross Bee Creek at 1 mile, and climb, looking for red oaks among the juniper. Pass a high point at 1.2 miles, from which Wolf Mountain is visible. Cross Mescal Creek at 1.8 miles, and come to a trail junction, where there is bear-proof storage and a path leading left. This goes to the primitive backcountry camping area and is a way to the Pedernales River. The area below the river bluffs is very pretty, though no camping is allowed there.

# Wolf Mountain Trail at Pedernales Falls State Park

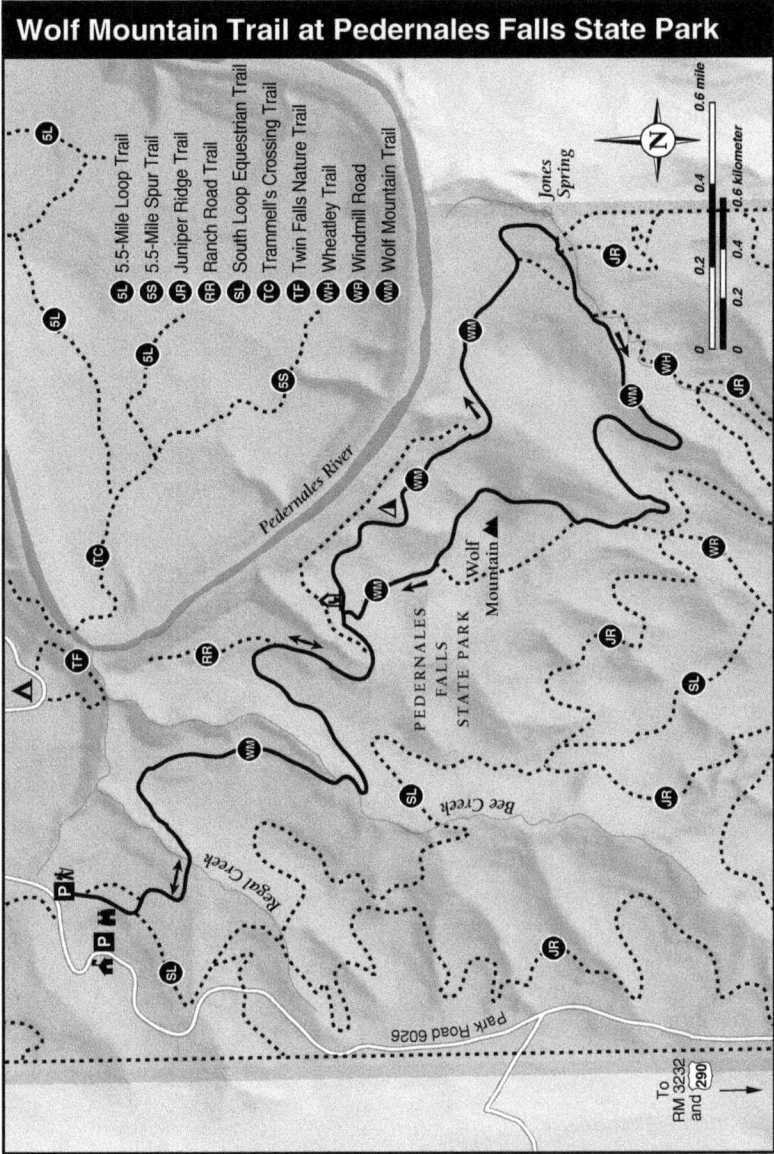

**5L** 5.5-Mile Loop Trail
**5S** 5.5-Mile Spur Trail
**JR** Juniper Ridge Trail
**RR** Ranch Road Trail
**SL** South Loop Equestrian Trail
**TC** Trammell's Crossing Trail
**TF** Twin Falls Nature Trail
**WH** Wheatley Trail
**WF** Windmill Road
**WM** Wolf Mountain Trail

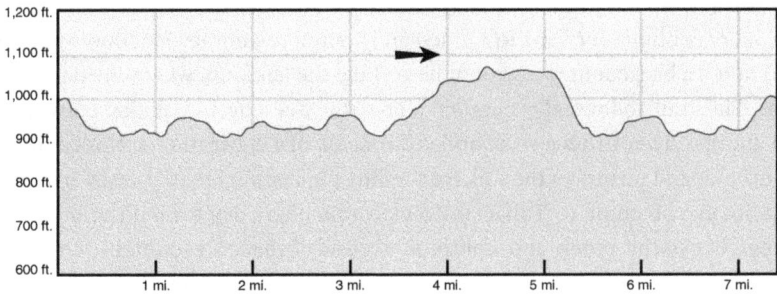

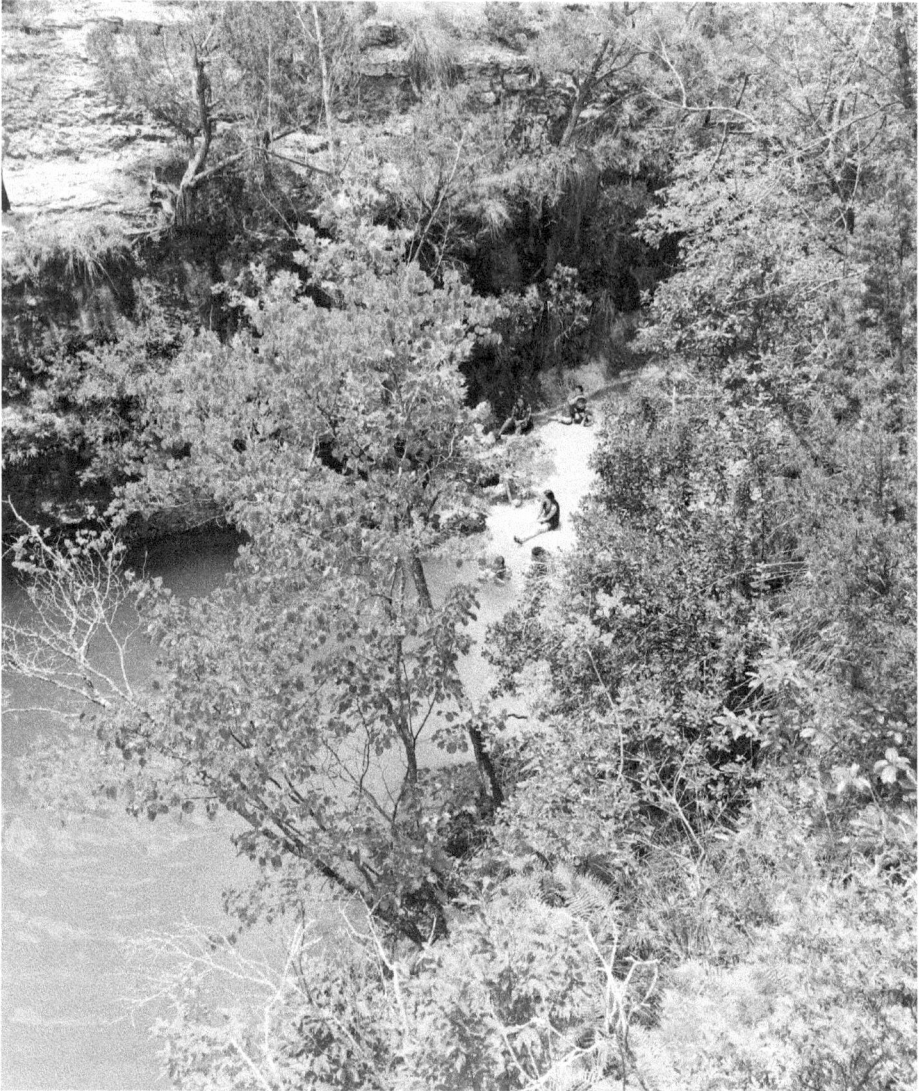

*The swimming hole on Bee Creek*

Day hikers continue forward to immediately come to another junction—the start of the loop. There's a backcountry restroom here. Take the left loop, where the path narrows somewhat. The trail follows the contour along the tree-covered slopes between Wolf Mountain and the river. Cross a wash under the shade of a cedar tunnel. Notice the subtle shifts in the color and texture of the soil, from sandy pink granite to rock-strewn limestone.

At 2.6 miles you come to Tobacco Creek, most likely dry even if the other creeks are flowing. Cross the creek and continue around Tobacco Mountain, coming to a meadow at the 3-mile mark. Cactus grows among the grasses, and live oaks mix with the cedar around the perimeter of the field. The path turns left and makes a big zigzag down the hillside to pass by Jones Spring, down a spur trail to your left. The spring is set in a creek bed. When it is flowing, the water tumbles down through a series of small tinajas. Ferns grow on the north bank of this creek bed, a nice place to rest awhile and perhaps eat lunch.

Return to Wolf Mountain Trail; ahead are the rock walls of an old homesite, undoubtedly situated here because of the close proximity to Jones Spring. The trail, now an earthen singletrack, goes through a gap in a rock wall, likely the result of hours of hard, lonely labor. Walk through a seep, and cross an unnamed creek, back into yet thicker forest. Look for tall, old cedar and red oak trees. This part of the trek, through the woods at the back of Tobacco Mountain, checks the "remote wilderness" box.

Cross the creek again, and walk alongside the muddy arroyo until, at nearly 4 miles, the trail turns away from the stream, climbing swiftly and steeply up over limestone *balcones* to a spur to the hike's high point, nearly 1,100 feet above sea level, where the cedar trees are shorter and the understory very rocky.

One more dip, and the trail picks up the roadbed at 4.6 miles. To the left is the park boundary and County Road 201. Go right, and come to a T-junction, where arrows point both ways. Either way takes you around the peak of Wolf Mountain, and your choice might depend on the angle of the sun. To the right, vistas quickly open up, and you can look out over the Pedernales Valley and beyond. Look for the winding blue-green ribbon that is the river. The route that takes in this shorter Wolf Mountain Loop is popular with mountain bikers. At 5.1 miles, meet the trail that came around the west side of the mountain. The road now makes a long descent down the northern spur of the mountain, returning to the start of the long loop at mile 5.4. Turn left, backtracking past the camping area, Mescal Creek, and Bee Creek. At Regal Creek, stop and admire the majestic live oak to the right of the trail. Lastly, don't miss the right turn back to the parking lot.

## **Nearby Activities**

At Pedernales Falls State Park, you can camp, fish, mountain bike, and swim and tube in the river. Try to fit in a trip to the falls and a dip in the river.

---

### **GPS TRAILHEAD COORDINATES**

#### **N30° 18' 28.6" W98° 15' 20.8"**

This state park is off US 290 at the Hays–Blanco county line, just west of Henly. It can be accessed from Austin via US 290 and from San Antonio via US 281 to US 290. Once at the county line, take Texas Ranch Road 3232 north 6.2 miles to the park entrance. From the park entrance station, keep forward 0.2 mile, and turn right at the sign for Wolf Mountain Trail to reach the trailhead.

# San Antonio (Hikes 36–47)

Guadalupe River

La Vernia

87

Cibolo Creek

90
10

6 miles
6 kilometers
0   2   4
0   2   4

N

35

Live Oak

LOOP 1604

LOOP 1604

181

Calaveras Lake

87

38

410

37

281

44

410

35

281

San Antonio

46

47

LOOP 1604

281

LOOP 13

281

LOOP 1604

90

410

Salado Creek

42

10   87

16   45

39   40

43

410

35

Leon Creek

Helotes

LOOP 1604

Macdona

16

36, 37, 41

Rio Medina

90

# SAN ANTONIO

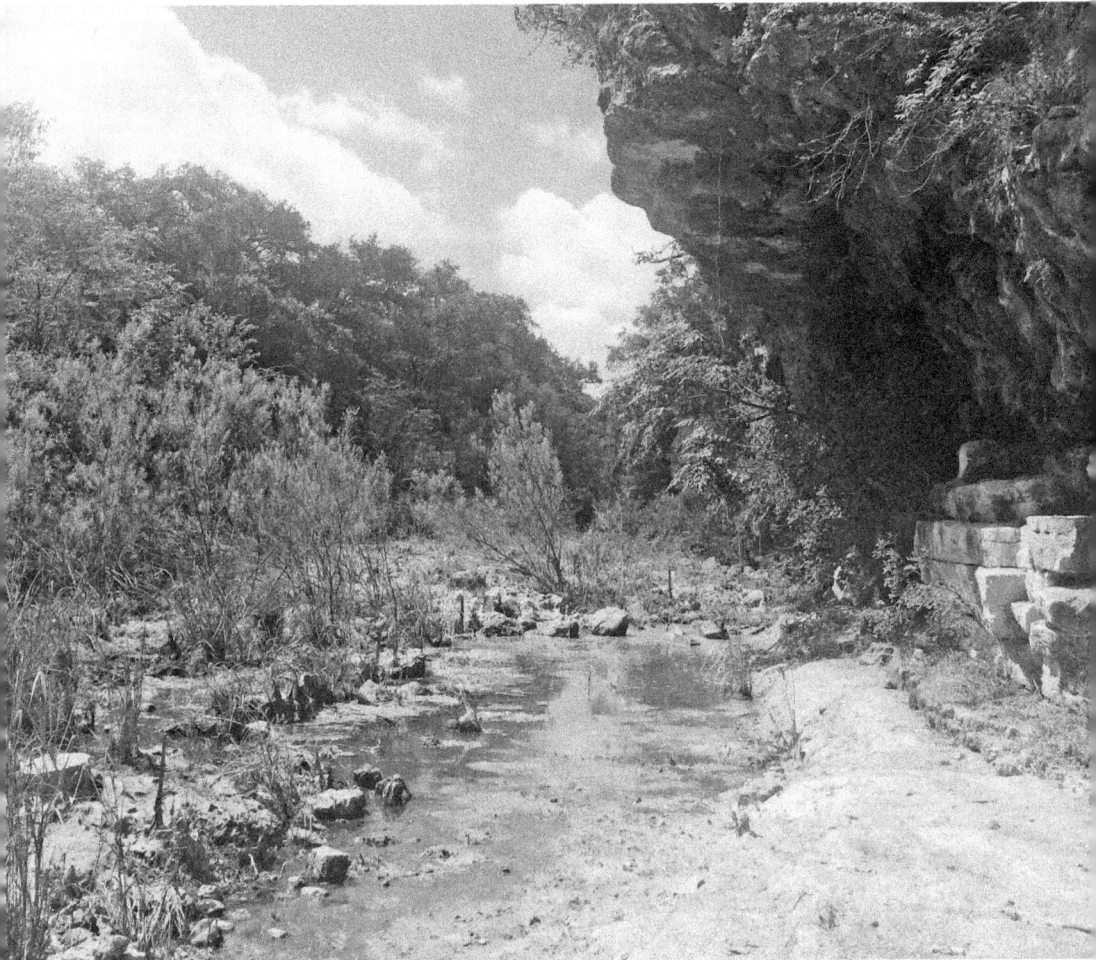

*Bluffs and springs at Government Canyon State Natural Area (see page 191)*

# 36 Bluff Spurs Overlooks

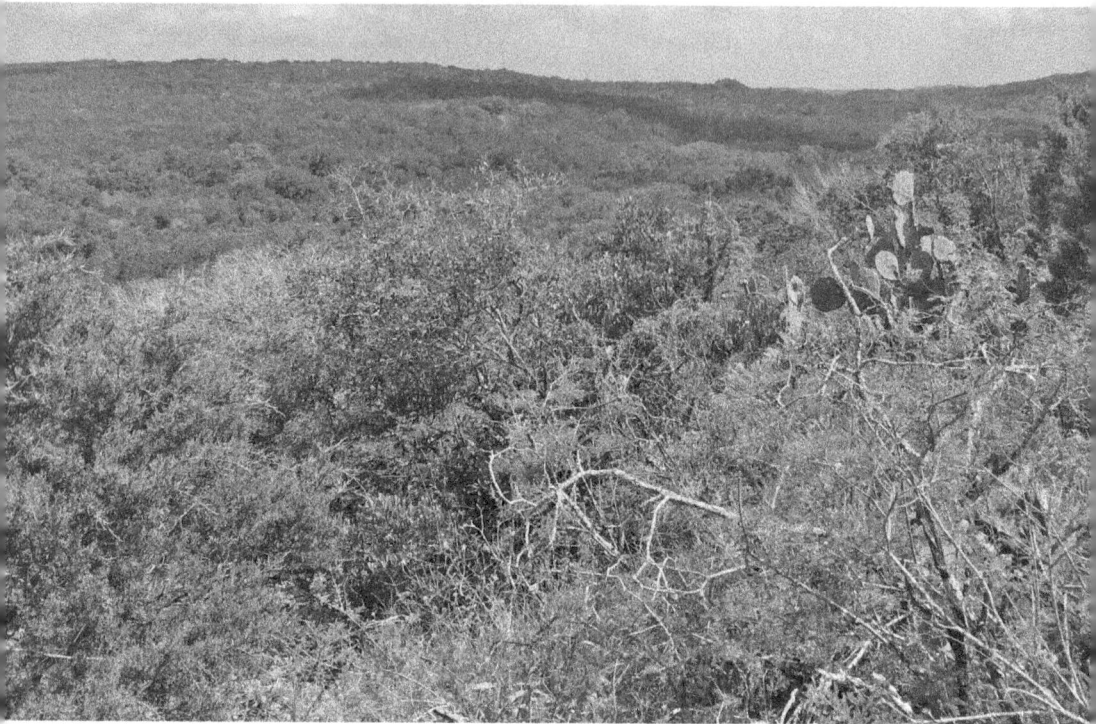

*The view over Government Canyon*

## In Brief

Get a workout on this hike climbing up rocky slopes to rewarding vistas. Government Canyon State Natural Area is the setting for a trek that briefly visits the boundary of hill and grassland before climbing onto rocky wooded prominences with extensive views of the Hill Country of northwest San Antonio.

## Description

San Antonio marches ever outward along its northwest frontier, and rows of houses are now popping up at the edge of Government Canyon State Natural Area, a place that felt remote when it first opened to the public in 2009. Let's be grateful that the state of Texas was persuaded to acquire these 12,085 acres of pristine Hill Country in 1993 as part of a plan to preserve areas that serve as a recharge zone for the Edwards Aquifer, the source of San Antonio's water. The hills in the preserve are karst, landscape that is formed when

| LENGTH: 4.1 miles | ACCESS: Friday–Monday, 7 a.m.–10 p.m.; $6 per person over age 13 |
|---|---|
| CONFIGURATION: Balloon loop with spurs | |
| DIFFICULTY: Moderately difficult | WHEELCHAIR ACCESS: No |
| SCENERY: Wooded hill country, oak savanna | MAPS: tinyurl.com/government canyonmap |
| EXPOSURE: Partly open | FACILITIES: Restrooms, water, picnicking, visitor center at trailhead |
| TRAFFIC: Busy on nice days | CONTACT INFORMATION: 210-688-9055; tpwd.texas.gov/state-parks/ government-canyon |
| TRAIL SURFACE: Rocks, roots, dirt | |
| HIKING TIME: 2.5 hours | |
| DRIVING DISTANCE: 25 miles from the Alamo | |

rainfall reacts with limestone and other rocks. The water has eroded the surface stone and carved out the system of caverns and underground streams that make up the aquifer. The preserve also protects the natural environment and offers a place of recharge and recreation for humans. Nature comes first here, so the park is only open Friday–Monday, and its furthest reaches are closed for much of the year. Pets are not allowed in the backcountry areas.

This hike travels an important fault line of the recharge zone and then climbs to overlooks that will add to your appreciation of the aboveground beauty and the aquifer below. From the backcountry trailhead, head north up the Joe Johnston Route, an old military road named after the route's surveyor. Brown plastic posts mark intersections on the route; each trail has its own logo. At 0.1 mile arrive at the junction with the Recharge Trail, and turn right. As the crow flies, this intersection is only 150 yards from the first overlook, but you must walk another 1.5 miles to get there.

The Recharge Trail briefly climbs back to the southeast over a mix of limestone, cedar, and cactus. It soon drops down again and jogs left to go east along the fault line that separates the Balcones Escarpment, which you are about to climb, and the plateau to your south. Walk along a ranch road with cedar on your left and a mix of shrubs, grasses, oaks, and mesquite to your right.

At 0.6 mile turn left onto the pedestrian-only Bluff Spurs Trail, which climbs the uneven karst through cedar on a narrow track. The lumps and slabs of limestone demonstrate the pitting that happens on contact with water. Often you must clamber over *balcones,* outcrops of harder stone that jut from the hillside. The landscape continually changes from open rock to cactus gardens to juniper thickets. Look for mountain laurel and cedar elm as you get higher. The path climbs more steeply and gets very rocky as it approaches the summit area.

Come to a trail junction at 1.1 miles. Turn left, southbound, on the level south spur. Descend to reach the edge of Government Canyon and a rock outcrop at 1.5 miles. The

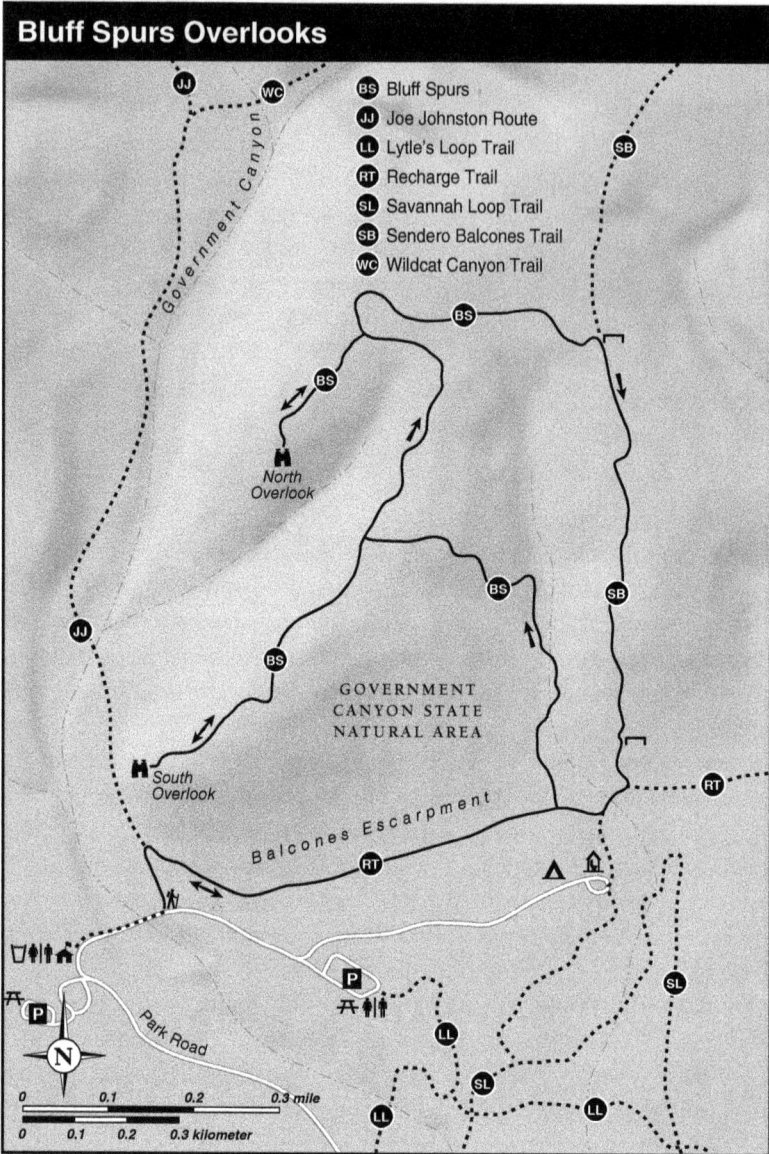

## Bluff Spurs Overlooks

- **BS** Bluff Spurs
- **JJ** Joe Johnston Route
- **LL** Lytle's Loop Trail
- **RT** Recharge Trail
- **SL** Savannah Loop Trail
- **SB** Sendero Balcones Trail
- **WC** Wildcat Canyon Trail

Government Canyon

North Overlook

South Overlook

GOVERNMENT CANYON STATE NATURAL AREA

Balcones Escarpment

Park Road

N

0     0.1     0.2     0.3 mile

0     0.1     0.2     0.3 kilometer

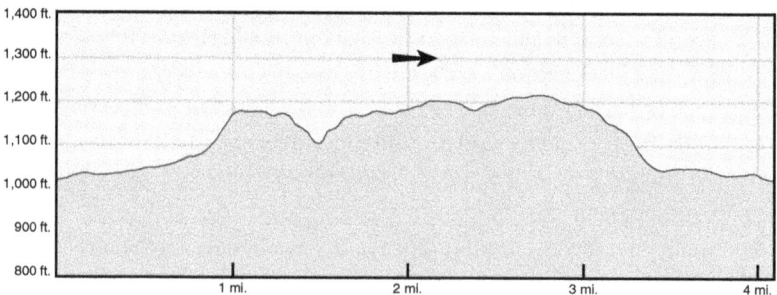

visitor center and attendant buildings are almost the only structures visible in a panoramic view.

Backtrack to the junction with the main trail, and travel north on a flat singletrack path in a mix of sun and shade, cedars, oaks, earth, and rocks. At 2.2 miles reach the north spur. This shorter trail leads through crowded tree thickets to a slightly less panoramic view, even though this overlook is 100 feet higher than the southern one. Rejoin the main loop, and follow it east through clearings to find the next junction at 2.9 miles. A bench here invites you to pause for a few moments. Turn right on the Sendero Balcones Trail, a hike-and-bike path, and travel southbound on this ridgeline track. Watch your feet, as the path is exceedingly stony. Views open to the south on the descent—another reason to go slow. Pass a bench under the spreading habit of an oak whose branches are hung with epiphytes, and shortly meet the Recharge Trail at 3.4 miles. Turn right, and trace the old roadbed west, passing a side trail leaving left to the park campground.

Complete the loop portion of your hike at 3.5 miles. Backtrack to the trailhead, and make your way back across the bridge to the visitor center and parking lot.

## Nearby Activities

Government Canyon State Natural Area offers tent camping, picnic facilities, 40 miles of hiking and biking trails, and regularly scheduled guided hikes.

---

### GPS TRAILHEAD COORDINATES

**N29° 33' 0.7"  W98° 45' 45.4"**

From the intersection of Loop 1604 and Shaenfield Road, northwest of downtown San Antonio and south of Braun Road, take Shaenfield Road west 1.6 miles to a traffic light. Continue through the traffic light, where Shaenfield Road becomes Galm Road. Keep west on Galm Road, and follow it 1.9 miles to the park entrance at a traffic circle. Drive to the parking lot and visitor center, and park your car. Once you have your permit, walk past the visitor center and over a road bridge across Government Canyon to find the backcountry trailhead.

---

# 37 Chula Vista Loop

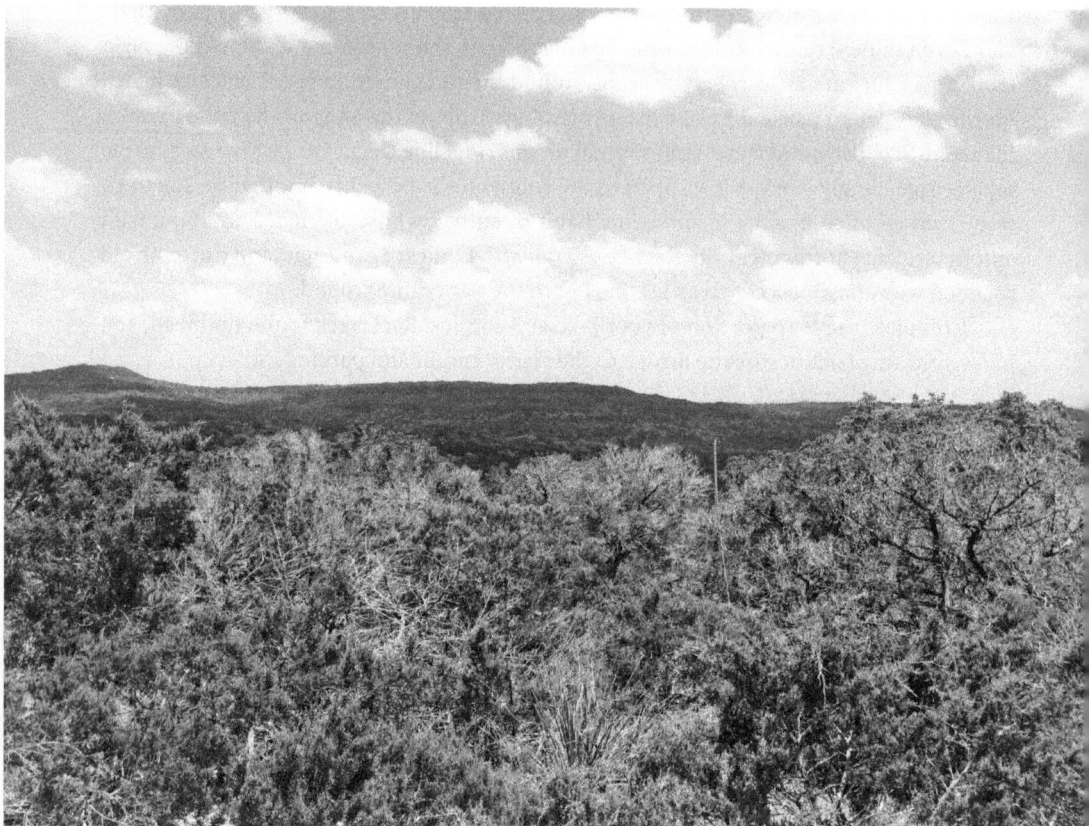

*Far-reaching Hill Country vistas can be found at Government Canyon State Natural Area.*

## In Brief

This lengthy loop explores high highs and low lows of the Government Canyon State Natural Area backcountry, heading up a wild and luxuriant canyon before climbing to breezy summits. Far-reaching views from two vista points are the reward here. The last part of the circuit visits the restored savanna of the frontcountry.

## Description

Government Canyon State Natural Area is big—more than 12,000 acres of rocks, cedar, oaks, and slopes crisscrossed by 40 miles of hike-and-bike trails. This long, wild trek doesn't cover even half of the park, but it will take you past ranching relics and up a feral

| | |
|---|---|
| **LENGTH:** 6.6 miles | **ACCESS:** Friday–Monday, 7 a.m.–10 p.m.; $6 per person over age 13 |
| **CONFIGURATION:** Loop | |
| **DIFFICULTY:** Difficult | **WHEELCHAIR ACCESS:** No |
| **SCENERY:** Open and wooded hill country, canyon | **MAPS:** tinyurl.com/government canyonmap |
| **EXPOSURE:** Partly open | **FACILITIES:** Restrooms, water, picnicking, visitor center at trailhead |
| **TRAFFIC:** Semibusy on nice days | |
| **TRAIL SURFACE:** Natural surfaces | **CONTACT INFORMATION:** 210-688-9055; tpwd.texas.gov/state-parks/government-canyon |
| **HIKING TIME:** 3–4 hours | |
| **DRIVING DISTANCE:** 25 miles from the Alamo | |

canyon and get your heart pumping as you climb above 1,300 feet. Rocky openings provide broad outlooks where you can see near and far. The views include downtown San Antonio and keep coming on your descent. The last portion straddles the margin between the hills and the level savanna area. The trail is open to bikers as well as hikers and is increasingly popular with runners.

Unless you are a Hill Country veteran, I recommend taking a few minutes to browse the exhibits outside the well-designed visitor center. Here you will learn interesting facts about the terrain you will be traveling and the flora and fauna you might see on the way. This knowledge will attune your eyes to the natural beauty around you. One thing to know about these crumpled hills is that they are what is known as a karst landscape. The pitted rock that is such a feature of the Balcones Escarpment is caused by a reaction between the stone and water. This reaction continues underground to create the caves and channels of the Edwards Aquifer, from which San Antonio gets its water. Although the stream and washes aboveground only flow occasionally, beneath you is a vast yet finite reservoir.

Make your way from the visitor center across Government Canyon itself to the backcountry trailhead, and head north on the Joe Johnston Route. As usual with old roadbeds, the hiking is easy but exposed for this first section. Cedars line the trail. Pass the junction with the Recharge Trail, and after 0.3 mile dip down to cross the lush, buzzing Government Canyon wash, where you will notice a wealth of hardwood trees, including persimmon, Mexican buckeye, and mountain laurel.

Cross a feeder branch at 0.7 mile, looking left for buildings that used to be the Wildcat Canyon Ranch. Bobcats and coyotes now patrol what once was cattle country. Ascend to reach a clearing and the singletrack Wildcat Canyon Trail. This is the 1-mile point. Turn right, cross Government Canyon—wider at the intersection with the side valley—and enter Wildcat Canyon. Hills flank the track, and live oaks, junipers, and scattered grasses border the trail. At 1.3 miles the path comes alongside the rocky wash at a confluence of drainages. Red oaks grow here among the juniper. The human world feels

## Chula Vista Loop

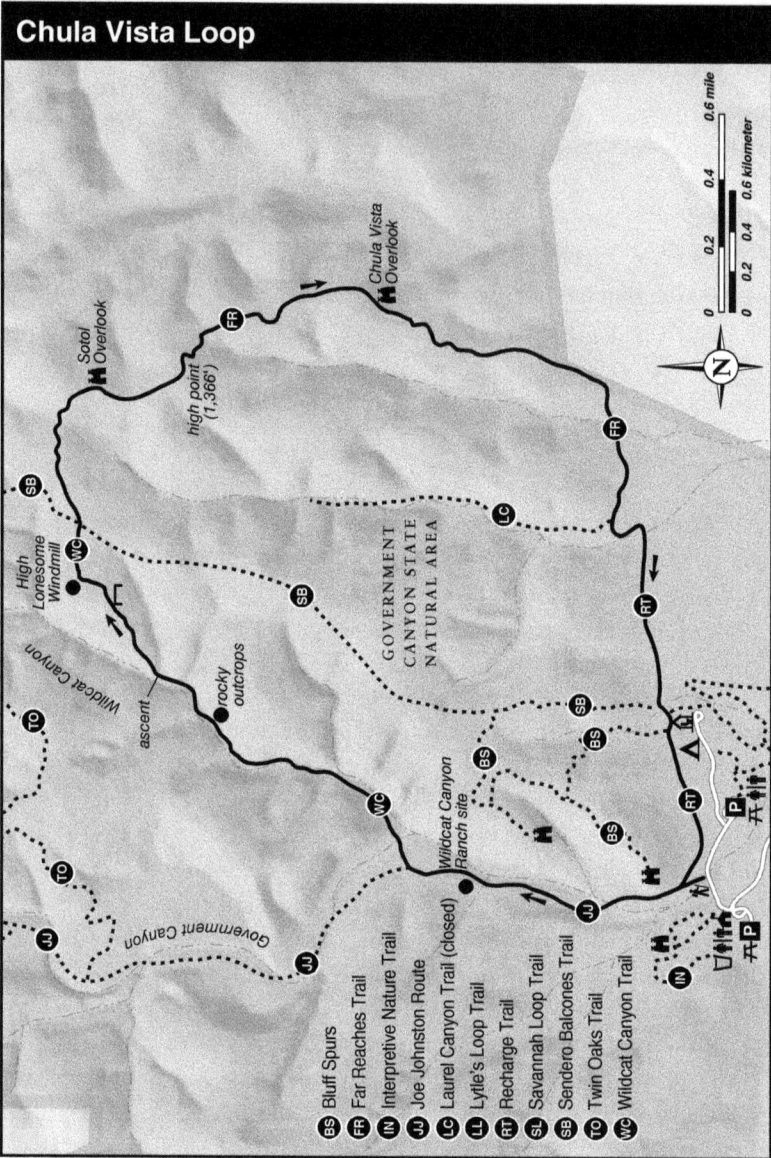

0.6 mile
0.4
0.2
0
0.6 kilometer
0.4
0.2
0

N

Chula Vista Overlook

Sotol Overlook

high point (1,366')

FR

FR

SB

WC

SB

LC

GOVERNMENT STATE CANYON NATURAL AREA

RT

SB

BS

BS

RT

High Lonesome Windmill

rocky outcrops

ascent

Wildcat Canyon

WC

Wildcat Canyon Ranch site

BS

JJ

TO

TO

JJ

Government Canyon

JJ

IN

BS Bluff Spurs
FR Far Reaches Trail
IN Interpretive Nature Trail
JJ Joe Johnston Route
LC Laurel Canyon Trail (closed)
LL Lytle's Loop Trail
RT Recharge Trail
SL Savannah Loop Trail
SB Sendero Balcones Trail
TO Twin Oaks Trail
WC Wildcat Canyon Trail

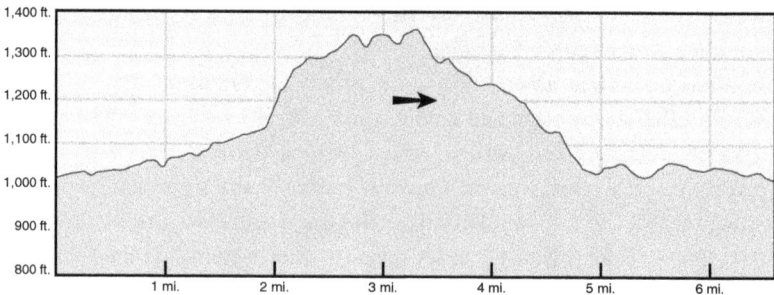

1,400 ft.
1,300 ft.
1,200 ft.
1,100 ft.
1,000 ft.
900 ft.
800 ft.

1 mi.     2 mi.     3 mi.     4 mi.     5 mi.     6 mi.

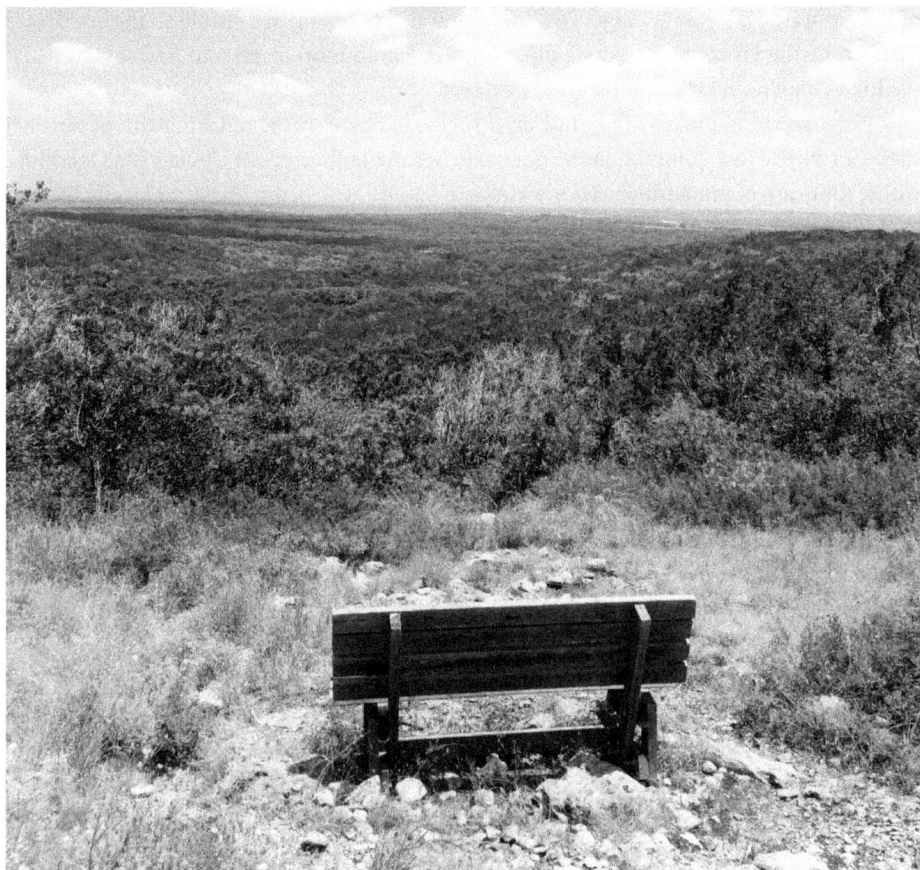

*A bench on the Chula Vista Loop offers a chance to take in the view.*

distant in the vibrant silence. The path continues up a gentle ascent in the intermittent shade of a thousand trunks and a million leaves, occasionally crossing a braid of washes on the way.

At 2 miles the trail turns away from the canyon bottom to climb a steep flank over a series of *balcones.* The drier environment is reflected in the size and diversity of the trees. The path levels out after a quarter of a mile or so, where a bench will let you catch your breath. Reach the aptly named High Lonesome Windmill at 2.3 miles. The blades are gone from the windmill, and the structure is now used as a park antenna tower. Continue wandering through a mix of grass and rock glens interspersed with evergreen patches.

Intersect the Sendero Balcones Trail at 2.5 miles. Tired hikers can shortcut the loop by heading south here. The main hike keeps forward, joining the Far Reaches Trail. Mexican buckeye, mountain laurel, and other shrubs proliferate among the grass and cedar as the trail climbs around the head of Laurel Canyon. Meet the spur trail leading left to Sotol Overlook at 3 miles. Sotols do indeed thrive around a bench that offers panoramic views of the natural area's vast acreage. Distant hills and civilization are visible to the south and east. Leave the vista point, cross a dip, and then climb more karst and *balcones* to reach the hike's high point at 3.3 miles and 1,366 feet.

Keep working mostly downhill on a rocky, exposed path, relishing the occasional shade. Primroses are common in the open patches. At 4 miles, reach Chula Vista Overlook, where there are commanding easterly views of San Antonio from the strategically located bench. From here, the stony path yo-yos down the grade to reach the flatlands at 4.8 miles. Turn right, west, traveling the fault line where water enters the Edwards Aquifer.

To your left, the savanna is under restoration to something approaching the bounty the first Europeans beheld. The grasslands that once stretched across Central Texas were what originally attracted settlers, who saw in the wavy meadows and prairies nourishment for their livestock. Sam Houston reported about Texas to Andrew Jackson: "I have no hesitancy in pronouncing it the finest country to its extent on the globe . . . there can be no doubt but the country east of the Rio Grande would sustain a population of ten million souls." Texas has more than doubled that. However, with the settling of the land came overgrazing, fencing, and fire suppression, which in the end altered the ecosystem from grassland to cedar and often to dirt and rock. The work the Texas Parks & Wildlife Department is doing here will protect the recharge zone and maintain habitat for the flora and fauna of the grasslands. Already the landscape is full of flourishing shrubs and bushes; this is one of the prettiest sections of the hike.

Bisect a dry wash at 4.9 miles, and shortly pass the end of the closed Laurel Canyon Trail. Curve south through woods, and meet the Recharge Trail at 5.4 miles, joining the westbound doubletrack. Intersect the Sendero Balcones Trail and then the Bluff Spurs Trail, reaching Joe Johnston Route at 6.5 miles to complete the loop. Backtrack to the trailhead.

## Nearby Activities

Government Canyon State Natural Area offers tent camping, picnic facilities, and guided hikes. Visit the Friends of Government Canyon website at friendsofgc.org for information about other events and volunteer opportunities.

---

**GPS TRAILHEAD COORDINATES**

**N29° 33' 0.7"  W98° 45' 45.4"**

From the intersection of Loop 1604 and Shaenfield Road, northwest of downtown San Antonio and south of Braun Road, take Shaenfield Road west 1.6 miles to a traffic light. Continue through the traffic light, where Shaenfield Road becomes Galm Road. Keep west on Galm Road, and follow it 1.9 miles to the park entrance at a traffic circle. Drive to the parking lot and visitor center, and park your car. Once you have your permit, walk past the visitor center and over a road bridge across Government Canyon to find the backcountry trailhead.

# 38 Comanche Lookout Loop

## In Brief

This hike travels up and around a historic hill in northeast San Antonio. A paved trail ascends to a medieval-looking tower and an overlook with stupendous views of the city.

## Description

This cedar-covered hill on the edge of northeast San Antonio has a long history. At 1,034 feet, it's the fourth-highest peak in Bexar County and overlooks the Cibolo Creek watershed. Apaches and Comanches scouted for game from this point, which later became a prominent landmark for travelers. The section of El Camino Real that led to Bastrop passed along what is now the busy thoroughfare of Nacogdoches Road. Once owned by Republic of Texas President Mirabeau Lamar, the hill in 1923 ended up in the hands of Colonel Edward H. Coppock, a fanciful man who built a compound on the hill. He intended the tower to be part of a castle that was never finished. Developers acquired the property after his death and tore down the compound but left the tower. The property was traded several times during the 1970s and '80s, but the bust meant that nothing was ever built, and in 1994 the land was saved from bulldozers by the efforts of a private group and transferred to the city for parkland.

The hike leaves the trailhead and follows a paved path up to the lookout, where you can inspect the four-story tower. From here, circle down and around the hill for a rewarding and invigorating hike. If the distance is too short for you, add the Library Loop to your hike. Benches appear at regular intervals along the route.

The concrete Comanche Loop leaves the trailhead and begins a rise through thick juniper laced with mesquite. A path soon leaves to the left. This is your return route. Keep following the trail uphill on asphalt. At 0.2 mile come to an X-junction. Keep forward on the asphalt path to take the Tower Loop. This path becomes concrete, goes around a circle, and passes by the old tower, now fenced in.

Keep along the ridgeline heading south. Live oaks are dotted across the summit, with picnic tables under their shade. A clearing at the south tip of the hilltop affords an excellent and far-reaching vista of greater San Antonio. Walk back along a concrete path, passing the lookout a second time.

Go right on the south section of the Tower Loop that zigzags downhill, returning to the X-junction. Keep straight again, taking a gravel trail that follows the shady downgrade, shortly passing Fox Run Elementary School on your right. Ignore two spur trails coming in from the left, and at 1.1 miles turn right onto Deer Loop, heading toward Rocky Creek Road and the edge of the park. Deer Loop passes through open grassland along the street before curving back into the low-lying but dense cedar and mesquite forest.

| | |
|---|---|
| **LENGTH:** 1.7 miles | **ACCESS:** Daily, 5 a.m.–11 p.m.; free |
| **CONFIGURATION:** Loop | **WHEELCHAIR ACCESS:** Yes, on paved part of hike |
| **DIFFICULTY:** Moderate | |
| **SCENERY:** Cedar forest, views | **MAPS:** tinyurl.com/comanche lookoutmap |
| **EXPOSURE:** Mostly open | |
| **TRAFFIC:** Moderate–busy on weekends | **FACILITIES:** Water fountain near tower, restroom at trailhead |
| **TRAIL SURFACE:** Asphalt, gravel, concrete | **CONTACT INFORMATION:** 210-207-7275; tinyurl.com/comanchelookout |
| **HIKING TIME:** 1.3 hours | |
| **DRIVING DISTANCE:** 16 miles from the Alamo | |

Keep forward at 1.4 miles, where Deer Loop comes back to Comanche Loop, and pass both ends of the Library Loop in quick succession at 1.5 miles. Keep curving around the hill through thick cedar. All too soon the path intersects the outward route close to the trailhead to complete the loop. Walk the few steps downhill back to the parking area.

## Nearby Activities

McAllister Park, 7 miles away, has more hiking and biking, a dog park, picnic tables, playgrounds, and athletic fields.

### GPS TRAILHEAD COORDINATES

**N29° 34' 57.5"  W98° 22' 0.3"**

From Exit 172 on I-35 north of San Antonio, take Loop 1604 west 1.9 miles to Farm to Market Road 2252, Nacogdoches Road. Head west on Nacogdoches Road toward San Antonio 1 mile. The trailhead at Comanche Lookout Park will be on your right.

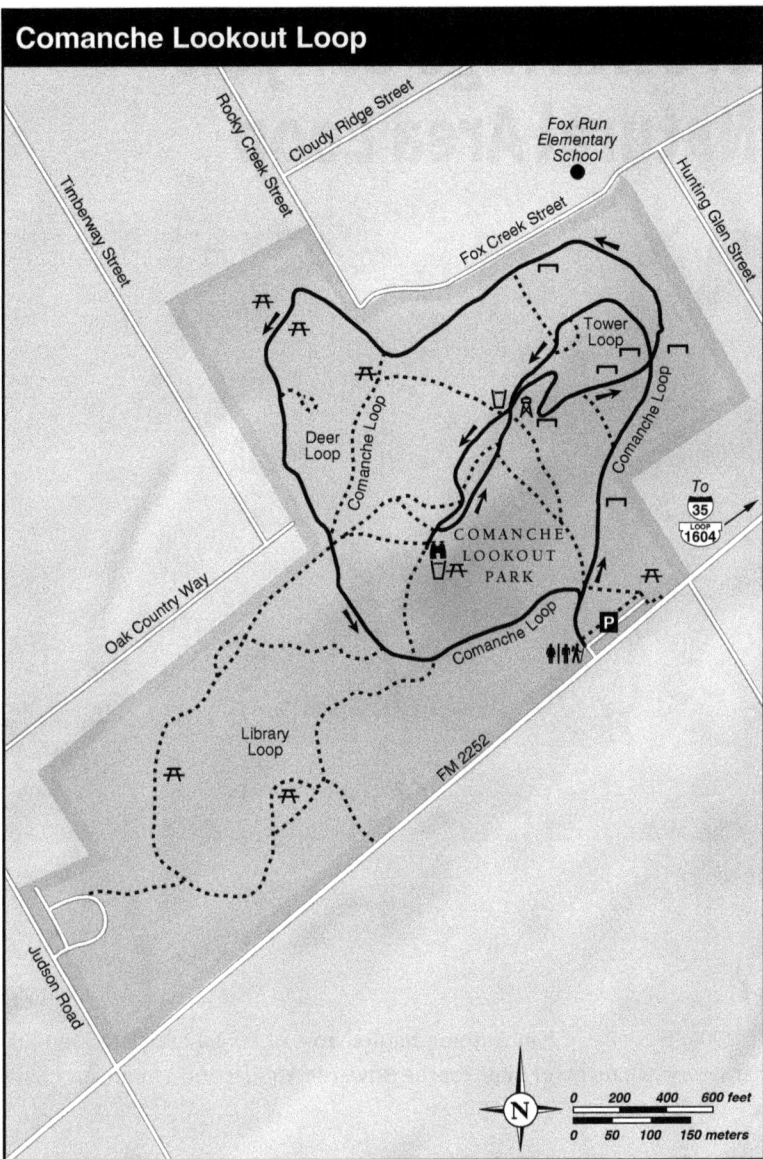

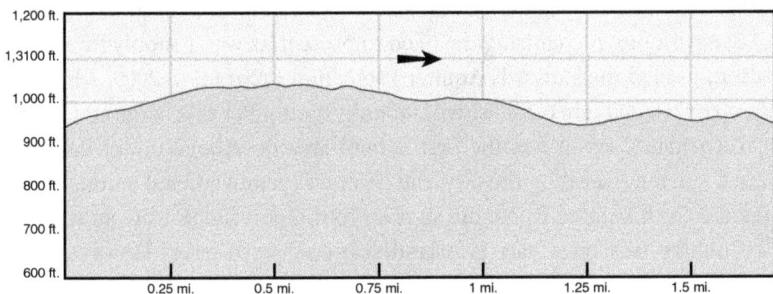

# 39 Crownridge Canyon Natural Area Loop

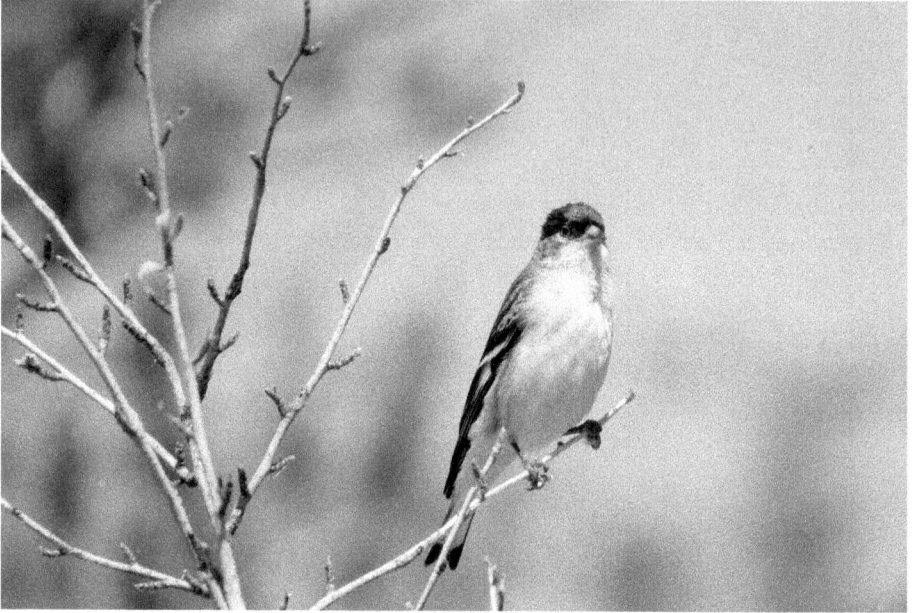

*Lesser goldfinch*

## In Brief

Opened in 2006, this city of San Antonio natural area offers an excellent loop hike in a canyon that serves as a recharge zone for the Edwards Aquifer and a home for native flora and fauna.

## Description

The city of San Antonio, recognizing the need to protect its water supply for an expanding population, funded the Edwards Aquifer Protection Program in 2000, which funded the acquisition of 250,000 acres of sensitive land over the aquifer's recharge zone. Formerly a dump, Crownridge Canyon was the first natural area developed under the program. After the land was purchased by the city, the trash was removed, and an ongoing effort began to restore the habitat to its condition prior to the arrival of European settlers. The Texas Hill Country was once vast grassland scattered with trees. However, fire was

| | |
|---|---|
| **LENGTH:** 1.9 miles | **ACCESS:** Daily (except Christmas Eve, Christmas Day, and New Year's Day), 7:30 a.m.–sunset; free; no pets allowed |
| **CONFIGURATION:** Loop | |
| **DIFFICULTY:** Easy | |
| **SCENERY:** Open and wooded hills | **WHEELCHAIR ACCESS:** Yes, on lower loop |
| **EXPOSURE:** Partly open | |
| **TRAFFIC:** Busy on nice days | **MAPS:** tinyurl.com/crownridgecanyon map |
| **TRAIL SURFACE:** Compressed gravel, natural surfaces | |
| **HIKING TIME:** 1.3 hours | **FACILITIES:** Restrooms, water, picnicking at trailhead |
| **DRIVING DISTANCE:** 19 miles from the Alamo | **CONTACT INFORMATION:** 210-207-7275; tinyurl.com/crownridgepark |

suppressed as settlements grew, allowing the oaks and junipers to take over. Fire, tree removal, and native plant restoration are being used in concert at Crownridge Canyon to restore the land to what it once was.

For hikers, the preserve provides a delightful stroll through various habitats: deciduous woodland, the rehabilitated savanna, and drier cedar-covered canyon slopes. The park's trail system consists of two interconnected loops. Red Oak Trail is the lower loop. The hard-packed surface allows wheelchair access for its entire length. Bear Grass Trail is a natural-surface upper loop that offers hikers a deeper look into the canyon. During wetter times, visitors can enjoy Bear Grass Falls, a cascade that drops over a stone lip into a rocky pool. No traffic other than pedestrian is allowed in the preserve.

At the entrance pavilion, a covered interpretive area explains the importance of places such as Crownridge Canyon and describes the flora and fauna you might see here. Take a moment to appreciate a mosaic, the work of artist Oscar Alvarado, that demonstrates graphically the movement of water from clouds to river.

Walk just a short distance, and come to an information booth, marking the start of the hike. Go left, switchbacking up the canyon's west side on an asphalt path. Cedars and oaks provide shade for some of the trail, occasionally making a tunnel of branches. The park is grassier than most because of the ongoing savanna restoration. Contemplation benches are scattered along the trails. At points, views of the Texas Hill Country open up, with houses at the uppermost reaches of the canyon. Persimmon and mountain laurel grow among the cedar. Continue up the trail, at 0.5 mile reaching Red Oak Canyon Bridge, a metal structure over a small but dramatic canyon that no doubt would become a raging torrent after a storm.

The surface turns to gravel after the bridge. The trail ascends with the canyon to your right and sotol all around to the junction with the Bear Grass Trail into the upper canyon, which you will reach at 0.7 mile. Take the narrower natural-surface trail straight; Red Oak Trail leads right to make a shorter loop.

Enter the upper canyon, going down steps into a drainage, and then ascend under a tight tree canopy on a stony path. The hike reaches its high point of 1,285 feet at 0.9 mile,

## Crownridge Canyon Natural Area Loop

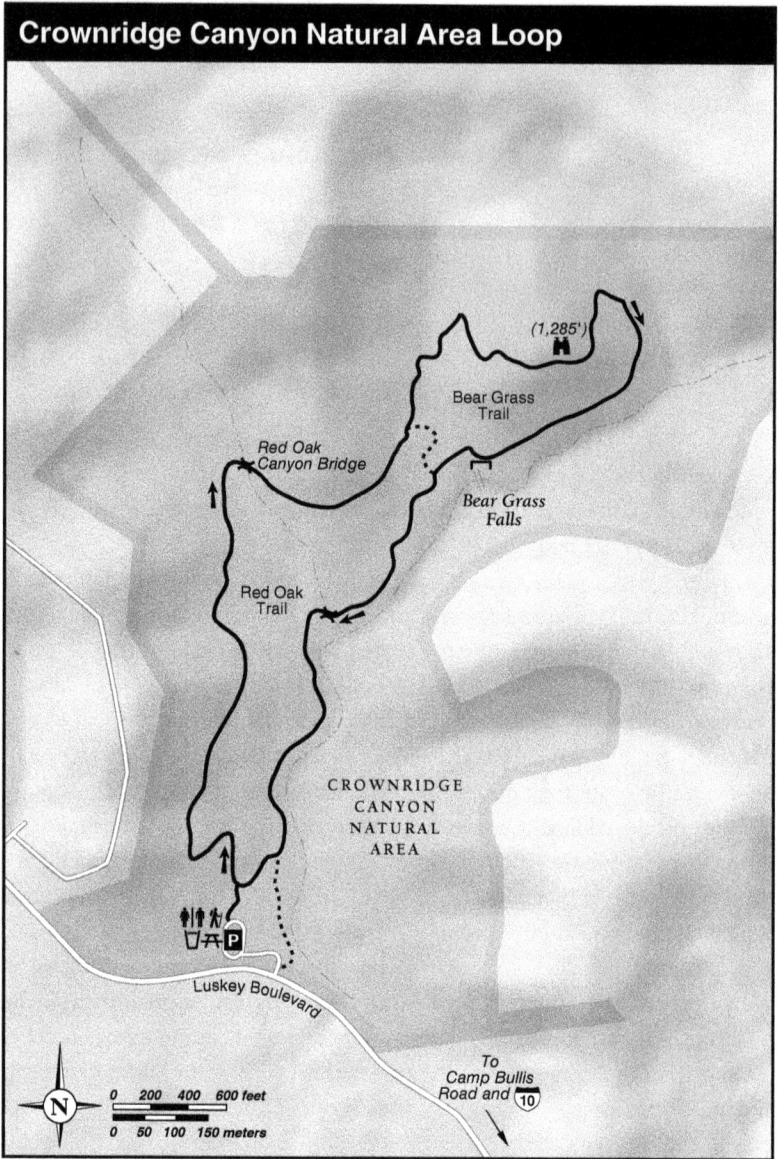

(1,285')

Bear Grass
Trail

Red Oak
Canyon Bridge

Bear Grass
Falls

Red Oak
Trail

CROWNRIDGE
CANYON
NATURAL
AREA

P

Luskey Boulevard

0  200  400  600 feet

0  50  100  150 meters

N

To
Camp Bullis
Road and 10

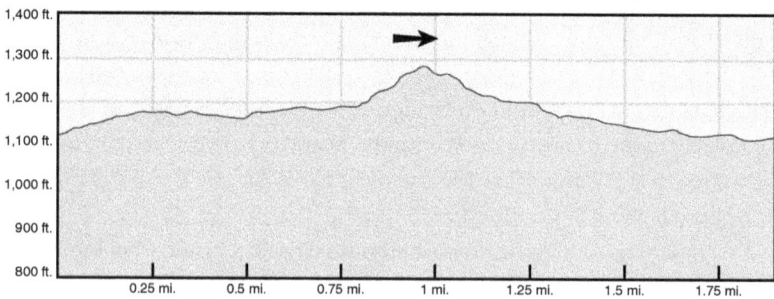

and there are views of the canyon and the expensive-looking houses along the opposite ridge. Sotol grows on open areas on the higher ground. At 1.1 miles the path turns right to begin the return to the valley floor. Enjoy the rugged trek as it cuts down the canyon amid buckeye and oaks.

A bench overlooks Bear Grass Falls at 1.3 miles, where a lip of stone protrudes over a pool some 40 feet below. The wild canyon is a riot of vegetation. If water is running, you will have to ford the stream above the lip. The trail widens and joins Red Oak Trail beyond Bear Grass Falls. Meander along the smooth path with the canyon bottom to your left and scattered grasslands to your right. Savanna restoration is taking place everywhere here, as well as the replanting of elm, walnut, and cherry trees and native grasses. Signs explain the work. Restoring the ecosystem to its natural state strengthens the habitat for native fauna, which depend on native plants and their fruits for food. At 1.6 miles cross Red Oak Canyon again, and continue drifting through a mosaic of grass and groves of trees before completing the hike at 1.9 miles.

## Nearby Activities

Friedrich Wilderness Park (page 186) and Government Canyon State Natural Area (page 191) offer longer hikes over similar terrain.

---

### GPS TRAILHEAD COORDINATES

**N29° 36' 59.9"  W98° 37' 49.9"**

Take I-10 west toward El Paso to Exit 554, Camp Bullis Road. Turn left on Camp Bullis Road, passing under the interstate, heading west. At 1.6 miles, turn right on Luskey Boulevard. It is a quick right onto a downhill before a bridge. Follow Luskey Boulevard 0.4 mile; then turn right into Crownridge Canyon Natural Area.

# 40 Friedrich Wilderness Park Loop

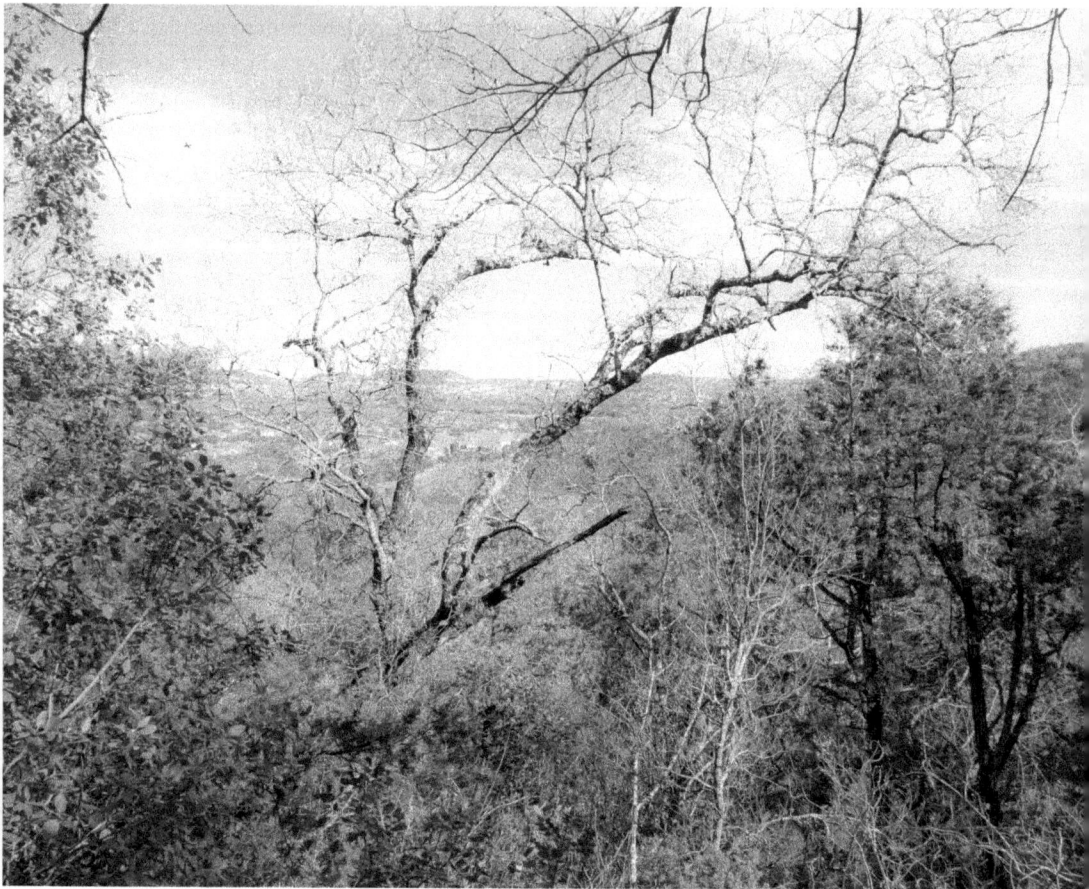

*Thick woods and steep canyons at Friedrich Wilderness Park*

## In Brief

The city of Leon Valley has expanded around Friedrich Wilderness Park, the setting for this loop, and the well-tended preserve gets heavy use, especially on weekends. Who wouldn't want to get their exercise in such a pristine slice of Hill Country? For hikers, this first-rate trek delivers steep climbs to high outcrops, varied environments, and an abundance of Central Texas plant life.

| | |
|---|---|
| **LENGTH:** 5.2 miles | **DRIVING DISTANCE:** 20 miles from the Alamo |
| **CONFIGURATION:** Loop | |
| **DIFFICULTY:** Difficult | **ACCESS:** Daily (except Christmas Day and New Year's Day), 7:30 a.m.–sunset; no fees or permits required |
| **SCENERY:** Thick hardwoods, limestone hills, restored savanna | |
| **EXPOSURE:** Shady–exposed | **WHEELCHAIR ACCESS:** Yes, for the first section |
| **TRAFFIC:** Moderate–heavy | **MAPS:** tinyurl.com/friedrichmap |
| **TRAIL SURFACE:** Concrete, dirt, roots, rock | **FACILITIES:** Restrooms |
| **HIKING TIME:** 2.5 hours | **CONTACT INFORMATION:** 210-207-8480; tinyurl.com/friedrichpark |

## Description

San Antonians have taken to the Friedrich Wilderness Park, enthusiastically using the preserve's nearly 6 miles of trails for running and walking, as well as hiking. We can imagine that Norma Friedrich Ward, who bequeathed the park's original 180 acres to the city in memory of her parents, would be happy to see the land both enjoyed and in good health. The preserve is a delicate ecosystem, and the rules require that it be treated as such. No pets or bicycles are allowed, and fires and smoking are also prohibited. As in all San Antonio city parks, the trails are rated for ADA accessibility from Level 1 (easy paved trails) to Level 4 (challenging paths for hikers only).

The park has expanded to 600 acres, and this hike takes in nearly all of that. The trek passes through backcountry, where land that was at one time to be a golf course is being restored. On the way out and back, you will journey up and down very steep slopes and visit thickly wooded canyons. Sparrows, cardinals, spotted towhees, and killdeers are common in the park. Check the kiosk at the trailhead for information about the park and a map of the trails, which are well signed and easy to follow.

Step into the woods, and head west on the concrete Entry Trail, rated Level 1. At the intersection with the Forest Range Trail, keep right to stay on the Entry Trail. The shade from the trees helps make this hike more bearable on a hot day. Frequent benches punctuate the beginning legs of the trail. Live oaks surround you but soon give way to juniper. Stay on the Entry Trail; the Forest Range Trail takes off to the right. Cross a wooden bridge, and reach a T-junction at 0.3 mile, where you turn left, starting the loop portion of the hike on the Main Loop, rated Level 3, a gravel path. Pass the junction of the Water Trail, a short but rugged detour to the right, which comes back to the Main Loop just before the Juniper Barrens Trail leaves to the left. Continue on the Main Loop, now rated Level 4, which climbs an increasingly shady but ever steeper flank to reach the hike's second-highest point at 0.9 mile.

This point is also the junction with the Vista Loop Trail. Turn left onto this rockier track, staying on the ridgeline, and shortly come to the Restoration Way Trail (part of the

# Friedrich Wilderness Park Loop

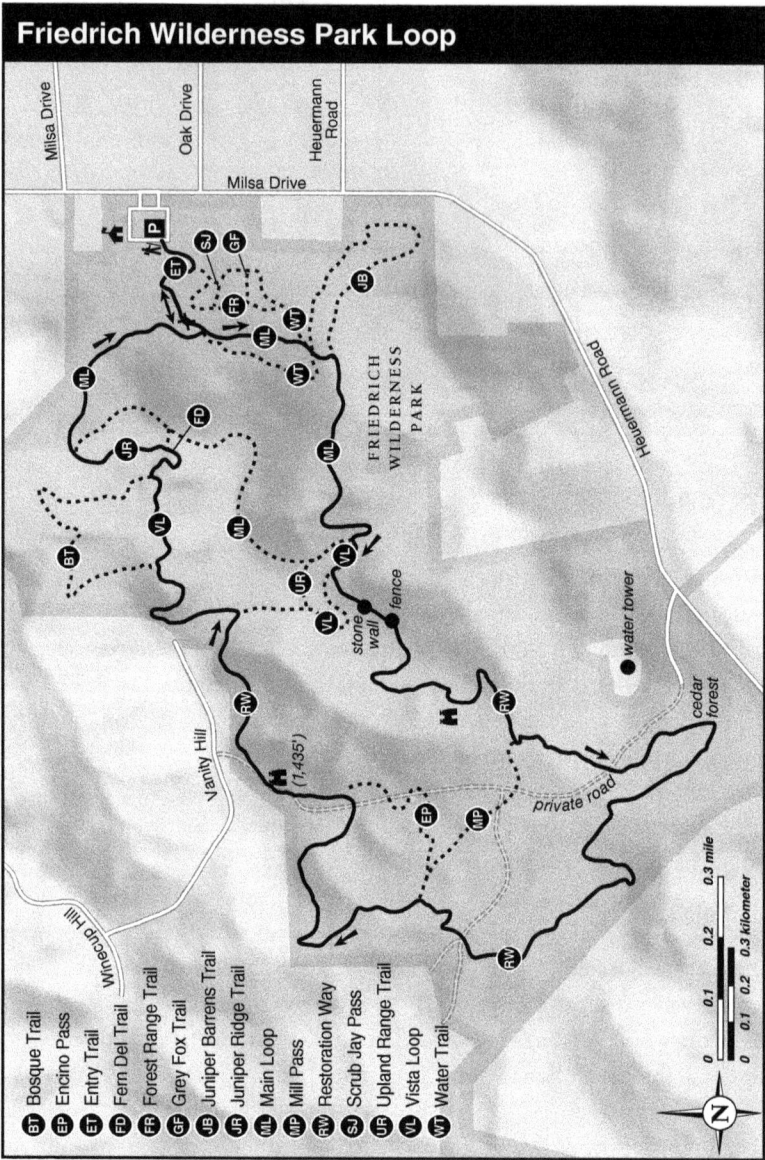

Milsa Drive · Oak Drive · Heuermann Road · Milsa Drive · Heuermann Road

FRIEDRICH WILDERNESS PARK

stone wall · fence · water tower · cedar forest · private road · Vanity Hill · (1,435') · Winecup Hill

0.3 mile · 0.3 kilometer · 0.2 · 0.1 · 0

**BT** Bosque Trail
**EP** Encino Pass
**ET** Entry Trail
**FD** Fern Del Trail
**FR** Forest Range Trail
**GF** Grey Fox Trail
**JB** Juniper Barrens Trail
**JR** Juniper Ridge Trail
**ML** Main Loop
**MP** Mill Pass
**RW** Restoration Way
**SJ** Scrub Jay Pass
**UR** Upland Range Trail
**VL** Vista Loop
**WT** Water Trail

N

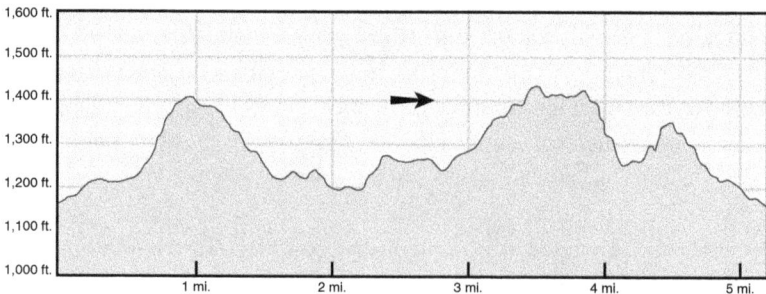

1,600 ft. · 1,500 ft. · 1,400 ft. · 1,300 ft. · 1,200 ft. · 1,100 ft. · 1,000 ft.

1 mi. · 2 mi. · 3 mi. · 4 mi. · 5 mi.

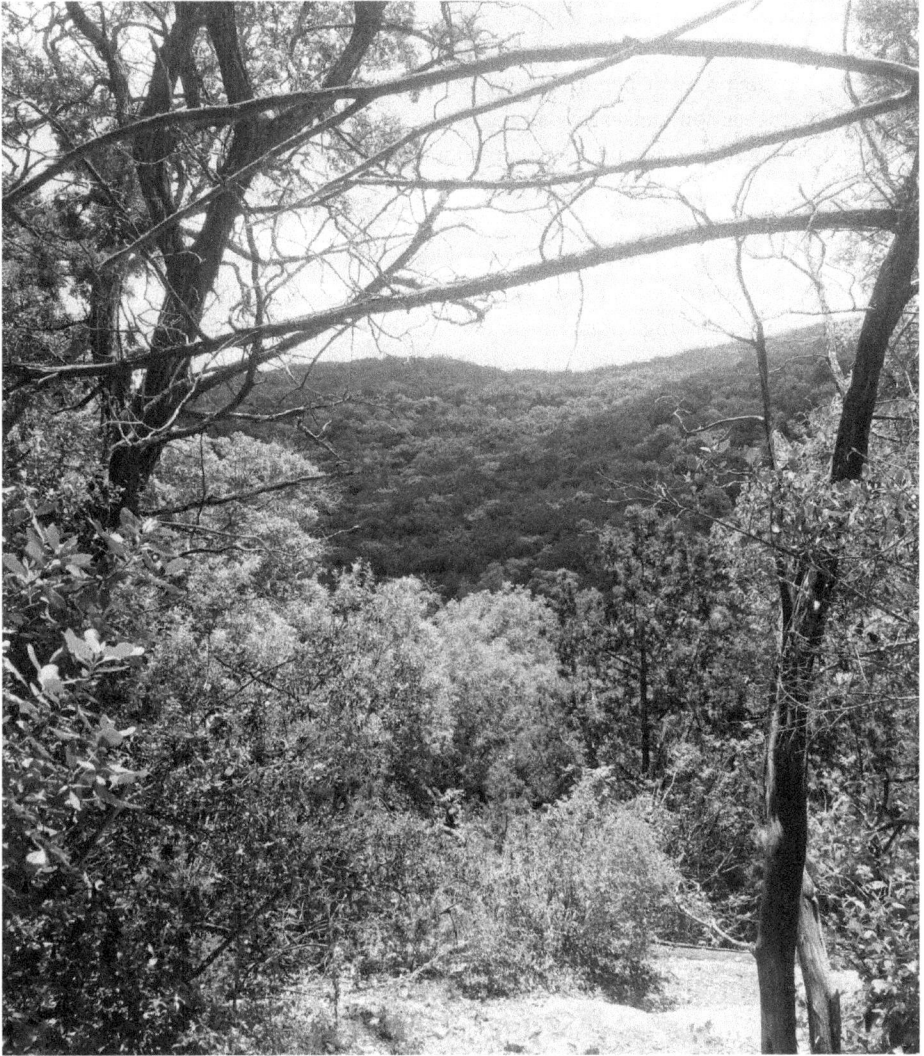

*Views abound at Friedrich Wilderness Park.*

Main Loop). Turn left here also, beginning the long and winding back portion of the hike, which wanders through the broken savanna in the western end of the park. Go through a gap in a stone wall, and views of the park's greenery and beyond—houses, a television mast, a large water tower—start to open up. Mountain laurel bushes proliferate on the heights. Pass through a metal fence several times as you descend into the valley in front of you through red oak and cedar.

At 1.6 miles turn left to stay on the Restoration Way Trail. To the right is the Mill Pass Trail, a shorter cutoff that passes an old windmill. Soon after this junction, the path moves suddenly into more-open areas. You can see around you that large tracts of the preserve have been cleared as part of an effort to restore the savanna to something approaching the original landscape of grasses and shrubs as habitat for wildlife. At 1.9 miles, there is a sharp right turn as you begin to head generally north. The route, which is mostly exposed on this section, makes its way across open meadow and through coppices, crossing an old road and a dry wash twice on the journey. The windmill remains visible across the valley.

A steep climb across a cleared area takes you to an intermediate peak at 2.4 miles, where sotol plants congregate among the scrubby trees. Drier cedar woods shade you here. At 2.8 miles the path comes to the other end of the Mill Pass Trail. Turn left, and begin the long ascent to the trek's high point. Eventually the track crosses the road again, and shortly the Encino Pass Trail leaves right, at 3.4 miles. Pick up the roadbed, and at 3.5 miles you arrive at 1,435 feet, the top of this hike, though there are no vistas from this spot.

Views do come soon, though. The next half mile of hiking features panoramas and a close-to-vertical descent. The trail passes through another section of chain-link fence and goes along a rocky and exposed outcrop, from which there are vistas to the south over a leafy canyon. Dip back into the woods to return to the Vista Loop at a T-junction. Turn left here, and begin the descent on a stony path alongside a rock wall. Shortly the path begins to go down the rock face at a dizzying grade. There's the occasional glimpse across the park as you make your way down into the heavily wooded canyon. The Bosque Trail leaves left at 4.1 miles, close to the bottom. You must climb up again to meet the Fern Del Trail. Turn right here, and make yet another ascent that, although short, is as steep as the descent you just made. This will bring you to the Juniper Ridge Trail. Turn left, and make your way along the summit line of the eponymous juniper-covered ridge.

Meet the Main Loop at 4.5 miles. Take the left fork, and go mostly downhill from this point. You'll be able to hear the traffic on I-10 again. The trail turns to cement as you approach the end. At 4.9 miles turn left onto the Entry Trail, and come back to the trailhead and parking lot.

## Nearby Activities

Government Canyon State Natural Area (page 191) and Crownridge Canyon Natural Area (page 182) offer similar hiking nearby.

---

**GPS TRAILHEAD COORDINATES**
**N29° 38' 26.4"  W98° 37' 33.7"**

Take I-10 west from San Antonio, and then take Exit 552 for Dominion Drive/ Raymond Russell Park. Stay on the access road 1.4 miles, and turn left at the TURNAROUND sign to head south on the access road. After 0.3 mile turn right on Oak Drive, just past North Park Volkswagen. Turn right on Milsa Drive at the T-junction, and the park is on your left. On weekend mornings, it is likely you will have to park on the street.

# 41 Government Canyon Loop

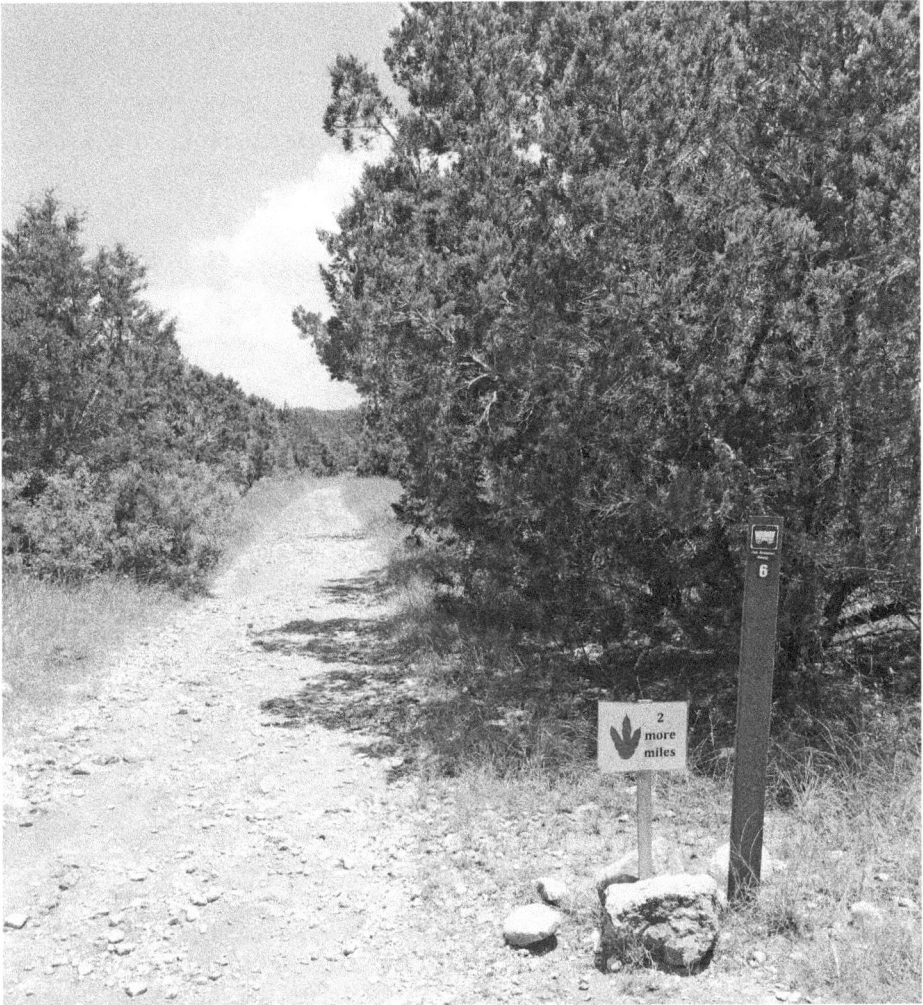

*The "government" road along Government Canyon*

## In Brief

This hike follows Government Canyon in the state natural area that bears its name to an overlook and old ranch house. Nearby are springs and dinosaur tracks. On the return journey, wander through a grove of live oaks hung with Spanish moss that was home to early inhabitants of the land.

| | |
|---|---|
| **LENGTH:** 6.2 miles | **ACCESS:** Friday–Monday, 7 a.m.–10 p.m.; $6 per person over age 13 |
| **CONFIGURATION:** Balloon loop | |
| **DIFFICULTY:** Moderate | **WHEELCHAIR ACCESS:** No |
| **SCENERY:** Wooded canyon, cedar uplands, springs, and bluffs | **MAPS:** tinyurl.com/government canyonmap |
| **EXPOSURE:** Partly open | **FACILITIES:** Restrooms, water, picnicking, visitor center at trailhead |
| **TRAFFIC:** Busy on nice days | |
| **TRAIL SURFACE:** Natural surfaces | **CONTACT INFORMATION:** 210-688-9055; tpwd.texas.gov/state-parks/ government-canyon |
| **HIKING TIME:** 3.5 hours | |
| **DRIVING DISTANCE:** 25 miles from the Alamo | |

## Description

This large swath of Hill Country was set aside to protect a critical recharge zone for the Edwards Aquifer, from which San Antonio gets its water. The preserve is also home to numerous species of plants and wildlife that thrive only among the crumpled limestone canyons and juniper- and oak-covered hills of the Balcones Escarpment. Finally, it allows San Antonians access to nature and the outdoors. Pets are not allowed in the backcountry. Most of this hike is open to bicyclists—it's a favorite of the city's off-road riders.

The route traces Government Canyon Creek, a rocky wash bordered by dense woods, grassy areas, and tall bluffs. On the loop portion, you will join a singletrack path as it climbs to an overlook from an overhanging cliff. The view extends up and down the canyon and into the Texas Hill Country beyond. The circuit winds around a side valley and comes to the Zizelmann House, a Texas-style stone dwelling situated near Government Canyon Springs. At the springs, there are tracks in the limestone left by a dinosaur at a time when the stone was mud. On your return trip, you'll visit the site of an aboriginal village whose inhabitants lived in a scenic live oak coppice with a magical coating of Spanish moss.

The trail up Government Canyon is called the Joe Johnston Route, after General Joseph E. Johnston, who surveyed the route when he was chief topographical engineer of the Department of Texas from 1848 to 1853. He became famous later as a Confederate general and survived the war to become friends with some of his Union counterparts. The road was known as "Old Joe Johnston Road," but locals referred to it as the government road, and the name was extended to the canyon itself.

Leave the parking area, and make your way to the well-designed visitor center, where you'll find interesting interpretive information and helpful staff. Take a moment to read the displays, as there is much information to enhance your hiking adventure. Head right, and join an artificial-surface path that soon joins Klepper Way, which crosses Government Canyon. The trailhead is immediately on the left after the bridge. Step onto the Joe Johnston Route, a northbound doubletrack wide enough for service vehicles. The

# Government Canyon Loop

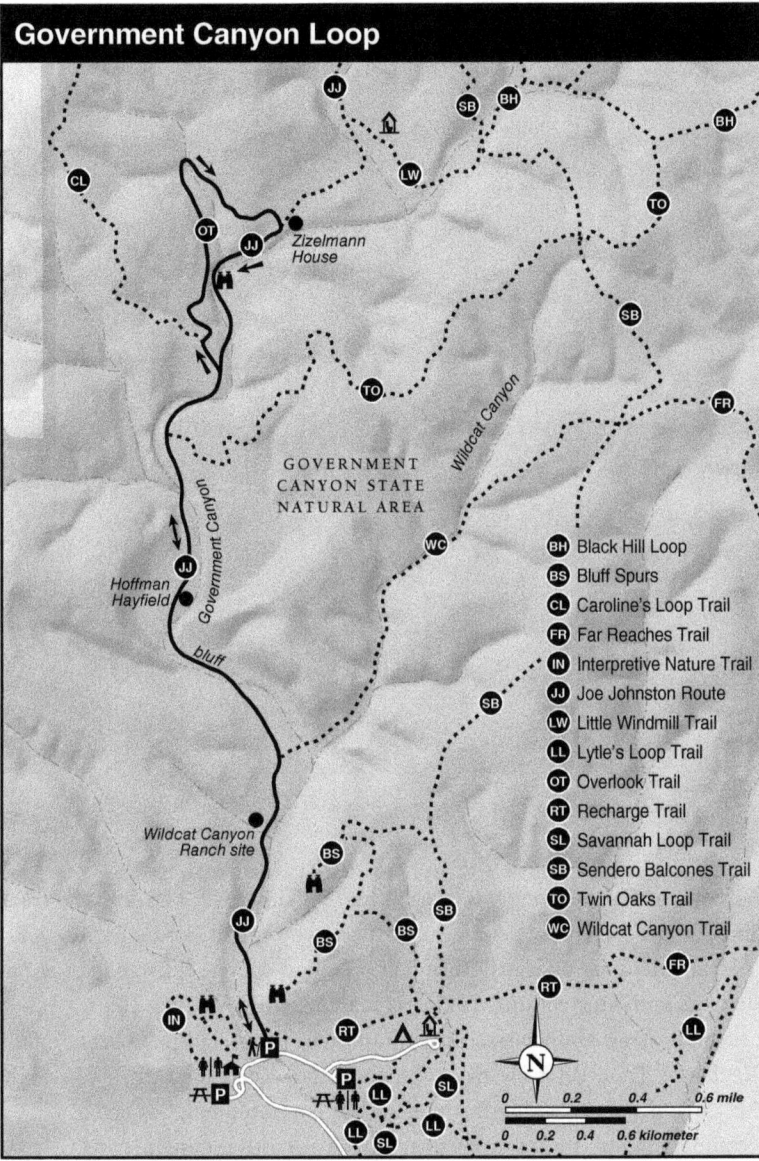

Zizelmann House

GOVERNMENT CANYON STATE NATURAL AREA

Wildcat Canyon

Government Canyon

bluff

Hoffman Hayfield

Wildcat Canyon Ranch site

BH Black Hill Loop
BS Bluff Spurs
CL Caroline's Loop Trail
FR Far Reaches Trail
IN Interpretive Nature Trail
JJ Joe Johnston Route
LW Little Windmill Trail
LL Lytle's Loop Trail
OT Overlook Trail
RT Recharge Trail
SL Savannah Loop Trail
SB Sendero Balcones Trail
TO Twin Oaks Trail
WC Wildcat Canyon Trail

N

0     0.2     0.4     0.6 mile
0   0.2   0.4   0.6 kilometer

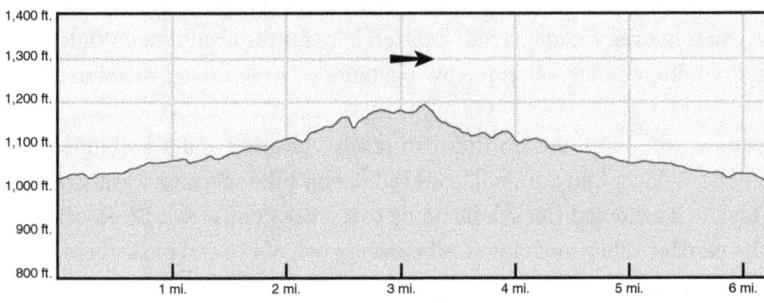

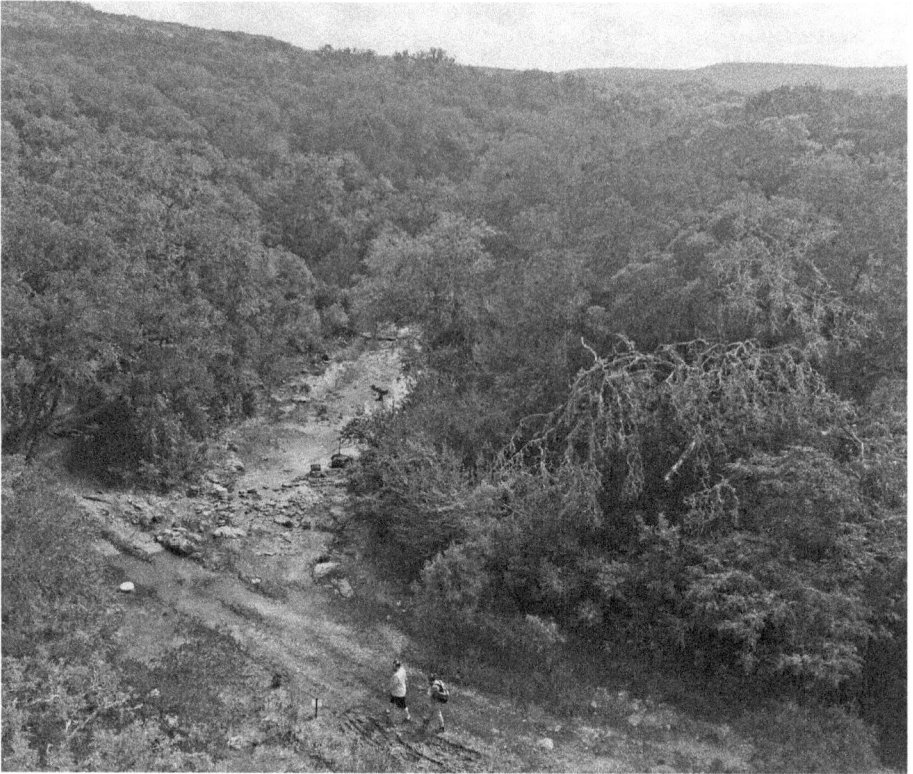

*Springs at Government Canyon State Natural Area*

first 2.2 miles of the hike are along this intermittently shady road. The dinosaur tracks are a recent find and perhaps draw people to the park who might not be regular hikers, as staff have placed encouraging signs every half mile that state the distance to the attraction. All the trails and intersections are clearly marked.

Walk through Ashe juniper laced with mountain laurel and persimmon, and soon pass the Recharge Trail, 0.1 mile from the trailhead. Keep forward, and at 0.3 mile traverse the canyon wash, passing through an impenetrable mass of cedar, elm, scrub oak, and mountain laurel. Intermittent streambeds cut into the main canyon across the historic road. The road is sometimes an easy-to-hike earth surface and sometimes rocky. At 0.7 mile you step over a feeder creek; look left here for the abandoned Wildcat Canyon Ranch buildings. Increasingly obscured by vegetation, the wood-and-metal structures are hard to pick out.

Continue up the Joe Johnston Route to reach a clearing and a trail junction at 0.8 mile, where the Wildcat Canyon Trail leads right. This hike keeps forward, crisscrossing the creek bed on a canopied track descending to a creek confluence. Steep canyon walls rise over the verdant valley to your left. The overgrown old Hoffman Hayfield lies below distant cliffs at 1.5 miles.

Gently rise to reach the Twin Oaks Trail at 2 miles; live oaks give way to cedar as you climb. Keep forward, crossing Government Canyon Creek yet again, and meet another junction at 2.3 miles. Here, Caroline's Loop and the Overlook Trail head left, while the Joe Johnston Route keeps forward. Stay left, and then split right with the hiker-only Overlook Trail at 2.4 miles. Climb over a scrabbly trail through scrubby cedar, sotol, and cactus, crossing small washes on the way to an open cliff top and the Canyon Overlook at 2.6 miles. Enjoy the view over Government Canyon, which should have water here at the springs and at the hilly wildlands beyond. No buildings are visible.

The surface changes from sandy to rocky as Overlook Trail falls into Government Canyon. Cross a few washes at the head of a feeder valley, and reach a flat meadow and a trail junction near the Zizelmann House at 3.4 miles. It is unclear if anyone ever lived in this sizable house, but the classic Central Texas stone ranch structure will hopefully be stabilized and open for exploration at some point. For now it's behind a fence.

From the Zizelmann House, turn right, heading southwest, back on the Joe Johnston Route. It isn't long before you enter a bower of live oak and Spanish moss, home to aboriginal Texans. A sign marks a midden while bemoaning past archaeological digging, apparently done with little care.

Come to the springs, situated at the bottom of the overlook, which is as stunning from this viewpoint as it was from the top. There are two sections of dinosaur tracks along the creek bed, both roped off to prevent damage. The main section is immediately upstream of the crossing, while another set is under the overhanging cliff to your right. They were made by an Acrocanthosaurus, a creature about the size of the better-known *Tyrannosaurus rex.*

Leaving the springs, cross Government Canyon Creek once more, and complete the loop portion of the hike at 3.9 miles. Backtrack 2.3 miles down the Joe Johnston Route to the trailhead.

## Nearby Activities

Government Canyon State Natural Area (page 191) offers drive-up tent and RV camping, backcountry camping, and picnic facilities. Visit friendsofgc.org for information about monthly hikes, other events, and volunteer opportunities.

### GPS TRAILHEAD COORDINATES
**N29° 33' 0.7"  W98° 45' 45.4"**

From the intersection of Loop 1604 and Shaenfield Road, northwest of downtown San Antonio and south of Braun Road, take Shaenfield Road west 1.6 miles to a traffic light. Continue through the traffic light, where Shaenfield Road becomes Galm Road. Keep west on Galm Road, and follow it 1.9 miles to the park entrance. Drive to the parking lot and visitor center, and park your car. Once you have your permit, walk past the visitor center and over a road bridge across Government Canyon to find the backcountry trailhead.

# 42 Hillview Natural Trail

## In Brief

This hike takes in the perimeter of Eisenhower Park in northwest San Antonio, a natural area that serves bikers, joggers, and hikers. Leashed pets can also enjoy this walk through Hill Country woodland. The goal is an observation tower with views of the city.

## Description

Northwest San Antonio is blessed with several wild places to run to on a weekend or after work, and Dwight C. Eisenhower Park is among them. Its special attraction is a wooden observation tower that was built by students from Churchill High School. From the tower, there are wide-ranging views of the Balcones Escarpment and the South Texas plains, whose boundary San Antonio has expanded to straddle.

The route heads west through sparse cedar, climbs over a ridgeline, and drops down before ascending to the tower. The return path makes a gentle descent back to the parking lot. The scenery is typical of the escarpment: cedar and rockier terrain on the exposed areas, with a greater variety of flora in cooler valleys. Camp Bullis, a military reservation, borders the park, so don't cross any fences. Watch for bicyclists as you hike. As with all the San Antonio city parks, the trail is well maintained and well signed.

The trailhead is at the north end of the parking lot, to the left of a large group picnic area. The Hillview Trail is both a short, accessible asphalt path and the longer hike that this entry describes, but they start out together on the paved surface. Go straight through the first junction, and then go right, stepping off the asphalt and onto the Hillview Natural Trail, rated Level 4 for accessibility, meaning that it is not suitable for wheelchairs. The hike follows this trail around the park. Immediately there is a climb up a little hill, and at 0.2 mile the trail turns left to head west, making its way around the back of the peak.

The surrounding hillside is typical of the terrain first encountered by settlers arriving in this area of Texas, and it looks deceptively fertile. However, the dense mesquite, hackberry, and cedar—as well as the thriving saw grass and yucca—hide the rocky soil, which is of little use for farming. The early settlers were forced into sheep and cattle ranching, as there is not much more this land will support.

Keep west on the trail to reach a junction just over 0.5 mile into the hike. The Shady Creek Trail to the left is a shortcut to the paved Cedar Flats Trail. Another branch of it will reconnect with this trail farther ahead. Stay on the path you're on, and stay right at a fork where the second Shady Creek junction joins the trail. The Hillview Natural Trail starts to climb the ridge that has dominated the view so far. It's a steep path with plenty of rocks and roots to step over, but it has the benefit of intermittent shade. Sotol and cactus

| | |
|---|---|
| **LENGTH:** 2.8 miles | **DRIVING DISTANCE:** 18 miles from the Alamo |
| **CONFIGURATION:** Loop | |
| **DIFFICULTY:** Moderate | **ACCESS:** Daily (except Christmas Eve, Christmas Day, and New Year's Day), 6 a.m.–sunset; no fees or permits required |
| **SCENERY:** Typical Hill Country woodland, wildlife, dog lovers | |
| **EXPOSURE:** Exposed | **WHEELCHAIR ACCESS:** For the first 0.2 mile of the route |
| **TRAFFIC:** Moderate | **MAPS:** tinyurl.com/eisenhowermap |
| **TRAIL SURFACE:** Cement, rock, asphalt, dirt | **FACILITIES:** Picnic tables, restrooms, water |
| **HIKING TIME:** 1.5 hours | **CONTACT INFORMATION:** 210-207-7275; tinyurl.com/eisenhowerparkinfo |

appear as you ascend. Ignore the spur trail that heads right at a sharp left turn, and reach the summit area, 1,330 feet high, at 0.7 mile. Wind around the cap of the peak, and then pick your way down a two-stage descent of the other side of the ridge, enjoying views over northwestern San Antonio as you go. The Yucca Natural Trail, a shorter route back to the parking lot, leaves right on this descent.

From the bottom of the valley, make another short climb, and come to a fork. You have hiked 1 mile. To the right, the Red Oak Trail adds half a mile to the hike, if you choose to take it. Go left on an exposed roadbed between wooded banks, and at 1.2 miles the Red Oak Trail returns from its adventure. The route climbs again over rock shelves, coming to a left turn at the top of the ascent. At 1.3 miles you join the asphalt Cedar Flats Trail near restrooms. Follow it as it bends right toward the observation tower. The trail circles the tower and two benches.

The Harmony Hills Optimist Club and students at Churchill High School built this wooden structure in 1984, and it shows minimal wear after all these years. Constructed of 4-inch beams, it looks like a climbing frame, and a staircase leads up two flights to the observation platform. The view from 1,290 feet takes in the rolling hills to the north and west, as well as San Antonio to the south and east. Loop 1604 and its traffic are visible 2 miles south of the park. Dust from a large quarry operation might be rising into the air.

When you are ready to move on, return down the Cedar Flats Trail to the junction with the Hillview Trail. If you wish, stay on the paved trail to go back downhill to the trailheads.

Our route follows the natural-surface Hillview Trail to the right, a longer route to the same destination that offers a chance to view more of the bird and animal life of the park.

Depending on the time of day, the chances of seeing white-tailed deer coming out of their hiding places are very good. Cottontail rabbits, roadrunners, and even wild hogs can also be seen among the yucca, mesquite, and prickly pear. Given the exposure and the better chance of seeing wildlife, I recommend making this hike in the early morning.

The Hillview Trail descends past sparse juniper. The Live Oak spur leaves to the left, connecting with the Cedar Flats Trail. The trail surface switches from rock to dirt at the

## Hillview Natural Trail

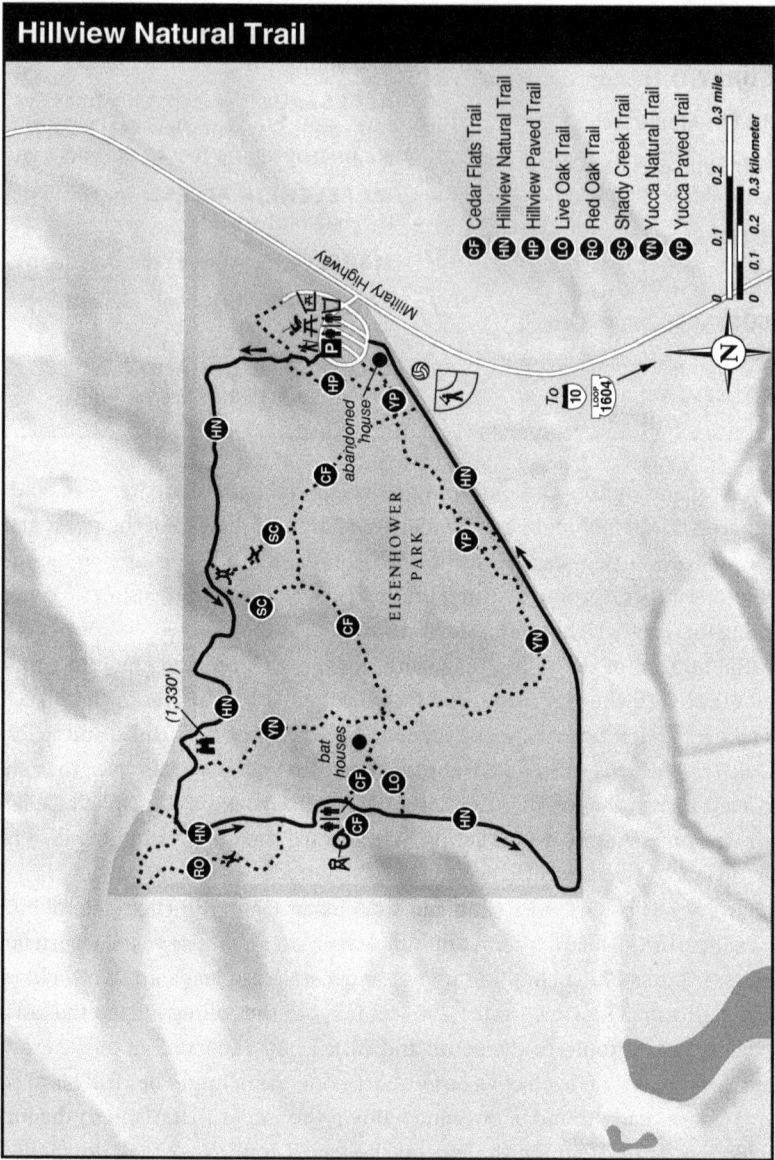

Legend:
- CF Cedar Flats Trail
- HN Hillview Natural Trail
- HP Hillview Paved Trail
- LO Live Oak Trail
- RO Red Oak Trail
- SC Shady Creek Trail
- YN Yucca Natural Trail
- YP Yucca Paved Trail

EISENHOWER PARK

Military Highway

abandoned house

bat houses

(1,330')

To 10  LOOP 1604

N

0    0.1    0.2    0.3 mile
0    0.1    0.2    0.3 kilometer

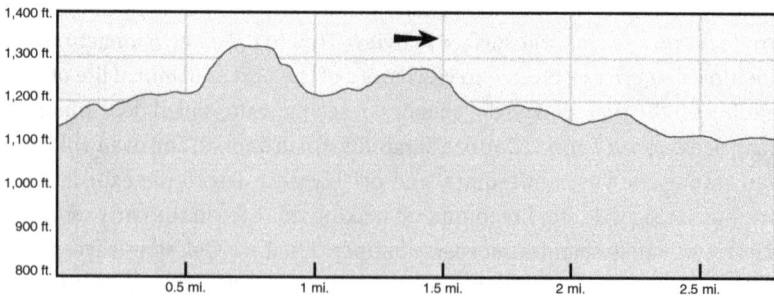

bottom and is very easy to traverse at this point. The hike meanders mostly downhill, gently undulating. Joggers and dog walkers just beginning their hikes start to appear from down the track.

At 1.9 miles the trail meets with a high fence bordering the quarry property, which it parallels for the remainder of the hike, and turns left. This begins the last leg, which is quite exposed. High-current power lines buzz overhead, carrying their load to a transformer station across the street from the park. Sotol grows among the cedar in this dry environment. At 2.4 miles, the Yucca Paved Trail appears alongside briefly. At 2.7 miles you'll see the park's baseball field to the right, south, on the other side of the fence. Pass an abandoned house on the left, and come to the end of the hike at a gate at the southern end of the parking lot.

## **Nearby Activities**

Friedrich Wilderness Park (page 186) and Crownridge Canyon Natural Area (page 182) are nearby.

---

### GPS TRAILHEAD COORDINATES

**N29° 37' 22.2"  W98° 34' 25.8"**

From I-10 and Loop 1604 in northwest San Antonio, go east on Loop 1604 to Northwest Military Highway. Go north on Northwest Military Highway and follow it 1.8 miles to Eisenhower Park, which is on the left just before Camp Bullis.

---

# 43 Leon Creek Greenway

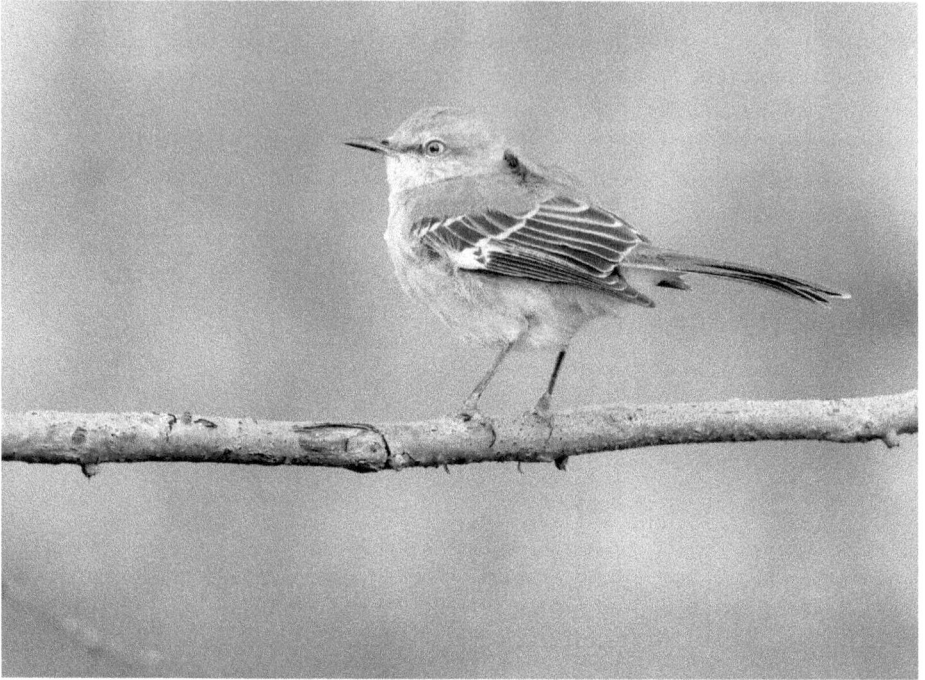

*You may see or hear a northern mockingbird along the trail.*

## In Brief

An easy stroll along a section of the leafy Leon Creek Valley in northwest San Antonio, the Leon Creek Greenway is part of San Antonio's popular Greenway system that now consists of nearly 50 miles of trails. It is justly popular with runners, cyclists, and walkers.

## Description

Former San Antonio mayor Howard W. Peak conceived the idea of a network of hike-and-bike trails along the city's creek floodplains when he was a councilman, and he followed through on his vision during his mayoral term. The Greenway system named after him now has 47 miles of paved trails along Leon Creek, Salado Creek, and the Medina River, with 32 more to come. This out-and-back hike takes in the section of the Leon Creek Greenway from the Buddy Calk Trailhead on Babcock Road to O.P. Schnabel Park, traveling along the creek banks through lush flora. Wildflower meadows, bluffs, and ancient deciduous woods await the hiker on an undulating descent.

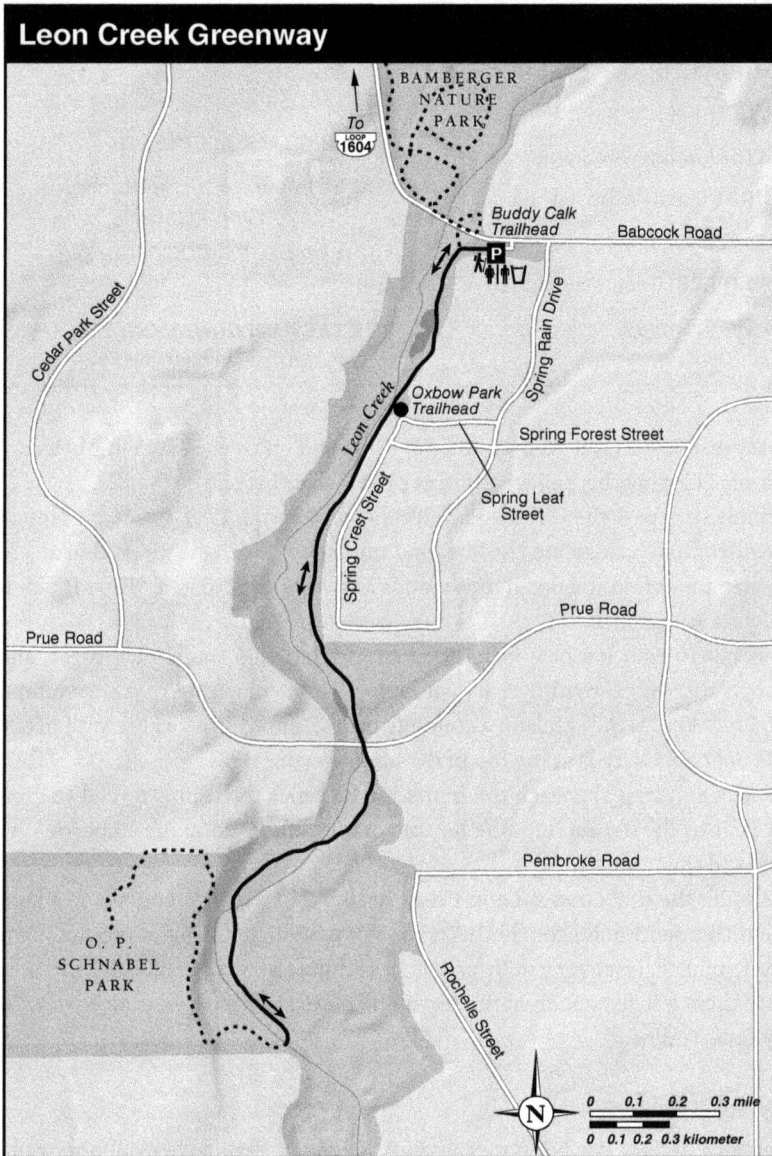

**Leon Creek Greenway**

Begin your hike on the concrete path that starts at the trailhead, and very shortly come to a junction. To the right, the trail leads to Bamberger Park and Loop 1604. Our hike goes left, heading toward Oxbow Park. Mesquite and cactus predominate on this section, which runs between backyards and the creek bed. The dense brush along the track generally restricts the view of the watercourse to brief glimpses.

At 0.2 mile the path skirts a small fishing lake, where the surface turns to asphalt. It will alternate between concrete and asphalt for the duration of the hike, making for

| | |
|---|---|
| **LENGTH:** 4.2 miles | **DRIVING DISTANCE:** 15 miles from the Alamo |
| **CONFIGURATION:** Out-and-back | |
| **DIFFICULTY:** Easy | **ACCESS:** Sunrise–sunset; free |
| **SCENERY:** Riparian woodland | **WHEELCHAIR ACCESS:** Yes |
| **EXPOSURE:** Mostly exposed | **MAPS:** tinyurl.com/lcnorthmap, tinyurl.com/lcparkingmap |
| **TRAFFIC:** Heavy | |
| **TRAIL SURFACE:** Concrete, asphalt | **FACILITIES:** Restrooms and water at trailheads |
| **HIKING TIME:** 2 hours | **CONTACT INFORMATION:** 210-207-8590; tinyurl.com/greenwaytrails |

smooth, easy walking. In the evening and morning, and on weekends, San Antonians will be out in force enjoying the trail, chatting as they hike or bicycle en famille.

At 0.5 mile you pass the Oxbow Park trailhead at Spring Leaf Street. Not long after, the creek widens and a ridgeline rises beyond the other bank. The forest thickens, and a patch of cedar appears in the deciduous woods as the trail approaches Prue Road, under which you pass at 1.3 miles.

The woods to your left past Prue Road are riddled with singletrack paths, and you may hear but not see off-road cyclists whooping as they navigate obstacles among the trees. At 1.5 miles cross the creek on a concrete bridge, entering a lovely swath of riparian forest. O.P. Schnabel Park is at the top of the bluffs to your right.

The creek and trail approach the bluffs. At 1.8 miles the trail is forced to cross the creek bed again as the stream hugs the bottom of the cliffs. Oaks and hackberries grow in the verdant and shady valley.

At 2.1 miles the trail crosses Leon Creek for the third time and comes to a junction. This is the turnaround point for this hike, though you might consider continuing to the Leon Vista Trailhead, just over a mile farther, or turning right and exploring O.P. Schnabel Park, where there is a vista point at the top of the bluffs. Otherwise, retrace your steps to the Buddy Calk Trailhead.

## Nearby Activities

Bamberger Nature Park has hiking trails; O.P. Schnabel Park has a concrete trail loop, rentable pavilions, and athletic fields.

### GPS TRAILHEAD COORDINATES
**N29° 33' 24.8"  W98° 37' 35.9"**

From Loop 1604 in northwestern San Antonio, take Babcock Road south 2.3 miles. The Buddy Calk Trailhead will be on the right.

# 44 McAllister Park Loop

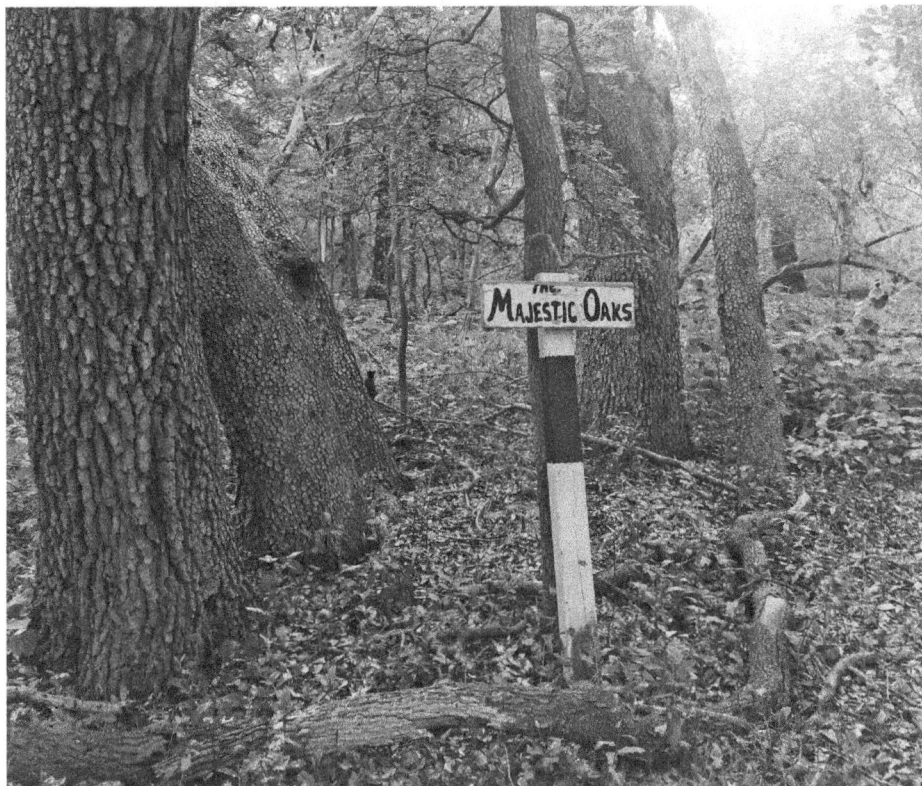

Ancient oak woods at McAllister Park

## In Brief

A large, popular city park with a number of athletic fields and picnic stations, McAllister Park has 15 miles of trails to tempt the hiker. This loop rambles through a mix of oak woods and South Texas scrub where you will likely come across deer and other wildlife.

## Description

Located on the north side of town near the airport, this well-maintained, 984-acre park features four pavilions, a dog park, and more than 50 athletic fields. It is very popular with bicyclists for the singletrack trails and for access to the Salado Creek Greenway, which is part of the excellent Howard W. Peak Greenway Trails System. (Both Peak and Walter W. McAllister were mayors of San Antonio.)

| | |
|---|---|
| **LENGTH:** 4.2 miles | **DRIVING DISTANCE:** 12 miles from the Alamo |
| **CONFIGURATION:** Loop | |
| **DIFFICULTY:** Easy | **ACCESS:** Daily, 5 a.m.–11 p.m.; free |
| **SCENERY:** Thick woodland, mesquite scrub, dam, wildlife | **WHEELCHAIR ACCESS:** Yes |
| | **MAPS:** tinyurl.com/mcallisterparkmap |
| **EXPOSURE:** Exposed–shady | **FACILITIES:** Restrooms and water fountains at the parking lot |
| **TRAFFIC:** Heavy | |
| **TRAIL SURFACE:** Asphalt, dirt | **CONTACT INFORMATION:** 210-207-7275; tinyurl.com/mcallisterpark |
| **HIKING TIME:** 1.7 hours | |

This almost entirely level route takes in the southern portion of the Blue Loop, passing through mesquite savanna and ancient oak groves on the far side of a high, grassy flood-control bank. The hike goes along the top of the berm and returns on the Red Trail, which shadows the Blue Loop through the woodland on the north side of the bank. The trails are designated as multiuse, but much of the route is on narrow singletrack, where you should be on the lookout for cyclists hurtling through the forest.

The unofficial trailhead for this hike is at the northwestern edge of the parking lot, where a track leads along the edge of the dog park toward a line of trees and a transmission line. Reach the treeline, and come to a trail junction where the Blue Loop crosses one end of the Red Trail. Look for the marker post, where blue and red arrows and colored bands identify the trails. These marker posts appear irregularly along the route.

Turn left here into the narrow strip of mesquite, hackberry, and cedar. The trail emerges briefly onto an access road underneath the transmission line, immediately dives back into the woods, and shortly comes out again onto a low, grassy berm, part of a long flood-control structure that will be a recurring feature of the hike.

At 0.4 mile there's a junction by a tiny coppice. The section of bank in front of you is reinforced with concrete. Turn left, and keep left to follow a jeep track along the south side of the dog park. Jets fly overhead, and the tall light towers of the athletic fields rise above the treetops. At 0.5 mile there is a fork; continue on the Blue Loop—the narrower path heading right into the scrub. Mesquite and oak savanna surround the now narrow track. Cross a cleared area under transmission lines. The Salado Creek Greenway is visible to your left. At 0.9 mile dip into a tree-lined wash by Wurzbach Parkway, and keep on the Blue Loop as it makes a right turn. Stay right at a fork, shadowing the creek.

The path moves away from the wash. You will pass under more transmission lines and approach the high, green bank that now rises to your right behind a fence. Cross another access road, and keep right at an unmarked fork. Continue under ever larger and more-ancient oaks. At 1.3 miles come to a dry creek bed deep in the forest. A handmade sign reads THE MAJESTIC OAKS, and it is not wrong.

Cross the creek here, and then turn right, walking parallel to a fence line between you and some soccer fields. The path goes right again and back over the creek bed before

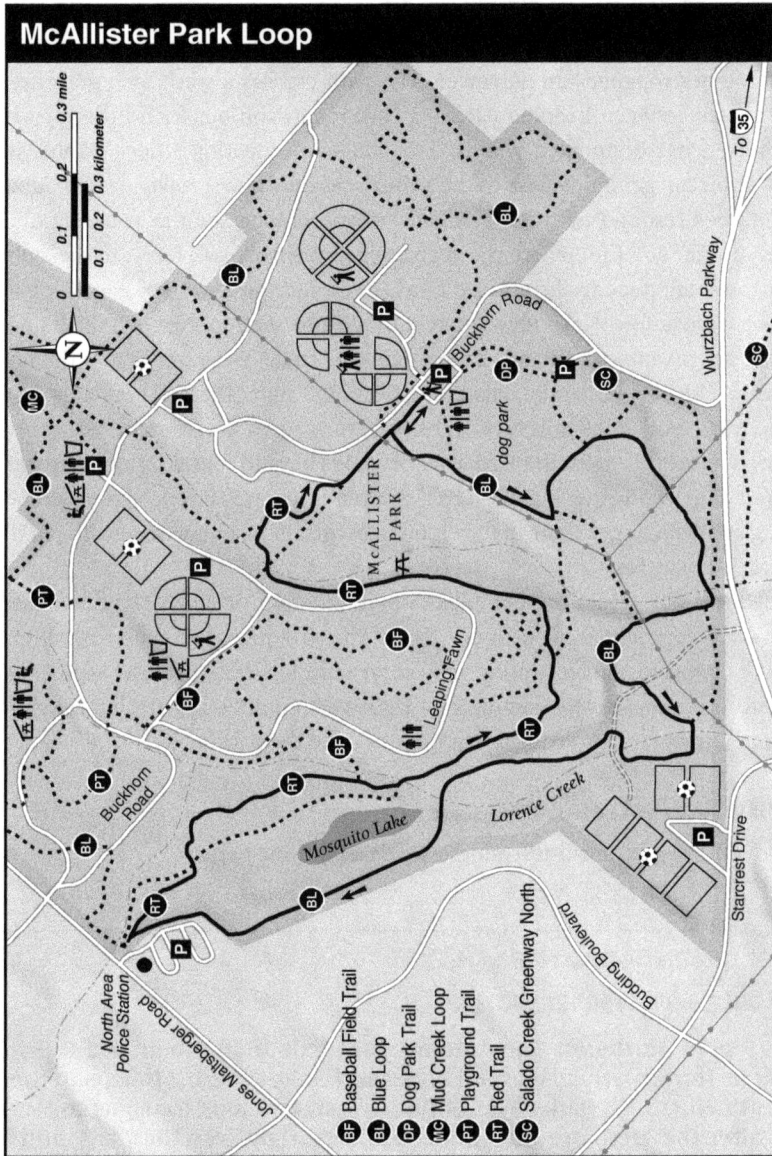

**McAllister Park Loop**

0.3 mile
0.2
0.1
0

0.3 kilometer
0.2
0.1
0

N

To 35

Buckhorn Road

dog park

Wurzbach Parkway

MCALLISTER PARK

Leaping Fawn

Lorence Creek

Mosquito Lake

Starcrest Drive

Budding Boulevard

Buckhorn Road

North Area Police Station

Jones Maltsberger Road

BF — Baseball Field Trail
BL — Blue Loop
DP — Dog Park Trail
MC — Mud Creek Loop
PT — Playground Trail
RT — Red Trail
SC — Salado Creek Greenway North

emerging from the forest and climbing up onto the top of the dam. For the next 0.5 mile or so, the route stays up on the berm in the open. The wind blows through the grama grass at the edge of the path. Mosquito Lake is to your right amid the thick mesquite and oak woods.

At 2.3 miles descend from the dam by a neighborhood, and pass a police station behind the park fence. Come to the junction with the Red Trail in a triangular open area, and turn right onto this asphalt path, which is mostly in the shade off the woods to your left. The path dips in and out of these woods, skirting Mosquito Lake, and comes to the junction with the Baseball Field Trail at 2.8 miles. Continue forward on the Red Trail, which becomes rougher and narrower. The path crosses a wash by a graceful oak and shortly passes between Leaping Fawn—a park road—and our friend the grassy bank to enter thicker, oak-dominated woods. The chance of meeting a deer on this section is high, and you can get quite close to the animals, as they have grown used to humans.

The trees resound with the cardinals' dive-bombing song as you continue. At 3.3 miles keep right at a fork where the vegetation shifts from oak forest to mesquite scrub. Shortly the singletrack trail runs into Mud Creek and turns north, shadowing the creek bed along a fence line. Keep forward at another intersection, through thick underbrush that slowly turns into woodland. Numerous spur trails lead right across the creek bed. Pass picnic tables set under the oaks along Leaping Fawn. The trail gradually comes level with the wash until at 3.8 miles there is a right turn and a short, rocky descent to a complex junction. At this point the Red Trail becomes hard to follow, as there are no marker posts and the woods are a maze of crisscrossing paths. If you have a phone with a mapping app, you might want to turn it on to ascertain that you are heading in the direction of the parking lot.

Head straight across the complex double junction, keeping right and then left in short order. Keep right at the next two forks. The path turns left, dips down into another wash, and comes to a deteriorating vehicle turnaround. Walk over the asphalt and come back onto the trail, shortly coming to a right-angle junction. Turn left here, and keep straight to return to the starting point at the edge of the parking lot.

## Nearby Activities

The park offers picnic facilities, athletic fields, and a dog park.

---

### GPS TRAILHEAD COORDINATES

**N29° 33' 13.9"  W98° 26' 43.2"**

From I-35 in northwest San Antonio, take Exit 167B (Thousand Oaks Drive/ Starlight Terrace). Head west on Thousand Oaks Drive 0.3 mile, and then turn left onto Wurzbach Parkway. Continue west, and look for signs to McAllister Park after the Wetmore Road junction. Turn right into the park, and follow the park road (Buckhorn Road) 0.6 mile to the paved parking lot on the left by the dog park.

# 45 Medina River Natural Area Loop

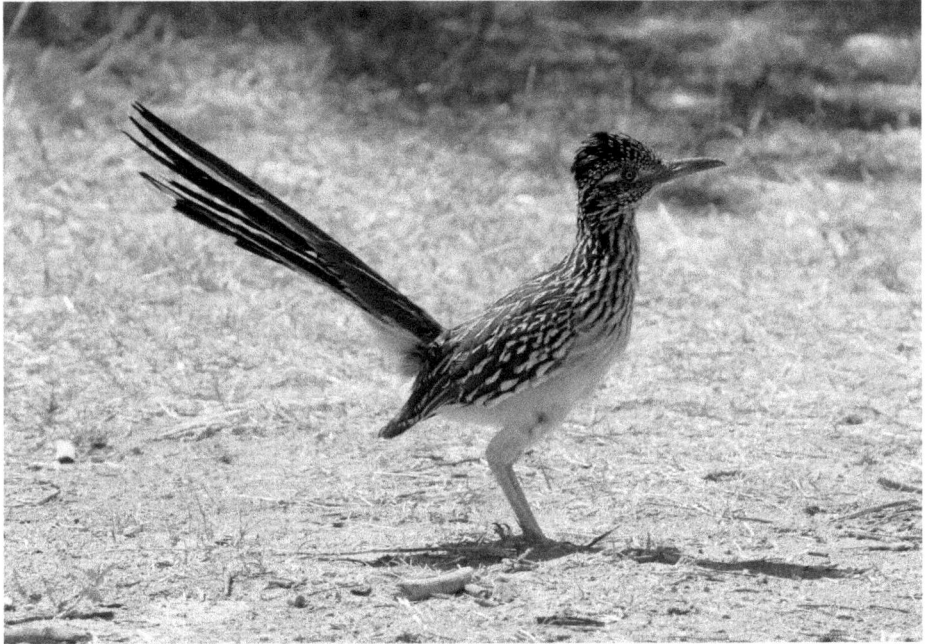

*Roadrunner*

## In Brief

This south San Antonio loop explores wooded bottomland along the Medina River where cypress and cottonwoods grow to mammoth proportions. The hike climbs onto mesquite-covered uplands and (optionally) explores historical sites along El Chaparral Trail, part of the 50-mile Howard W. Peak Greenway Trail system.

## Description

What is now the Medina River Natural Area was once going to be a reservoir, but thankfully that did not happen. Instead we have this 511-acre natural area not far from the Toyota plant. Opened in 2005, it protects a bottomland corridor along the river that hikers can explore on 10 miles of trails. El Chaparral Trail, a concrete hike-and-bike path also known as the Medina River Greenway, runs for 7 miles east of the park proper and passes some fascinating historical sites.

| LENGTH: 2.3 miles or 6.5 miles | HIKING TIME: 1.2 hours |
| --- | --- |
| CONFIGURATION: Loop | DRIVING DISTANCE: 15 miles from the Alamo |
| DIFFICULTY: Easy | |
| SCENERY: Wooded river bottom, open upland | ACCESS: Daily, 7:30 a.m.–sunset; free |
| | WHEELCHAIR ACCESS: Yes, along El Camino and El Chaparral Trails |
| EXPOSURE: Mostly shaded, open areas exposed | MAPS: tinyurl.com/medinarivermap |
| TRAFFIC: Moderate | FACILITIES: Restrooms, water, picnicking at trailhead |
| TRAIL SURFACE: Concrete, natural surfaces | CONTACT INFORMATION: 210-207-3111; tinyurl.com/medinariverna |

The wide swath of river bottom contains gigantic cypress, cottonwood, and pecan trees that you have to see to believe. As you hike, you can enjoy these big trees and the brown Medina River as it flows to meet the San Antonio River. The route moves through the dappled forest and then climbs up to the exposed mesquite and shrub uplands covered with all kinds of grasses and forbs—flowering plants that are not grasses. At the junction with the Greenway, you can turn left and return to the trailhead or go right and see an old jacal—a ranch house made out of wooden poles—and the site of a river crossing on El Camino Real de los Tejas, the road from Texas to Mexico City.

Concrete trails lead away from the main trailhead near the park police office. Look right for the El Camino Trail, which descends by switchbacks into the Medina River valley. Pass a large picnic pavilion, and reach a trail junction at 0.2 mile. El Camino Trail keeps straight to dead-end at the river's edge. This river flows from springs on the west side of Bandera County. It passes through Medina County, where it is dammed as Medina Lake and Medina Diversion Reservoir, and flows through Castroville and into Bexar County to meet the San Antonio River, not far downstream from the Medina River Natural Area. It is named after Pedro Medina, a Spanish engineer, and was once the border between Coahuila and Texas.

Admire the immense cypress trees lining the banks. Retrace your steps to the junction, and turn right onto a gravel track—the Rio Medina Trail—surrounded by hackberry and a multitude of other hardwoods. Spur trails lead to fishing spots; the river is renowned for catfish. (A permit is required for fishing.) Mostly the waterway sometimes flows quietly, but occasionally it gathers in noisy rapids. At 0.5 mile there is a junction where the Rio Medina Trail splits. A short spur trail leads down to a gravel bar at the river's edge. Turn right and then left, staying with the path closest to the river.

You are now in bona fide bottomland, among tall deciduous trees that have been allowed to flourish undisturbed. As you walk along the river, admire the cottonwoods, sycamores, pecans, ashes, willows, and vines that thrive here. Because this is bottomland, the trail can be muddy in places, especially after rains. Watch for deer or their tracks.

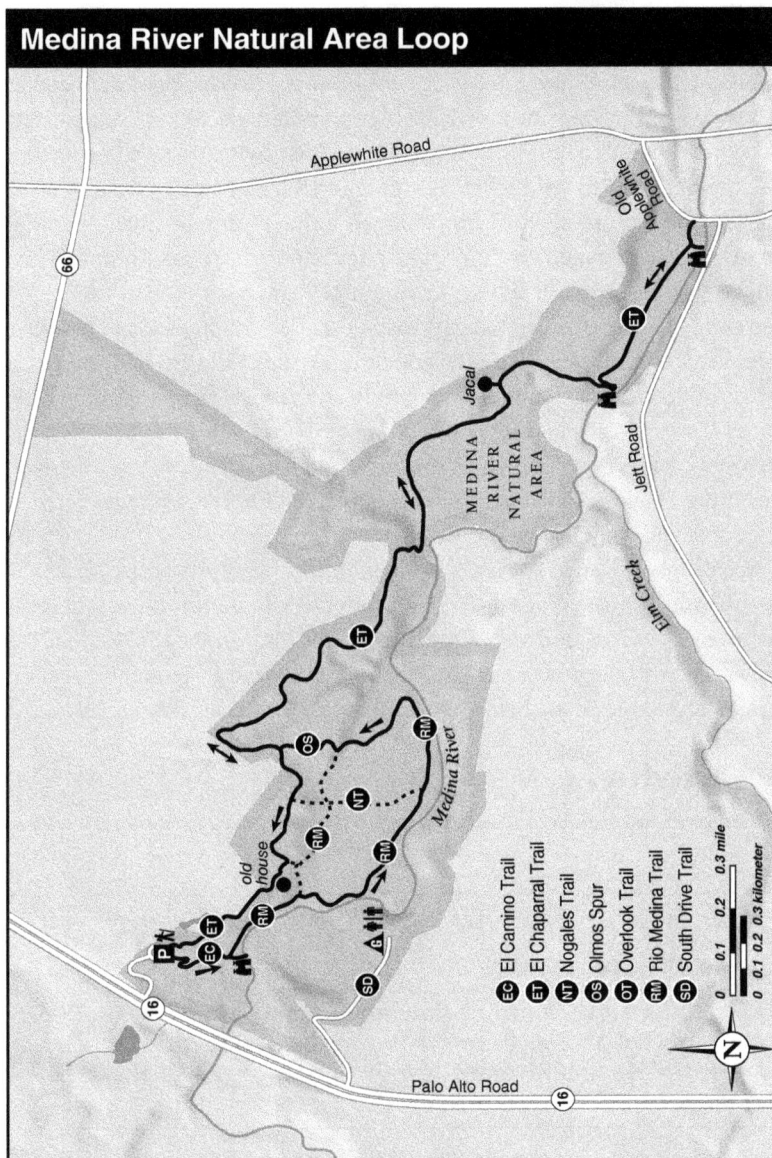

**Medina River Natural Area Loop**

Applewhite Road

Old Applewhite Road

Jett Road

Elm Creek

Jacal

MEDINA RIVER NATURAL AREA

Medina River

old house

Palo Alto Road

**EC** El Camino Trail
**ET** El Chaparral Trail
**NT** Nogales Trail
**OS** Olmos Spur
**OT** Overlook Trail
**RM** Rio Medina Trail
**SD** South Drive Trail

0  0.1  0.2  0.3 mile
0  0.1  0.2  0.3 kilometer

At 0.9 mile the Nogales Trail leaves left. Keep along the Medina, noting bluffs across the river. Shortly turn away from the waterway, northbound. Cross channels that flow only during floods. At 1.4 miles turn right on the Olmos Spur, and make a short, steep climb up some steps into another world—uplands where mesquite trees grow amid a smorgasbord of smaller flora.

Meet El Chaparral Trail, a concrete path also known as the Medina River Greenway, at 1.6 miles. If you are making the shorter loop, turn left and return to the trailhead for a 2.3-mile hike. Otherwise, gird your loins and keep right, crossing a drainage and then walking through lush open meadowland. At 2.3 miles a series of sharp switchbacks returns you to the wooded bottoms. At 2.9 miles similar switchbacks climb back up to the top. Look to your right to see the fenced-off Pérez Rancho jacal, a traditional structure with walls of wooden poles. No doubt it played a role in the livestock operation based here that belonged to Lieutenant Colonel Juan Ignacio Pérez, a San Antonio native with a reputation for cruelty who was interim governor of Texas from 1816 to 1817.

Keep going, returning down the steep bank to the river bottoms, and pass Overlook 2 at 3.3 miles. At 3.7 miles you arrive at Overlook 1, the site of El Paso de Dolores, the name of the crossing where a segment of El Camino Real, the royal road to Mexico City, forded the Medina. Traces of the old camino are still visible between here and the Pérez jacal.

The overlook is very close to the trailhead at Old Applewhite Road. The road crosses the river on the Donkey Lady Bridge, where, as legend has it, a poor woman who was horribly burned and went insane terrorized unlucky passersby.

Retrace your steps, and return to the junction with the Rio Medina Trail at 5.9 miles. Pass the other end of the Nogales Trail and a power line at 6 miles. The trail passes through mesquite, cactus, and yucca, meeting a connector to the Rio Medina Trail at 6.2 miles. Stay right with the greenway. The concrete trail passes a pond and a pair of chimneys marking an old ranch site before returning to the trailhead at 6.5 miles.

## Nearby Activities

The Medina River Natural Area features a group camping area available by reservation.

---

**GPS TRAILHEAD COORDINATES**

**N29° 15' 48.5" W98° 34' 41.6"**

From Exit 49 on I-410 south of downtown San Antonio, take TX 16 (Palo Alto Road) south 4.2 miles to turn left into the natural area, just before the bridge over the Medina River. Follow the entrance road a short distance to the parking area.

# 46 San Antonio Botanical Garden Trail

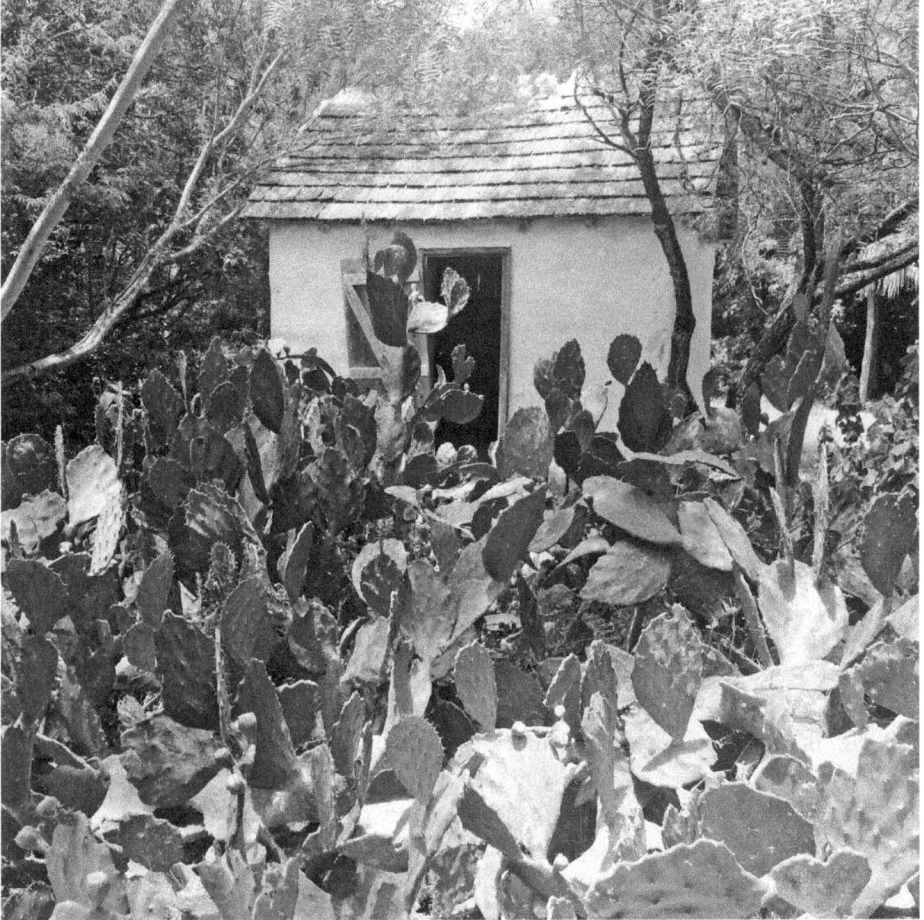

*The South Texas section of the San Antonio Botanical Trail*

## In Brief

Close to downtown San Antonio, the botanical garden is perfect for a simple nature recharge and lunch, though one might easily spend a day here studying the flora of Texas and the world. Formal gardens, a grand conservatory, and the Texas Native Trail are among the attractions.

| | |
|---|---|
| **LENGTH:** 1.4 miles | **ACCESS:** Daily (except Thanksgiving, Christmas Day, and New Year's Day), 9 a.m.–5 p.m.; $10 adults; $7 children ages 3–13; $8 seniors (ages 65 and older), active military, and students |
| **CONFIGURATION:** Loop | |
| **DIFFICULTY:** Easy | |
| **SCENERY:** Local and exotic plants | |
| **EXPOSURE:** Shady | **WHEELCHAIR ACCESS:** Yes, on cement trails |
| **TRAFFIC:** Moderate | |
| **TRAIL SURFACE:** Cement, flagstone, dirt, mulch | **MAPS:** sabot.org |
| | **FACILITIES:** Restrooms, gift shop, restaurant |
| **HIKING TIME:** 1.5 hours | |
| **DRIVING DISTANCE:** 3 miles from the Alamo | **CONTACT INFORMATION:** 210-207-3250; sabot.org |

## Description

At one time a quarry, and then a reservoir, the San Antonio Botanical Garden was a long time in gestation—imagined in the 1940s, the preserve eventually opened in May 1980. It was worth the wait. The formal gardens are an ever-changing delight, and the Lucile Halsell Conservatory, designed by Argentinean architect Emilio Ambasz, is one of the city's finest buildings. Several smaller structures have been moved to the garden and serve as examples of homesteads from Texas's settler days.

For hikers and nature lovers, the Texas Native Trail is a must-see, especially if your tree-identification skills start at cedar and end at "I think that's a live oak." It is in fact three short trails that circle through re-creations of Hill Country, East Texas, and South Texas ecosystems. Trees and shrubs are clearly labeled, so if you want to know the difference between guajillo and huisache or sweetgum and sugarberry, this is the place to come.

The guest center is the Daniel J. Sullivan Carriage House, which was built in 1896 for the Irish immigrant, soldier, and banker. It was moved stone by stone from its original location downtown to the garden. The carriage house now contains the Carriage House Bistro and the Garden Gate Gift Shop. This is where you pay your entry fee.

From the back of the carriage house, head up a wide set of stairs (there is a ramp for wheelchairs and strollers beside the stairs). You'll see a plaque at the top with a map of the park—the same map shown in the brochure. A signpost with arrows points to the various attractions. Our hike takes in almost everything in the garden, though because this is more of a stroll than a true hike (with no possibility of getting lost), feel free to ditch these instructions at any time and wander where you will.

Turn right at the top of the steps—heading for the Conservatory—and walk through the Wisteria Arbor to the Fountain Plaza, an experience as delightful as it sounds. In front of you to the right is the Kumamoto En, a garden built by craftsmen from Japan and Texas that was a gift from San Antonio's sister city Kumamoto. To your left is the entrance to the conservatory. Its glass pyramids tower over the surrounding plazas and terraces. Farther left, a gazebo on a little hill provides an overlook.

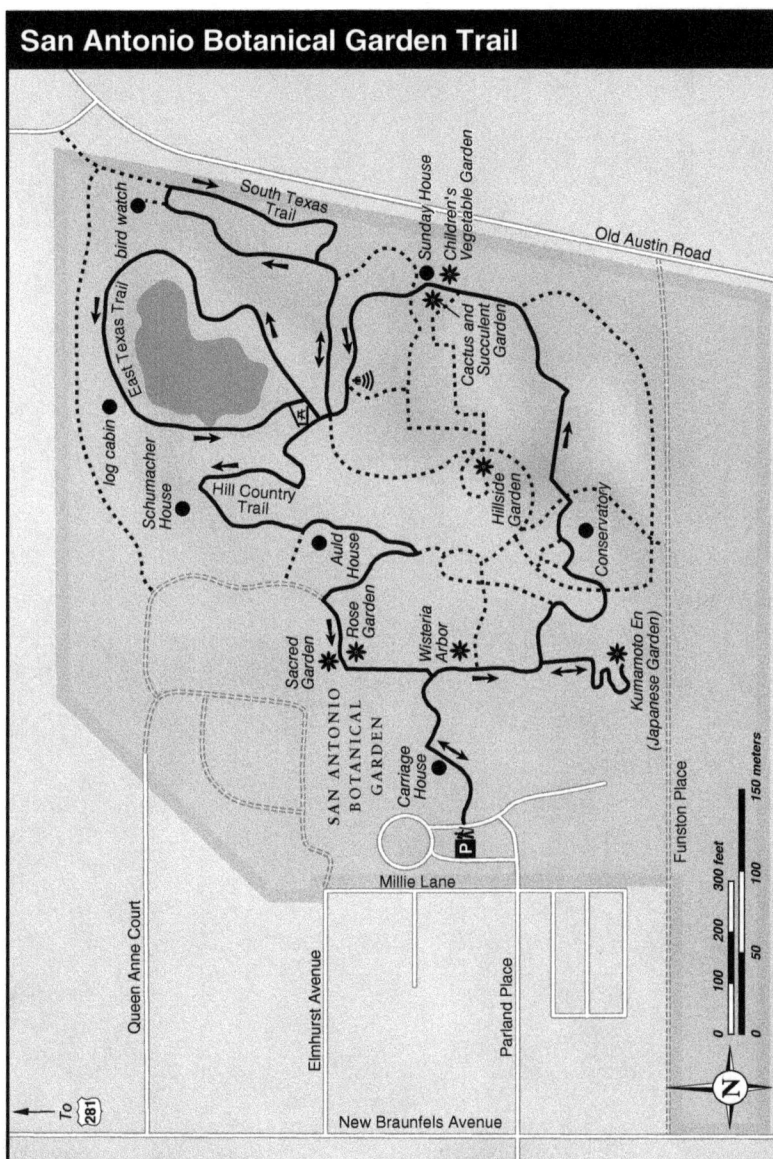

**San Antonio Botanical Garden Trail**

Walk around the Japanese garden, and then make your way to the conservatory, which has been constructed as five separate rooms around a large, open atrium. Only the glass roofs are above ground level. The fern grotto is particularly lovely. Linger and admire plants from all over the world.

Steps lead out of the northern side of the atrium. Turn right at the top, walking over the sunken courtyard toward the Cactus and Succulent Garden. The beds are full of cacti and other desert plants. Pass the Children's Vegetable Garden and Sunday House on your

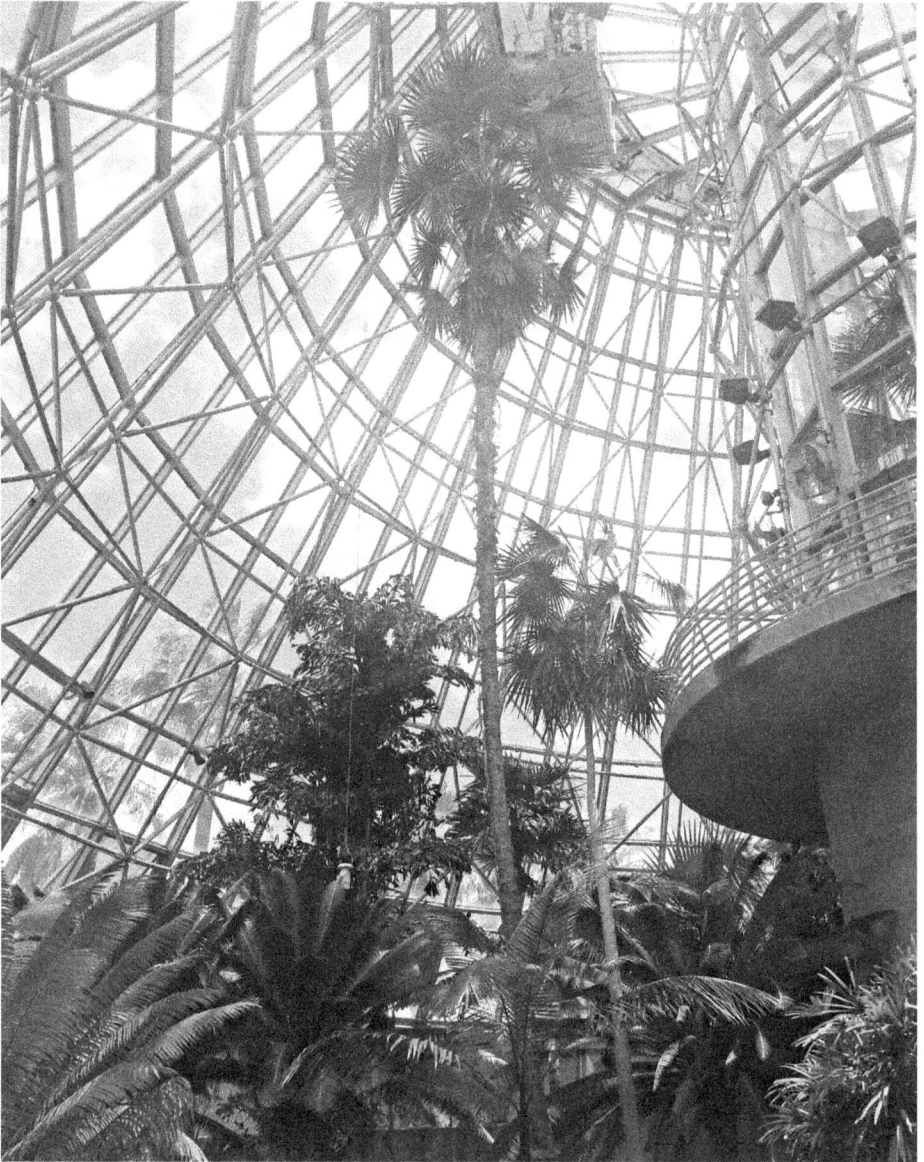

*The Conservatory at the San Antonio Botanical Garden*

right, keeping straight at an intersection. The path bends left and comes to another junction. To your left is the amphitheater, once a reservoir for San Antonio's water supply. The portico at the entrance to the Texas Native Trails is a few steps to the right.

The South Texas exhibit area showcases the trees and shrubs found in the southern part of the state, such as mesquite, blackbrush, and ebony. There is a small adobe house on this path and a bird-watching shelter at the far end.

The East Texas Trail circles a small lake under the shade of tall deciduous trees typical of that area. It passes a log cabin with a corral and barn where you can imagine life in the thick forests before they were cut down in the early 1900s. There is even a garden with tomato and pepper plants. Back then, a small plot to grow corn and vegetables and a few pigs foraging in the woods were all it took to have a plentiful existence for a family.

Finally the Hill Country Trail wanders past cedar and mountain laurel, a limestone water feature, and two houses. Built in 1849 from wood, mud, and sand, the Schumacher House was relocated from Fredericksburg. The next building on the trail, the Auld House, was reconstructed from a cabin in Leakey and is available for rental. ("Auld" is the name of the family that lived in the original and not a description of the structure's age.)

Exit the Texas Native Trail past the Auld House, and turn right at a fork on a concrete path. Pass the entrance to WaterSaver Lane, a row of tiny, colorful cottages set in drought-tolerant native landscaping, and come to the Sacred Garden amid the scent of jasmine. Turn left here, and wander through the Rose Garden to come back to the top of the steps leading down to the Carriage House. Enjoy lunch in the Bistro.

## Nearby Activities

The San Antonio Botanical Garden offers bird walks, classes, camps, and other events. Visit sabot.org for details.

---

**GPS TRAILHEAD COORDINATES**

**N29° 27' 31.6" W98° 27' 31.8"**

**From US 281 in San Antonio, just north of I-35, exit on East Hildebrand Avenue. Turn right on New Braunfels Avenue, and then take a left on Funston Place. The garden is on the left.**

# 47 San Antonio Mission Trail

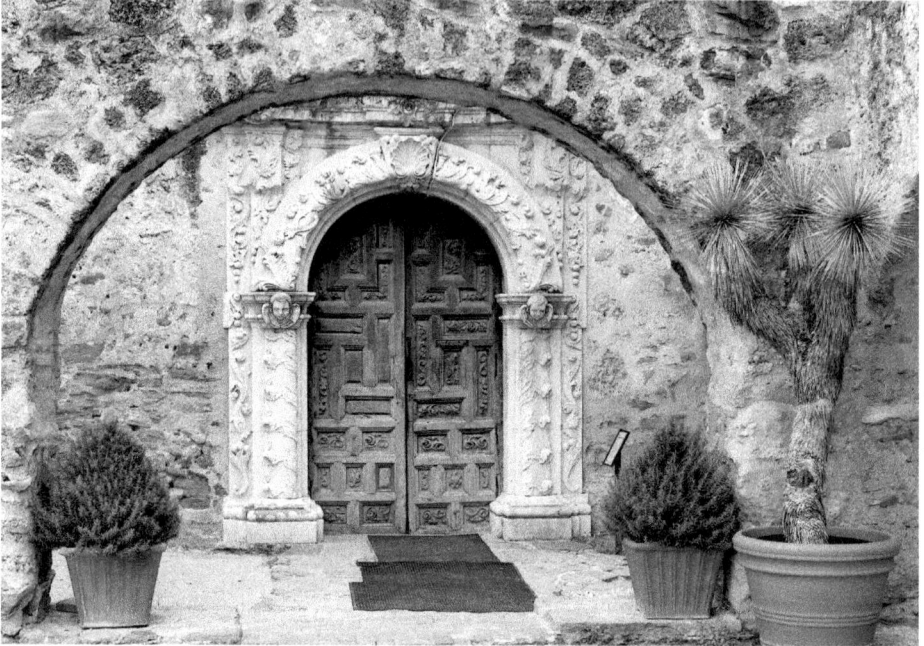

*Mission San José*

## In Brief

Visit two historic missions as part of a stroll along the historic and surprisingly lush San Antonio Mission Trail, part of the San Antonio River Walk Hike and Bike Trail.

## Description

San Antonio Missions National Historic Park consists of a chain of four missions along the San Antonio River: San José, San Juan, Espada, and Concepción. These structures, in conjunction with the Alamo, form the oldest chain of Catholic missions in North America. Originally lured here by rumors of wealth and the encroaching French from Louisiana, Spaniards established these missions in east Texas hoping to take advantage of local riches. Failing this, they set about converting the locals to Catholicism.

The first mission built in the area served as a waypoint between the missions in Louisiana and those in east Texas and New Spain (Mexico). This was Mission San Antonio de Valero, later known as the Alamo. Two years later, in 1720, Fray Antonio Margil de Jesús established a second mission, San José, for the purpose of converting the native

| | |
|---|---|
| **LENGTH:** 6 miles | **DRIVING DISTANCE:** 6 miles from the Alamo |
| **CONFIGURATION:** Out-and-back | |
| **DIFFICULTY:** Very easy | **ACCESS:** Daily (except Thanksgiving, Christmas Day, and New Year's Day), 9 a.m.–5 p.m.; no fees or permits required |
| **SCENERY:** Historic Spanish missions, San Antonio River | |
| **EXPOSURE:** Open | **WHEELCHAIR ACCESS:** Yes |
| **TRAFFIC:** Moderate–heavy | **MAPS:** tinyurl.com/samissionsmap |
| **TRAIL SURFACE:** Asphalt | **FACILITIES:** Restrooms, gift shop, and picnic areas with barbecue pits |
| **HIKING TIME:** Walking time is about 1.5 hours, but allow extra time to explore the missions. | **CONTACT INFORMATION:** 210-932-1001; nps.gov/saan |

Coahuiltecan tribes. In the meantime, the east Texas missions failed; three of these missions were relocated to the San Antonio area. The missions soon became not only religious centers but also cultural and economic centers, complete with fortified walls, farms with an irrigation system, and herds of sheep and cattle. Though considered historical sites, the missions are still active worship centers. The park service asks that you respect services and parish staff.

The San Antonio River Walk connects the Brackenridge Park to Mission Espada, with 15 miles of continuous trail available. This well-maintained and easy path along the river attracts many hikers, bikers, and joggers. The visitor center and park headquarters are located at Mission San José, where this hike begins.

Before starting your hike, explore the remains of the old mission at a leisurely pace. The size of Mission San José led to its being known as the "queen of the missions." The center of village life and source of its defense, the mission, with its large walls, helped resident American Indians fend off attacks by Apache and Comanche tribes.

The beginning of the hike is very open. There is no reason why children couldn't enjoy this trail, and a stroller would be easy to push along. Many families venture along the path on bicycles. Leave the visitor center, and head southeast across the parking lot area, following Napier Avenue to reach Padre Drive. Cross Padre Drive, and turn right, picking up the trail as it parallels the road.

The trail widens and you arrive at the first of four footbridges; another lies just ahead. The path reaches the San Antonio River at just over 0.5 mile and continues south beside it.

Pass under Military Drive and then arrive at Espada Park 1.8 miles into the trail, where you'll find parking spaces, picnic tables, and grills set up for public use. A short way south of the park, the path separates from the road, which crosses the river at Espada Dam and continues along the west bank of the river.

The trail is wide and in very good shape, and it's more pleasant for leaving the traffic behind, albeit briefly. Shortly after leaving the road, you'll come to a third footbridge, at which point the trail stands about 40 feet above the river at normal levels. As you walk

## San Antonio Mission Trail

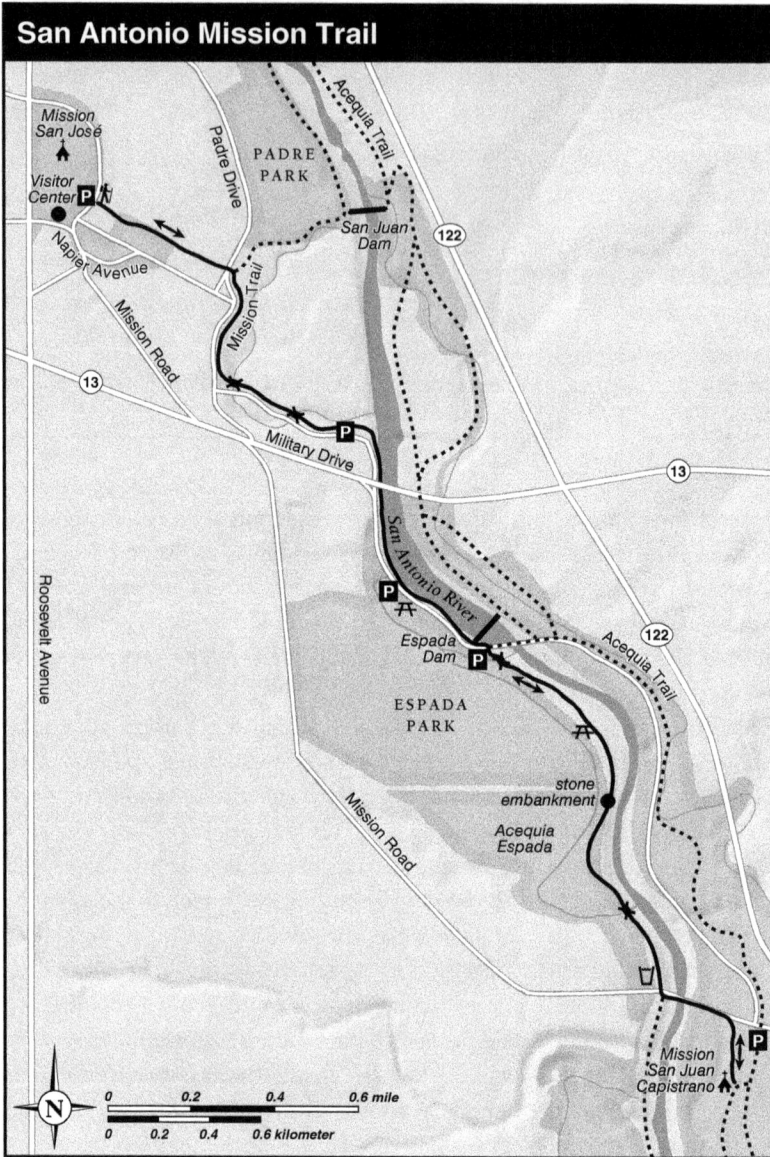

along this section, look to the right, and you can see portions of the Acequia de Espada, the remains of a gravity-flow ditch system. These acequias remain as part of a larger system of dams and aqueducts that were used to irrigate the missions' fields for agricultural use. Espada Dam still diverts water into the Acequia Madre, or "mother ditch," which is carried over Sixmile Creek by the oldest Spanish aqueduct in North America, the Espada Aqueduct. This system still provides water to nearby farms.

Continuing southward, you'll reach a stone embankment on your right that prevents further erosion; shortly thereafter, the fourth and final footbridge crosses another feeder creek. At 2.6 miles the trail joins Mission Road. Turn left onto the road, and go over the bridge. Just across the river, turn right and walk into the parking lot for the San Juan mission.

Mission San Juan Capistrano was originally established as San José de los Nazonis in east Texas. Relocated to this spot in 1731, it oversaw a rich agricultural area and orchards that supported not only the mission but also the nearby settlements and presidio. Take the time to explore the old building before heading back up the trail to Mission San José. An alternative route back follows the trail network up the eastern bank of the river.

## Nearby Activities

Restaurants and hotels line the portion of the River Walk where it loops through the center of town close to the Alamo, still Texas's top tourist destination.

---

**GPS TRAILHEAD COORDINATES**

**N29° 21' 37.4" W98° 28' 43.2"**

From I-37, exit at East Southcross Boulevard. Proceed west on Southcross to Roosevelt Avenue. Turn left, and proceed south on Roosevelt until it intersects Napier Avenue. Turn left. The visitor center is on your left.

---

# North of San Antonio (Hikes 48–60)

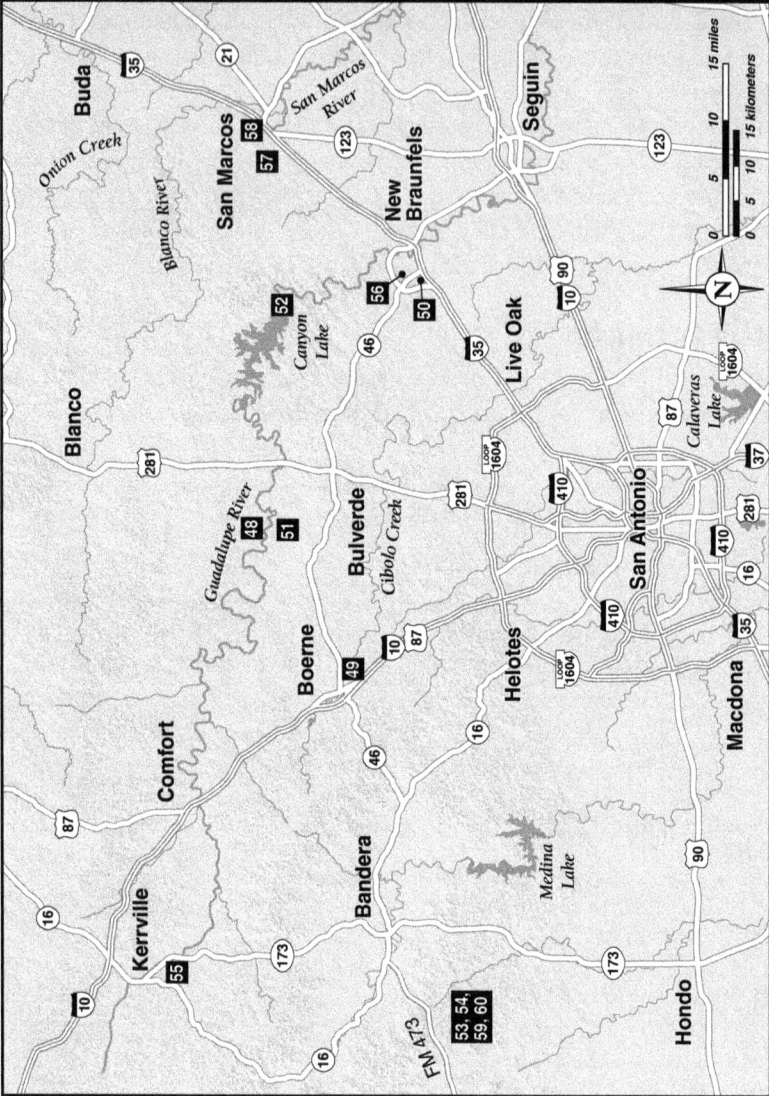

# NORTH OF SAN ANTONIO

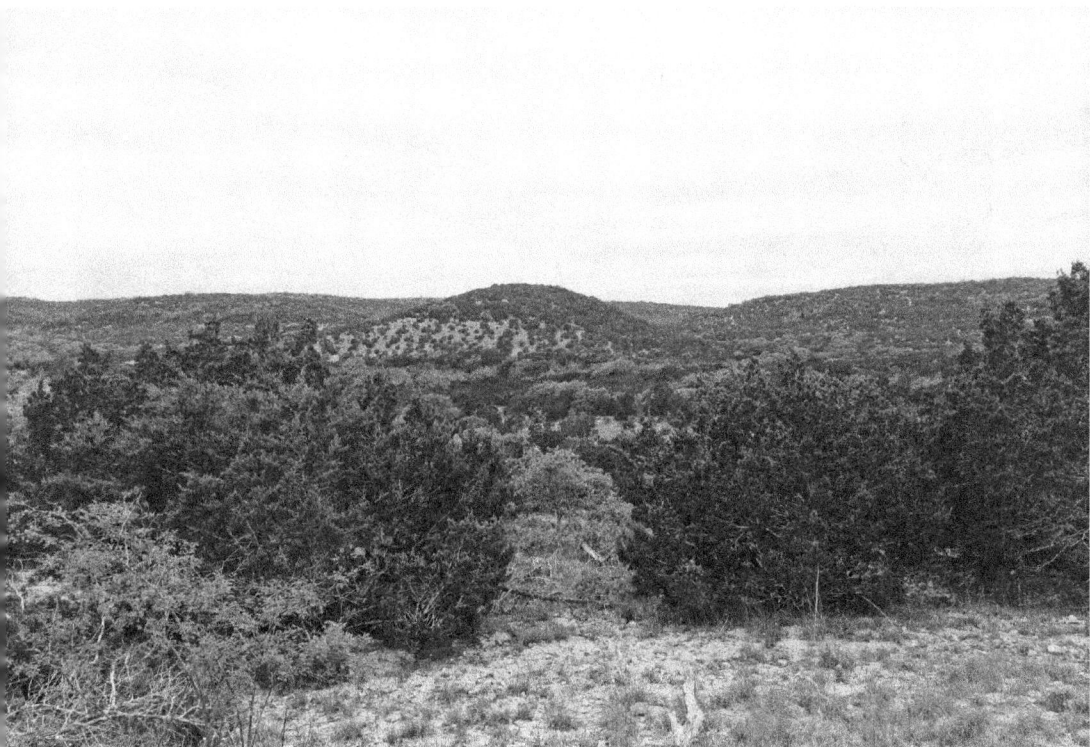

*Hill Country State Natural Area (see page 247)*

# 48 Bamberger Trail

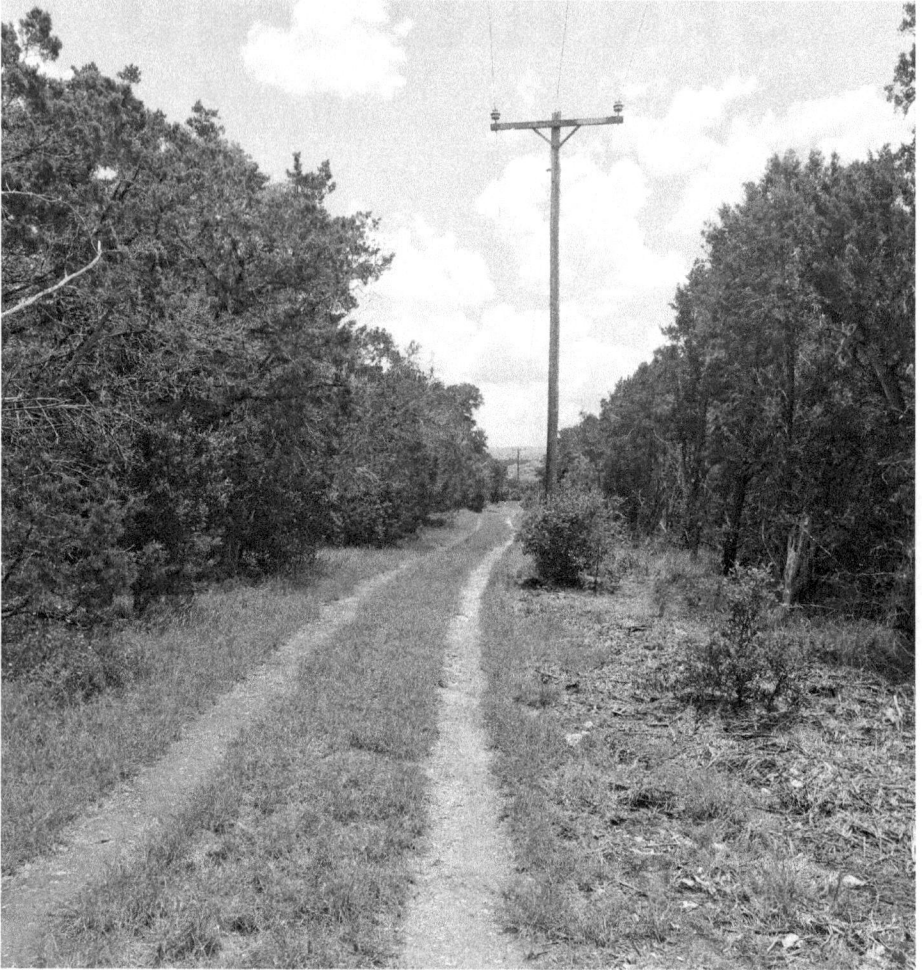

*A jeep track, part of the Bamberger Trail*

## In Brief

This hike through the Bauer Unit of Guadalupe River State Park takes you into virgin Ashe juniper woodlands, descends to a grove of ancient oaks, and then loops around a grassy meadow. This still little-known section of the otherwise popular park has no river access and is moderately hard to get to, which means it's perfect for a quiet trek through nature.

| | |
|---|---|
| **LENGTH:** 4.8 miles | **ACCESS:** Daily, 8 a.m.–10 p.m.; $7 entrance fee per person over age 13 (bring cash for self-pay station); closed for public hunts |
| **CONFIGURATION:** Figure eight | |
| **DIFFICULTY:** Easy | |
| **SCENERY:** Juniper forest, grasslands, oak grove | **WHEELCHAIR ACCESS:** None |
| **EXPOSURE:** Some shade, mostly exposed | **MAPS:** At information board or tinyurl.com/grspmap |
| **TRAFFIC:** Light to moderate | **FACILITIES:** None |
| **TRAIL SURFACE:** Dirt, rocks, gravel road | **CONTACT INFORMATION:** 830-438-2656; tpwd.texas.gov/state-parks/guadalupe-river |
| **HIKING TIME:** 2 hours | |
| **DRIVING DISTANCE:** 41 miles from the Alamo | |

## Description

Unmentioned on the park's website, the Bauer Unit is 661 acres of untouched juniper forest and savanna north of the Guadalupe River and deep in the ranching country on the border of Comal and Kendall Counties. The unit's remote location and lack of facilities are a deterrent to casual park visitors who simply want to unwind by the river. But for hikers and off-road bikers, it is an exciting destination. From the parking lot, you will follow the Bamberger Trail through cedar, then walk down a jeep track to a low tongue of land at a bend in the river, where you will find old oaks and bluestem grassland.

The trailhead, information board, and self-pay station are by the gravel road that runs through the unit. This is the Bauer Trail, your return route for the last half mile of the hike. Step onto the road and around the metal gate. Look for the start of the Bamberger Trail on your left, leading off into the dappled shade of cedar trees. The first half mile of the hike undulates through the forest. Shade and birdsong accompany you through pristine nature.

A slight descent and a switchback bring you into a long, narrow field of grasses, broken only by the occasional cedar. It must have been cultivated relatively recently, as cactus and mesquite have yet to reclaim the meadow. The path, a jeep track, leads toward a deer blind at the far end of the field. Go through a gap in a fence line, reentering the forest, and in another 0.2 mile come to the junction with the Golden Cheeked Warbler Trail. Turn left here.

The landscape stays the same until, at 1.2 miles into the hike, the tracks veer right to follow a line of telephone wires down the hillside to a wash. Juniper trees crowd up against the fence to your left. Despite woods to the left and right, the trail is mostly exposed and will remain so for the rest of the hike. The last part of the descent is moderately steep but not rocky. Toward the bottom of the hill, you might hear the sounds of park visitors enjoying themselves in the river, which is very close at this point. You can

## Bamberger Trail

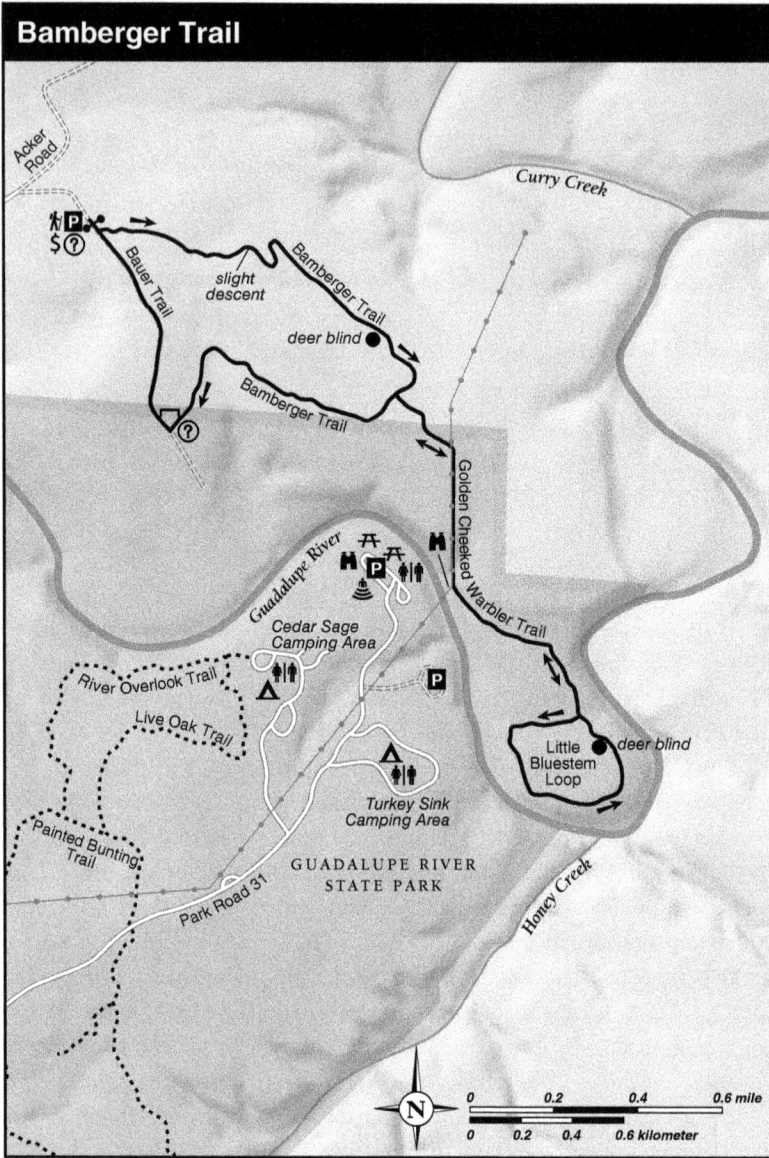

Curry Creek

Acker Road

Bauer Trail

slight descent

Bamberger Trail

deer blind

Bamberger Trail

Golden Cheeked Warbler Trail

Guadalupe River

Cedar Sage Camping Area

River Overlook Trail

Live Oak Trail

Little Bluestem Loop

deer blind

Turkey Sink Camping Area

Painted Bunting Trail

Park Road 31

GUADALUPE RIVER STATE PARK

Honey Creek

N

0     0.2     0.4     0.6 mile

0     0.2     0.4     0.6 kilometer

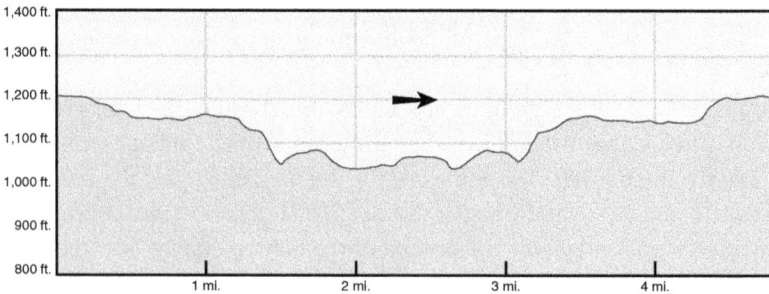

1,400 ft.
1,300 ft.
1,200 ft.
1,100 ft.
1,000 ft.
900 ft.
800 ft.

1 mi.     2 mi.     3 mi.     4 mi.

overlook the action from a bluff. The trail veers left, passing through live oak savanna at the bottom of the slope as it goes around the end of the hill.

Large boulders and more trees announce a change in ecosystem from savanna to riverside forest. Pass through the grove of ancient oaks, whose gnarled black trunks have twisted into monstrous shapes. Moss hangs from the branches. Dead trees lie rotting on the forest floor. At 2 miles emerge into the open, and turn right at the junction of the Little Bluestem Loop. Look for the bluestem grasses on the rise to your left as you head west on the first section of this loop.

Make a sharp left in a scrubby patch of cedar, and climb slightly onto the meadow proper, a flat field where butterflies, grasses, and flowering plants of all kinds flourish. The Guadalupe River is to your right, tantalizingly out of reach at the bottom of a wooded bank.

Cross a shallow drainage just before you come to the end of the Little Bluestem Loop, and turn right to retrace your steps up the hill to the junction with the Bamberger Trail. Turn left here. The trail follows a jeep track, the woods opening up here and there on either side. At 4.3 miles you will arrive at the grand junction with the Bauer Trail, the gravel road, where there are benches and another information board. Turn right here, and follow the road for the half mile or so back to the parking lot.

## Nearby Activities

The main section of Guadalupe River State Park has camping, picnic areas, and access to the Guadalupe River. Call the park to sign up for a tour of the adjacent Honey Creek State Natural Area, offered on Saturdays at 9 a.m.

---

**GPS TRAILHEAD COORDINATES**

**N29° 53' 7.1"  W98° 29' 46.1"**

From I-10 N, south of Boerne, take Exit 550 to Farm to Market Road 3351 north. Continue 15.3 miles, and turn right onto Edge Falls Road. After 2.3 miles turn right onto Acker Road, and follow it 2.2 miles to the park entrance, which will be on your right.

# 49 Cibolo Nature Center Hike

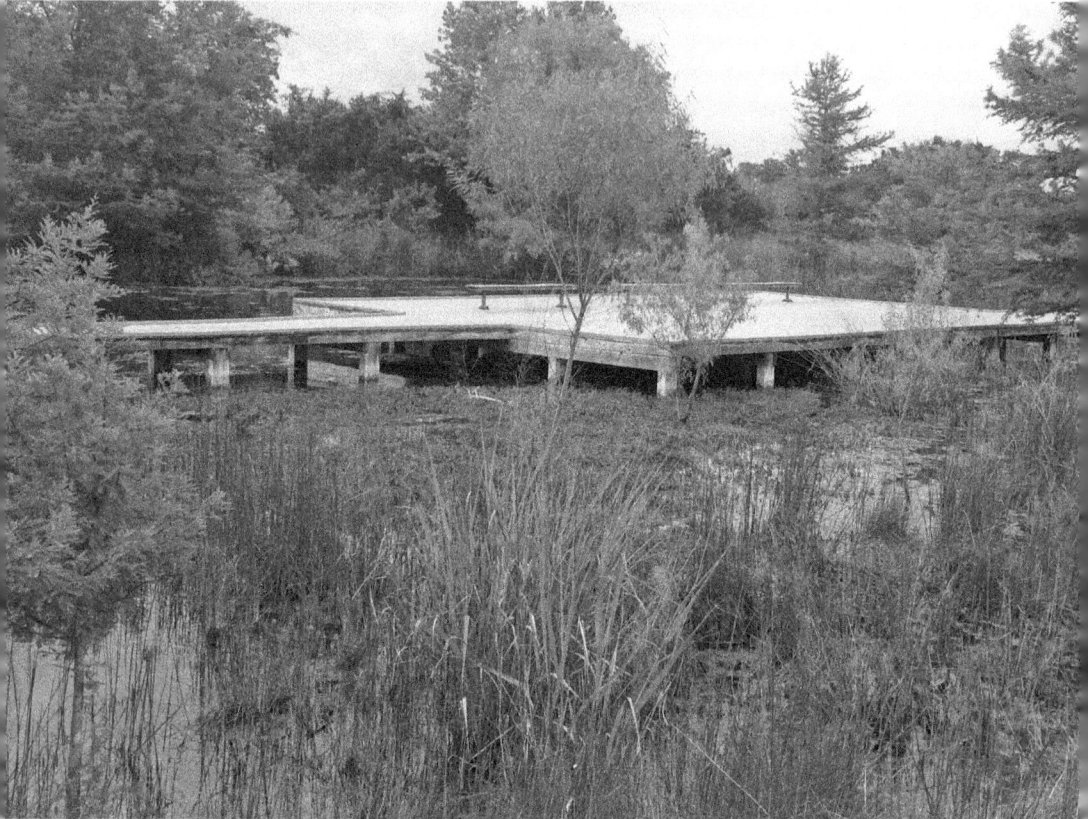

*A boardwalk at the Cibolo Nature Center*

## In Brief

A success story on every level, Boerne's Cibolo Nature Center protects 100 acres of wetland and riparian forest while welcoming more than 100,000 visitors a year. Education programs are available for adults and for children, who will love the wetland boardwalk and dinosaur tracks.

## Description

Never doubt the difference a few committed people can make. The Cibolo Creek Nature Center opened in 1990, thanks to the efforts of Carolyn and Brent Evans and some of their friends, and it now welcomes many thousands of visitors a year. The visitor center informs

**LENGTH:** 2 miles

**CONFIGURATION:** Loop

**DIFFICULTY:** Easy

**SCENERY:** Wetlands, prairie, creek, and woodlands

**EXPOSURE:** Very sunny–very shady

**TRAFFIC:** Moderate

**TRAIL SURFACE:** Grass, dirt, boardwalk

**HIKING TIME:** 1.5 hours

**DRIVING DISTANCE:** 31 miles from the Alamo

**ACCESS:** Daily, 8 a.m.–sunset; no fees required, but donations welcome

**WHEELCHAIR ACCESS:** Yes, in some sections

**MAPS:** At visitor center and trailheads

**FACILITIES:** Restrooms and picnic tables; water and gifts available at visitor center

**CONTACT INFORMATION:** 830-249-4616; cibolo.org

visitors about the area's distinct ecosystems and sells lists of birds found in the area as well as nature books on Texas. Programs for children and adults, including gardening workshops, help spread knowledge and understanding through the community.

Hikers can experience at least four different environments on a fairly short walk, from wetlands to wild creekside forest. This is a great place to bring friends you would like to introduce to hiking and the outdoors—it's the perfect introduction to the natural world. One word of caution: Until you reach the creekside forest, this hike is completely exposed to the elements, so be sure to wear or bring appropriate protective clothing.

You will pass the visitor center toward the end of the hike, but go there first if you want to get some more information about the hike before you start. Otherwise, find the trailhead to the right of the restrooms close to the parking lot. Plaques here display a map of the trail system, give ecological information, and explain the dinosaur tracks in front of you.

The Dinosaur Trackway is an exact copy of tracks that were uncovered in 1997 at a spillway at Boerne Lake after a flood. The spillway is inaccessible to the public, so Peggy Maceo, an Austin-area artist, was commissioned to make these copies for public view. Molds were made of the original prints and then cast in concrete and arranged to replicate the spillway site. The carnivore *Acrocanthosaurus* made the tracks—the same species that left tracks at Glen Rose and at Government Canyon in Helotes.

Walk past the trackway to a wooden bridge, and cross Spring Creek. Turn right, and head toward the wetlands. To your left, the tallgrass prairie stretches to the line of cypress trees along Cibolo Creek. Benches and nesting boxes have been placed in the field. Look for a bat house on the right.

At 0.1 mile keep right to make the Marsh Loop Trail. A sign announces this as the Wrede Marsh just before you step onto the boardwalk, which was built by students from the local high school. It leads to a deck standing over the pond. Three benches allow for contemplation of the aquatic life. The marsh area is home to cattle egret, redwing blackbirds, and kingfishers. Small cypress trees are the most prominent flora. The boardwalk

## Cibolo Nature Center Hike

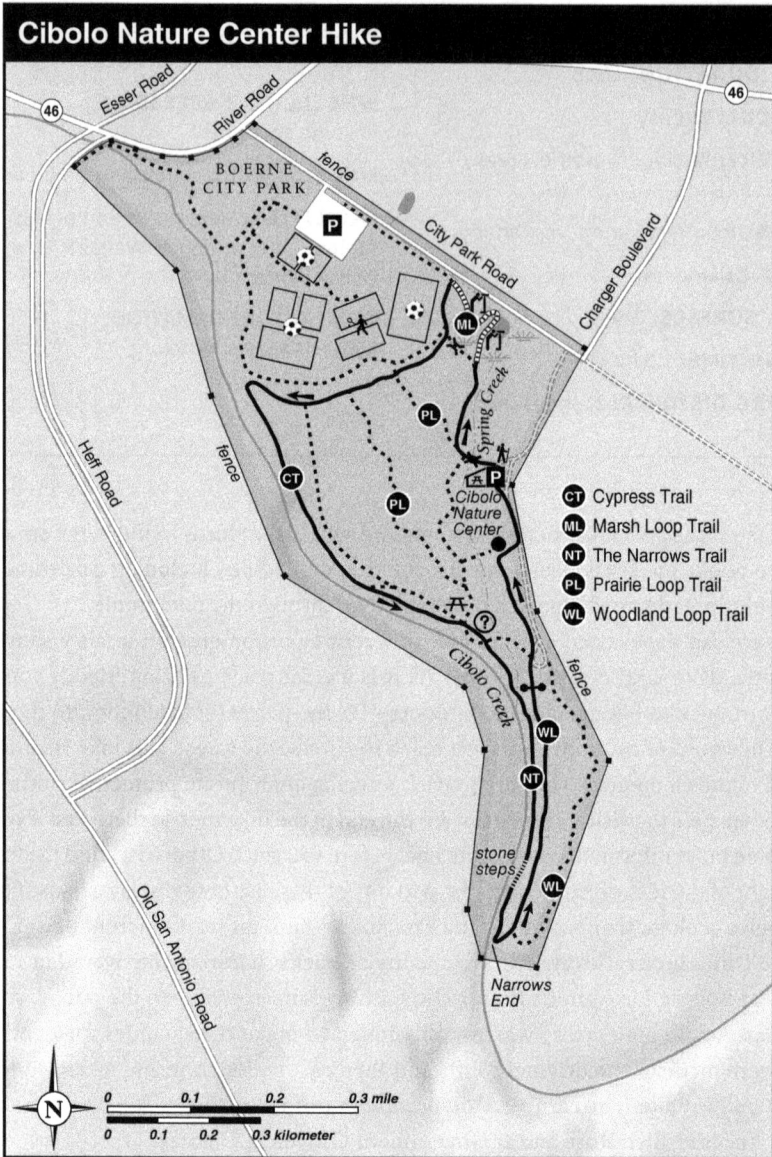

CT  Cypress Trail
ML  Marsh Loop Trail
NT  The Narrows Trail
PL  Prairie Loop Trail
WL  Woodland Loop Trail

loops around to another platform and ends by Boerne City Park. Turn left back toward the prairie, and briefly enjoy the intermittent shade of trees along the path.

Pass a bank on the right, and turn right toward the line of cypress trees. This part of the trail is called the Tree of Life Arboretum, and the bank has been planted with a variety of tree species. Follow the trail to the creek, passing the end of the Prairie Loop Trail and crossing a jeep track. Just before you turn left onto the Cypress Trail, look for an area at

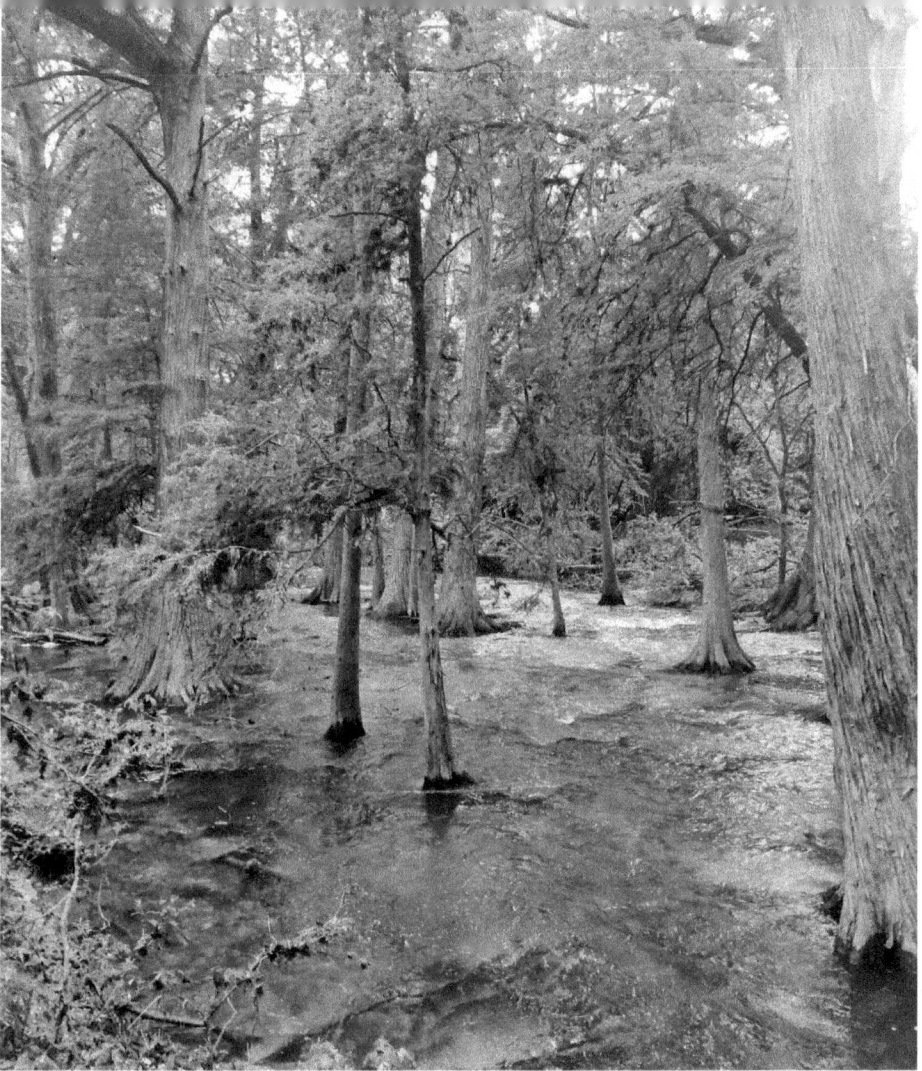

*Cibolo Creek*

the edge of the sports facility where an astonishing array of shrubs and flowering plants are growing; I saw mesquite, lavender, and lantana, to name but three.

The Cypress Trail follows the creek a few yards from the water, which is hard to glimpse behind the trees. These bald cypresses are giants, towering above the prairie. At 0.9 mile keep right at a fork, and keep on through the picnic area. Go left at the next fork, and pick up the jeep track. The jeep track shortly veers left; keep right on a dirt track, heading into the woods on The Narrows. You will notice a circle of stone seats on the left, seemingly awaiting some robed guru and his acolytes. This series of instructions reads as more complicated than it is; on the ground, you simply follow the creek and head into the forest.

For 0.4 mile the trail follows the creek edge through the woods—no problem seeing the water from this path. The scenery and terrain along The Narrows are surprisingly wild, and you will find yourself ducking under branches, pushing through overgrown vegetation, and scrambling over rocky areas. The creek tumbles over a series of pretty falls, and huge bald cypresses rise out of the water, which you will notice is very clear. The creek area is monitored by the Texas Stream Team and other groups and is regularly checked for quality as a critical source of recharge for the Edwards Aquifer. Anglers come here hoping to catch bass or catfish.

At 1.3 miles there is a grove of cypresses in a pool at a point where the creek splits to go around an island, a breathtakingly beautiful spot. It's not far from here to the end of the trail at the fence that marks the start of the Cibolo Preserve. Climb up the bank, and come to the Woodland Loop Trail. This level, gravel-covered trail leads back to the visitor center along the creek bluff, through shady oak and juniper woods. Look for American beautyberry and Mexican buckeye in the verdant underbrush. You might also glimpse deer and an armadillo, and you will certainly hear birds around you. You'll notice the high fence protecting the Cibolo Preserve to your right.

At 1.7 miles you will walk through a wooden gate that looks out of place and then come to a road at the end of a loop. The road's left fork goes down to the picnic area you passed earlier, and the right fork leads to the visitor center and parking lots, but there is a hiking trail between the two. Take this trail; it passes another picnic table and arrives at the main complex of buildings, including the administrative offices and the Education Center. Stop at the visitor center for a cold drink, and maybe sign up for an educational program or to volunteer.

## Nearby Activities

Cibolo Nature Center offers numerous continual outreach programs, and the facilities are available for rental. Boerne City Park offers soccer, swimming, and tennis.

---

### GPS TRAILHEAD COORDINATES

**N29° 46' 57.7"  W98° 42' 33.7"**

Follow I-10 west to Boerne, and take Exit 540. Turn right onto TX 46 East (West Bandera Road). Follow TX 46 for 2.4 miles, turning left at Business 87 (South Main Street), right at River Road, and then right again on City Park Road. After 0.2 mile, turn right and shortly arrive at the Nature Center.

# 50 **Dry Comal Nature Trail**

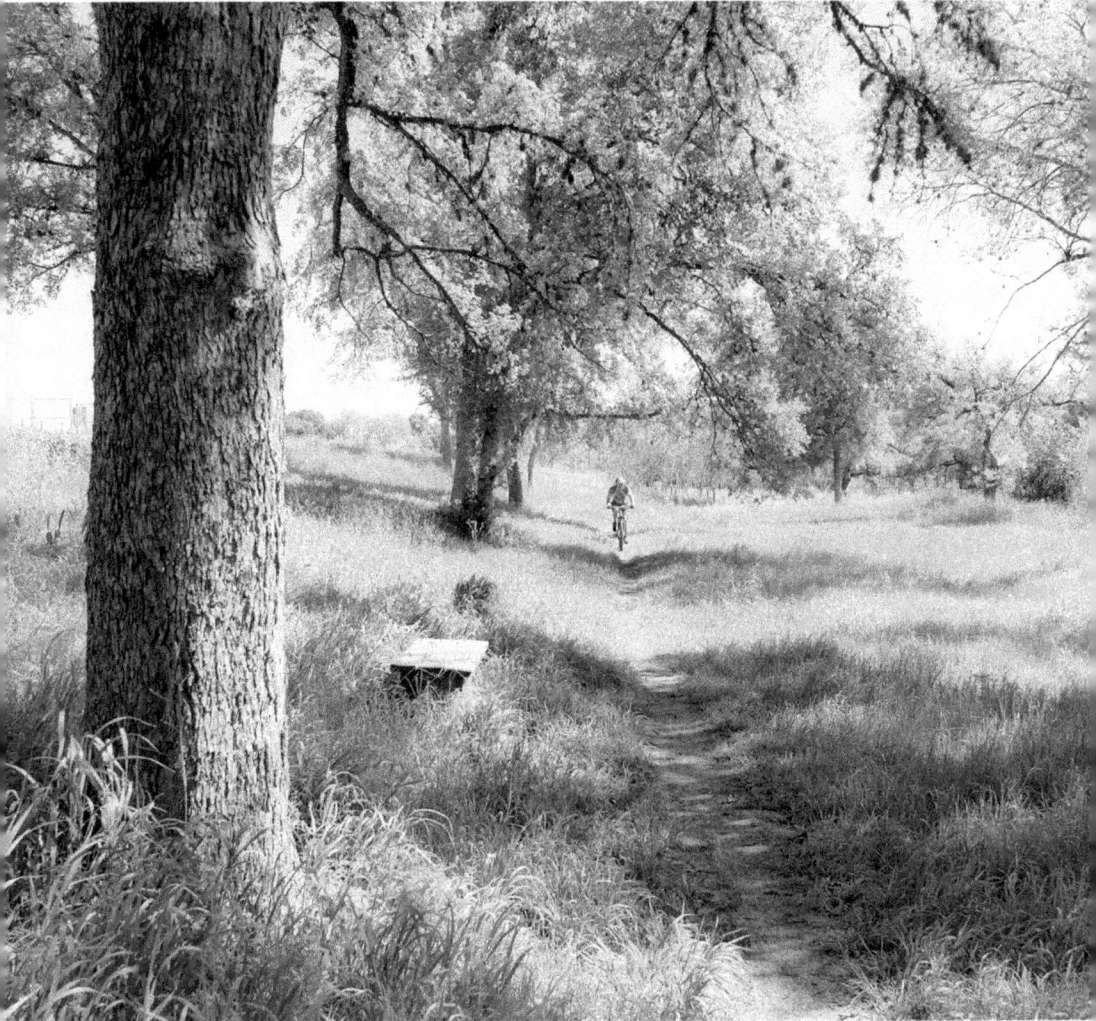

*Cyclists share the Dry Comal Nature Trail with hikers.*

## In Brief

This trail makes the most of the odd-shaped tract of land surrounding the Little League field. Hikers and bikers can wander along the creek and through dense woodland where the birdsong can be louder than the traffic on Landa Street.

| | |
|---|---|
| **LENGTH:** 1.6 miles (2.5 miles of track available) | **HIKING TIME:** 1 hour |
| **CONFIGURATION:** Balloon loop | **DRIVING DISTANCE:** 30 miles from the Alamo |
| **DIFFICULTY:** Easy | **ACCESS:** Daily, 6 a.m.–midnight; free |
| **SCENERY:** River bottom and woodland | **WHEELCHAIR ACCESS:** No |
| **EXPOSURE:** Mostly shady | **MAPS:** tinyurl.com/drycomal |
| **TRAFFIC:** Moderate | **FACILITIES:** None |
| **TRAIL SURFACE:** Natural surfaces | **CONTACT INFORMATION:** City of New Braunfels, 830-221-4000 |

## Description

Don't be put off by the large and unlovely Little League parking lot—step past the welcome sign, and follow the trail down and to the left; you will immediately be on a singletrack that follows the flat river bottom of Dry Comal Creek. Large clusters of reeds growing along the riverbank on your right are an example of the riverbed flora found in this part of the trail, which goes through at least three distinct habitats, as if the park were deliberately designed to showcase different environments found in the Hill Country.

The hike as described is 1.6 miles long, but there are a total of 2.5 miles of trail snaking the park. The wooded area in particular is crisscrossed by interconnected tracks by which you could extend or shorten your hike. Given that you can always see the baseball field or hear nearby traffic, it would be almost impossible to lose your way, but watch out for mountain bikers whizzing through the woods along the singletrack paths.

The creek wasn't dry when I last visited in the spring, and the valley was a lush grassland where birds flitted in and out of the bushes and trees dotting the meadow. The city has set wooden benches at intervals along the trail, where you can sit and observe the activity. The welcome sign mentions painted buntings, who live in Texas in the summer and like the deep brush along riverbanks, but many other species can be spotted here.

After 0.2 mile there's an easily missed junction. The left fork is the route by which you will return, so keep going straight along the widening creek valley for another 0.1 mile until you come to the edge of a creek—a tributary to the Dry Comal that flows in from the woodlands at the north end of the park. The trail turns left to follow the rocky bed of this watercourse. Larger trees shade the path, and a grass-covered bank slopes up toward the baseball field. At 0.3 mile you cross the stream under a big oak and step into the dappled shade of the forest, where you might imagine yourself many miles from any city. This deciduous wood is a delight for hikers and a haven for wildlife, including deer and many birds. Keep left at the next fork, and at 0.6 mile you will see a side trail that takes you to a bench located at the center of the woods. A sign invites you to listen for warblers, sparrows, kingbirds, and chickadees. I'm not sure which of these I was hearing on my visit, but their song was all around, and the purple flowers and strong scent of mountain laurel filled the woods.

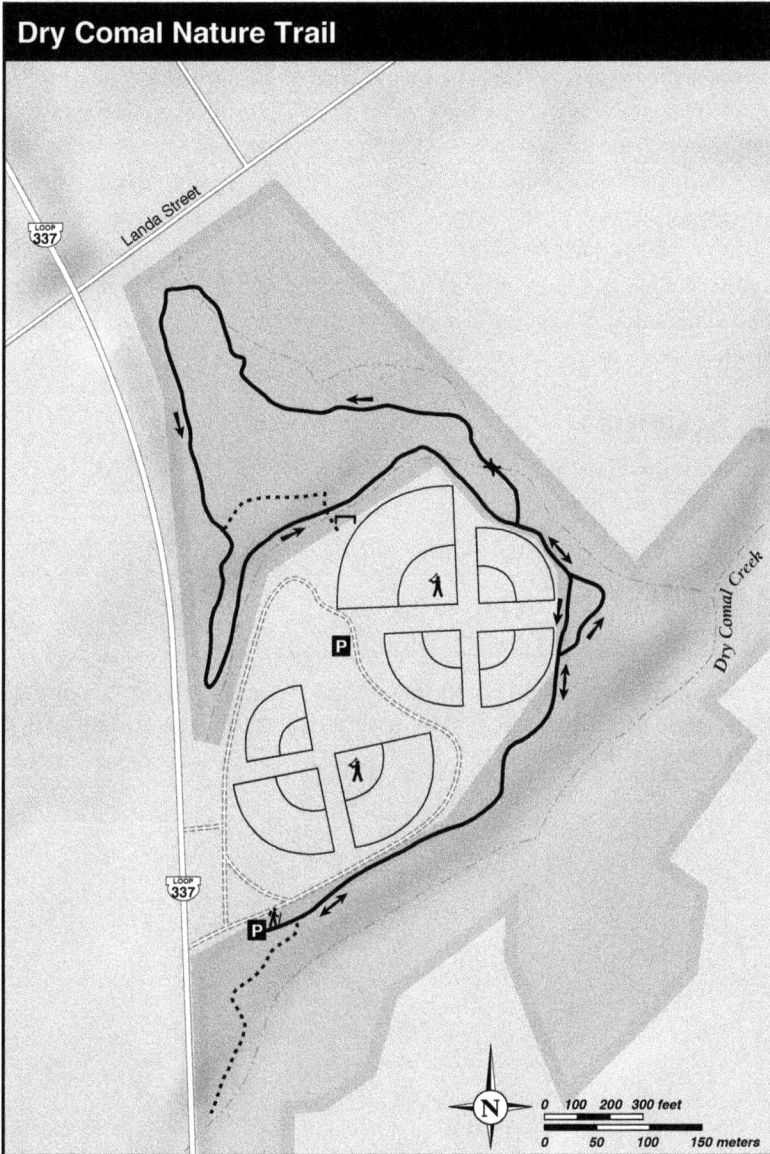

**Dry Comal Nature Trail**

It's not far from the bench to the loop's apex at Landa Street. At the next fork, take the right-hand track to stay on the perimeter of the park. Shadow TX Loop 337 as you head back toward the sports complex, crossing a shallow dip before making a right fork onto a short but quick descent into the narrow triangle of rockier ground at the western side of the parking lot. The grove of cedar and smaller trees signifies a change of habitat. The loop makes a sharp 180-degree turn at its point to exit out of this area. Climb back up the bank, keeping right at the next fork, and you soon come across a few benches placed between rock borders to fashion a little picnic area. To the right, a track leads across a wooden bridge back to the northern end of the parking lot.

Take the right-hand fork from the picnic area, and follow the edge of the baseball field. After 500 feet, keep right at the fork to walk right next to the perimeter fence, where you have a great vantage point if a game is in progress. Once past the field, you cross the top of the bank that slopes down to the creek on your left, walk through a glade of cedar elm trees to reenter the river bottom, and pick up the trail for the last 0.2 mile back to the parking lot.

Easily accessible and with options for undemanding hikes of different lengths, this network of trails offers a wonderful way to immerse yourself in nature whenever you need a quick pick-me-up.

## Nearby Activities

New Braunfels is home to the famous Schlitterbahn water park, and water lovers can also go tubing in the Comal River.

---

**GPS TRAILHEAD COORDINATES**

**N29° 41' 22.4"  W98° 9' 15.4"**

From San Antonio, take I-35 north to Exit 184. Head north on TX Loop 337 for 1.4 miles, and turn into the Little League parking lot. The trailhead is at the southern end of the lot.

---

# 51 Guadalupe River State Park Loop

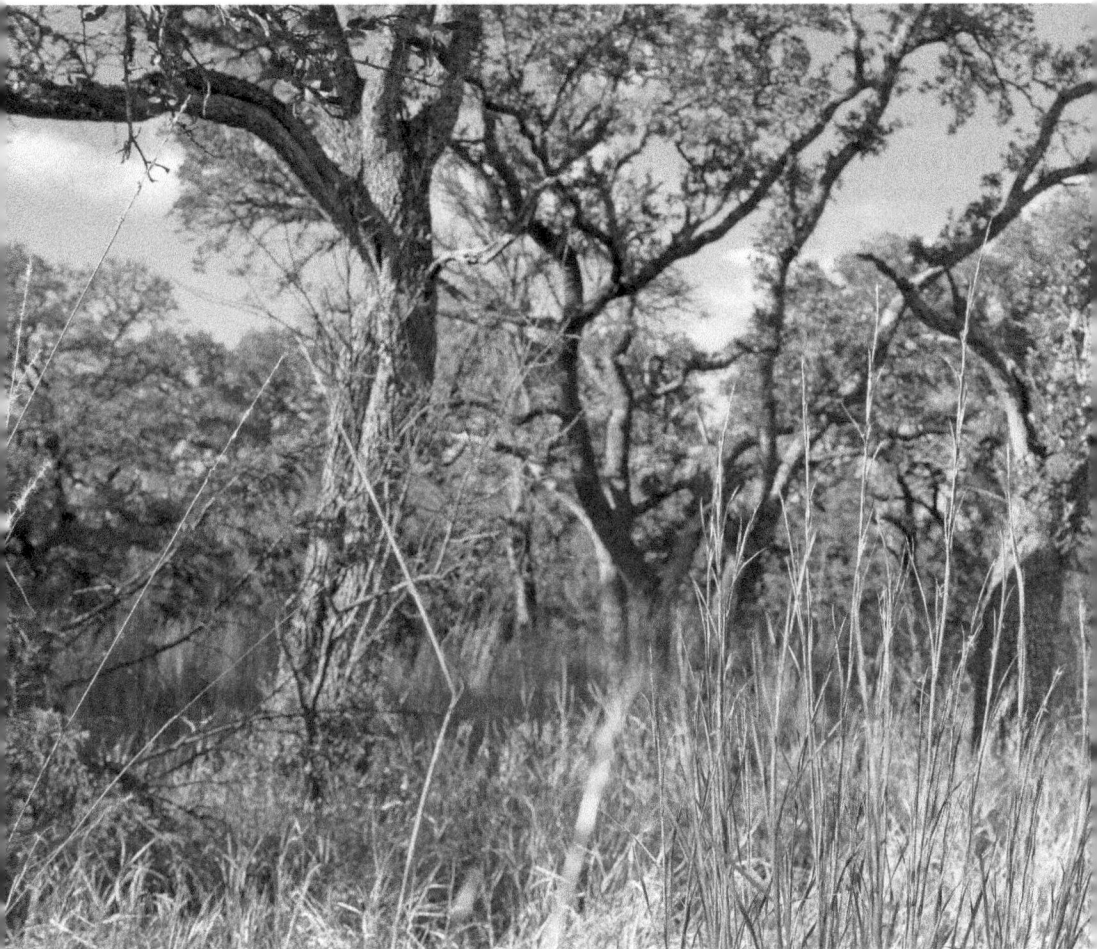

*Grasses and oak trees at Guadalupe River State Park*

## In Brief

Central Texans flock here to cool off in the Guadalupe River, but the park also offers easy hiking on multiuse trails that loop through live oak savanna and along bluffs above the river.

| | |
|---|---|
| **LENGTH:** 2.7 miles | **ACCESS:** Daily, 8 a.m.–10 p.m.; $7 entrance fee per person over age 13; closed for public hunts |
| **CONFIGURATION:** Loop | |
| **DIFFICULTY:** Easy | **WHEELCHAIR ACCESS:** No |
| **SCENERY:** Open and wooded hills, river bluff | **MAPS:** tinyurl.com/guadaluperiver loopmap |
| **EXPOSURE:** Mostly open | **FACILITIES:** Restrooms, water, and picnicking in park; none at trailhead |
| **TRAFFIC:** Moderate, busy on weekends | |
| **TRAIL SURFACE:** Natural surfaces | **CONTACT INFORMATION:** 830-438-2656; tpwd.texas.gov/state-parks/ guadalupe-river |
| **HIKING TIME:** 1.5 hours | |
| **DRIVING DISTANCE:** 37 miles from the Alamo | |

## Description

A popular spot for all types of outdoor enthusiasts, Guadalupe River State Park retains its rugged beauty in spite of the large number of visitors it receives. The park includes 4 miles of river frontage, multiple campsites, and day-use areas. During the summer months, it is almost sure to be full to capacity because of the allure of the cold river. The best times to visit during this season would be early in the week and as early in the morning as possible.

While most park visitors will be down by the water, the trail system mostly stays on the less-visited live oak savanna, and this loop is no exception. The hike does take in views of the river from high bluffs. These uplands are wooded grassland, and the trails are stony. The paths are open to mountain bikers and equestrians, though the equestrians have their own separate trailhead near the park entrance station.

From the parking lot a half mile beyond the entrance station, head north on the Painted Bunting Trail, traveling on wide doubletrack amid scattered oaks and the occasional stand of juniper. Cacti grow among the grasses. Before long, you pass the first of many hunting blinds. Public hunts in the fall and winter control the native white-tailed deer population and help eliminate exotic species such as wild hogs and axis deer, an Asian native. Be sure to check the dates if you plan to visit during those seasons.

Soon you come to a telephone line and the boundary fence, which the path follows north for a while, beginning the overall downgrade that continues to the farthest point of the hike. Tunnel through a coppice of live oaks, whose widespread branches shade the path. At 0.4 mile the path veers right through an open meadow, where it meets the River Overlook Trail, another jeep track. Turn left on the River Overlook Trail, keeping north toward the Guadalupe River through a mix of oak groves and stony meadows, shadowing the fence line. A little climb takes you away from a wash.

At the 1-mile mark, you reach the bluff above the Guadalupe River. The rocky track curves right, keeping the river to your left. You are heading downstream—the water flows

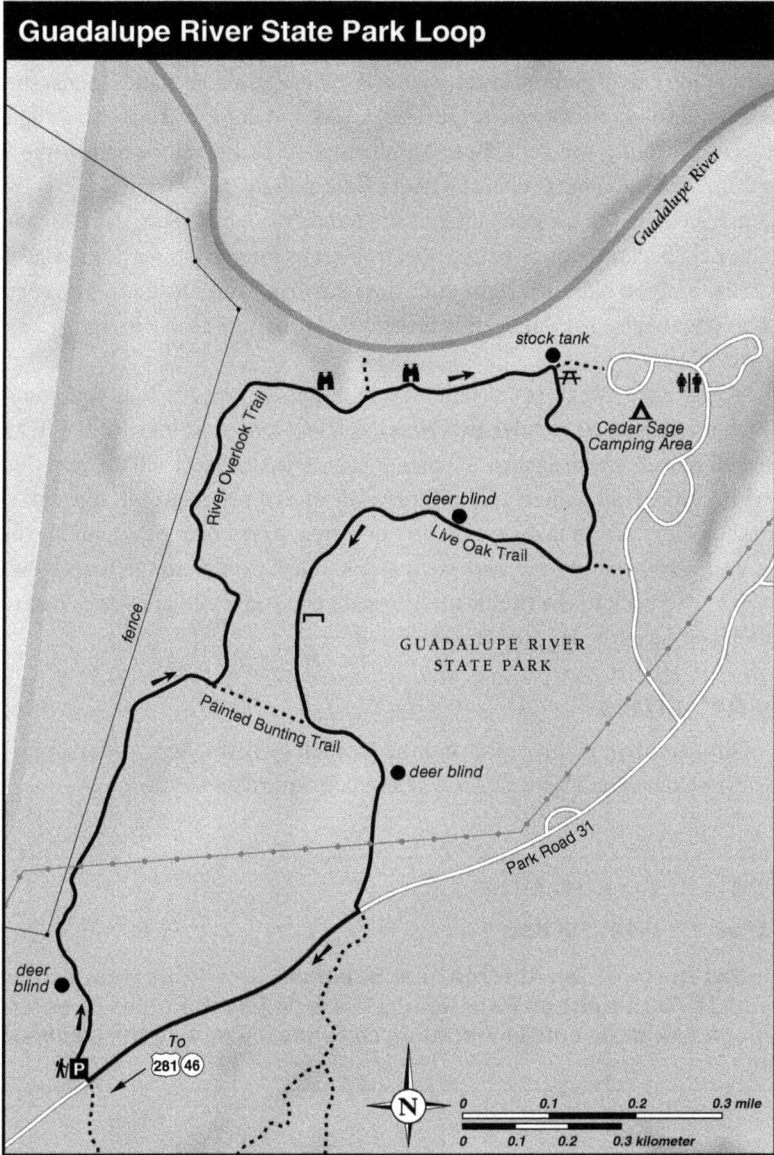

## Guadalupe River State Park Loop

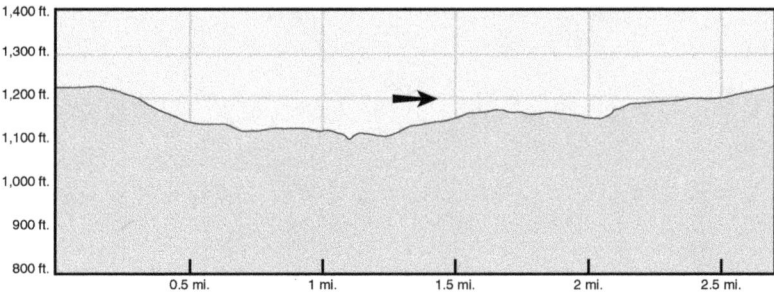

east 100 feet below. Spur paths lead to wooded dark outcrops with views of the winding Guadalupe, though signs remind you to stay on the marked trails. Cypress trees line the banks below, while gravel gathers in the shallows. Fallen boulders stand against the flow, which has eroded these bluffs over centuries. Hawks and vultures soar along the edges, and swallows flit around the rock face. An abandoned ranch stands across the water, accessible from the Hofheinz Trail in the Bauer Unit of the park.

At 1.3 miles you will see a stock tank. A shaded picnic table, set under the canopy of a gnarled live oak, beckons you to pause. The trail keeps forward to reach the Cedar Sage Camping Area, but you will turn right onto the Live Oak Trail for the return portion of the hike. This path begins to climb gently toward the main park road through grassy glens and dense woodlands.

Turn sharply right, west, at 1.5 miles, picking up the jeep track as you come back onto the higher savanna. At 2 miles two benches allow a modest view of the Texas Hill Country. A rail to lean a bike against is a nice touch. At 2.1 miles reach the junction with the Painted Bunting Trail, where you will turn left onto a rougher path through an oak motte. Another short ascent takes you to an open area, past a deer blind, under the telephone line again, and then to the park road at 2.4 miles. Complete the loop by walking along the park road back to the trailhead. Alternatively, you could cross the road to continue around the rest of the Painted Bunting Trail.

## Nearby Activities

The park offers camping, picnic areas, and the Guadalupe River. Sign up for a tour of the adjacent Honey Creek State Natural Area, offered on Saturdays at 9 a.m.

---

### GPS TRAILHEAD COORDINATES

**N29° 51' 38.5"  W98° 29' 59.1"**

From US 281 north of San Antonio near Bulverde, take TX 46 west 7 miles to Park Road 31. Turn right on Park Road 31, and follow it 3 miles to enter the park. Once beyond the entrance station, continue 0.6 mile to the trailhead on your left.

---

# 52 Guadalupe River Trail

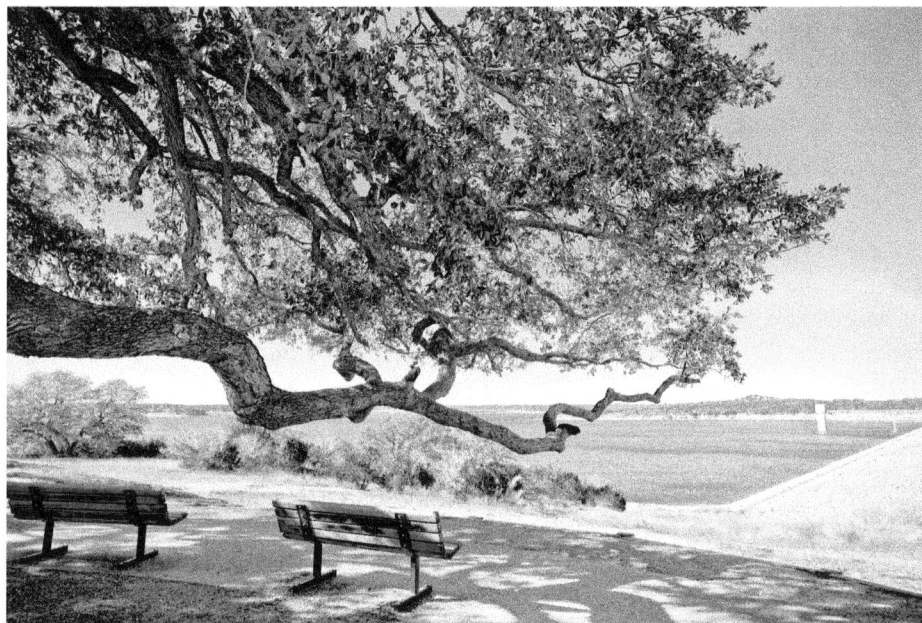

*Overlooking Canyon Lake along the Guadalupe River Trail*

## In Brief

The Canyon Lake Tailrace offers anglers the best fly-fishing in the state and hikers a quiet getaway through the woods along the Guadalupe River. The walk offers a chance to learn the names of various species of riparian flora.

## Description

Cold water roars out of the bottom of the Canyon Lake spillway, cold enough that rainbow trout can live here throughout the year. As such, the tailrace is extremely popular with fly-fishers, but apart from that solitary breed, most visitors stay in the parking lot to gaze from the fence at the mesmerizing flow. As such, this unlikely trail close to one of the state's busiest recreation areas is not much used. It offers respite from summer heat as well as river access, and because it doesn't really go anywhere, it is perfect for an unstructured amble through the woods. For birders and nature watchers, it is a small oasis of tranquility located in one of the busiest summertime getaway spots in the state. It's also an interpretive trail—you can find the guide to the numbered signs at tinyurl.com/guadalupetrailsguide.

**LENGTH:** 2 miles

**CONFIGURATION:** Out-and-back

**DIFFICULTY:** Moderate

**SCENERY:** Lush woods, Guadalupe River

**EXPOSURE:** Shady

**TRAFFIC:** Light

**TRAIL SURFACE:** Gravel, dirt, roots

**HIKING TIME:** 40 minutes

**DRIVING DISTANCE:** 57 miles from the Alamo

**ACCESS:** Daily, sunrise–sunset; no fees or permits required

**WHEELCHAIR ACCESS:** No

**MAPS:** tinyurl.com/guadalupetrailsmap

**FACILITIES:** None

**CONTACT INFORMATION:** 830-964-3341; www.swf-wc.usace.army.mil/canyon

I recommend using the guide because this short hike is the perfect opportunity to brush up on your tree knowledge. It has one note that you will want to know about: "The interrupting sound of a siren indicates that the water level may be altered and a detour up the hill may be necessary."

The path begins at the sign at the far end of the parking lot. Only the wooden frame remains, and a nearby bench is missing its seat, but the trail itself is well maintained, at least for the first part. A gravel path bordered with wooden beams descends some steps into the shade of the trees. The path stays in the dense riparian woodland along the riverbank for most of its length, and though the river is barely visible through the tangle of leaves and trunks, the sound of water is always present. From the guide you can learn to identify pecan, cedar, hackberry, buckeye, persimmon, and Mexican buckeye as you make your way through the forest.

At the bottom of the first descent, there is a bridge over a sheer earth ravine that looks torn open. The wooden bridge has been damaged, so you must use the diversion around it. It's hard to imagine the force of the water that has carved such a gash in the few yards between the floodplain and the river.

The trail continues down the steep riverbank. Spur trails lead off to good angling spots, no doubt. Shortly you come to the river's edge at a wooden boardwalk. On my last visit, soon after the floods of 2015, water was lapping over the end of the boardwalk, and a section of the trail was underwater. Because there is an established unofficial track connecting to the point where the trail resurfaces, it seems that this is not an unusual occurrence.

At just over 0.1 mile there are three benches set at a river overlook. This might be as far as you want to go; it's very peaceful sitting here enjoying the sounds of the birds and the flowing water, watching wading birds and anglers play in the river. You will see squirrels, cardinals, and possibly deer feeding along the path.

From here, the path loses the gravel for a natural surface, though the retaining logs stay. A wooden bridge over another wash is the lowest point of the hike, before some steps mark the beginning of an ascent away from the riverbank. There's another bench at the top of this climb and the sound of wind chimes from a house across the river. The

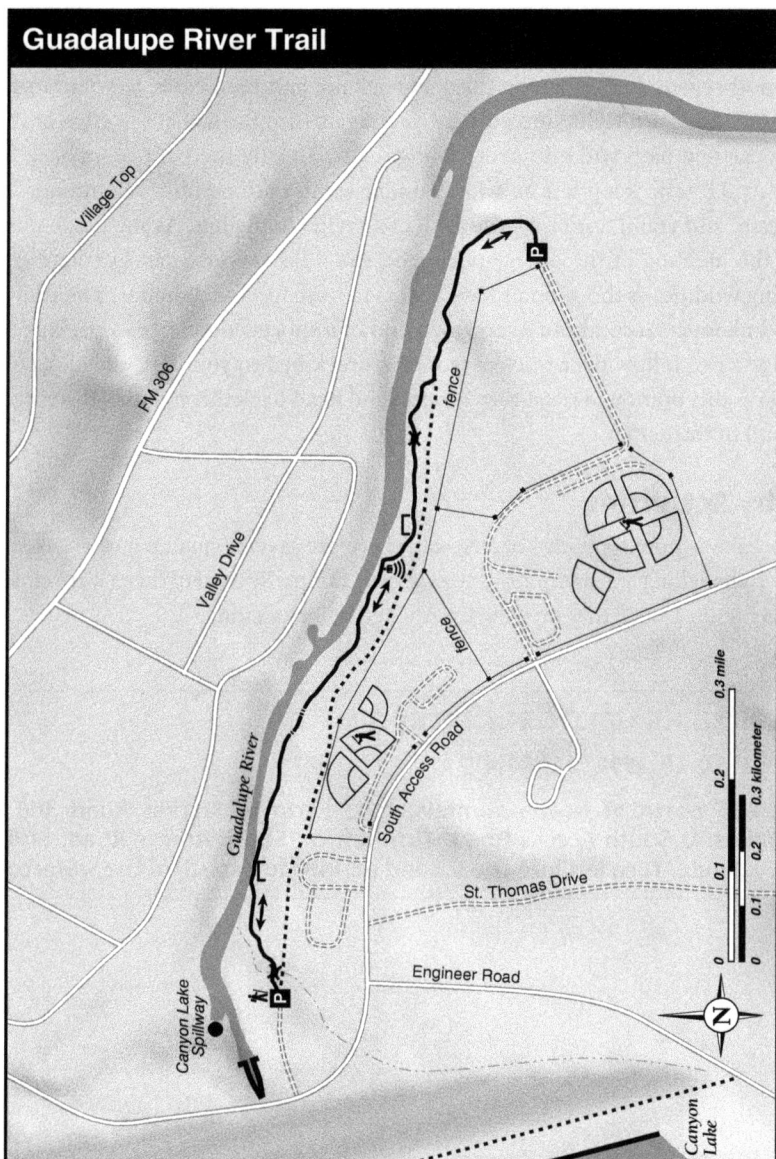

Guadalupe River Trail

lawns and terraces lining the other bank seem to belong to another world compared to the tangle of impenetrable creepers and limbs on this side.

At the half-mile point, you pass a huge cypress, and the path climbs again. A side trail leads back to the right at the top of some wooden steps. Take it a few yards, and you'll find a disused open-air amphitheater or lecture hall. A few benches are arranged above an overlook that makes a small stage—what this setup was for, I have no idea.

The trail steps out of the woods at a bench. A jeep track runs along the edge of the field, but our path makes another plunge back into the forest down yet more steps. Cross another wooden bridge on the way back up, and then come to some stone steps at a T-junction. Turn right, and emerge once again into the sun at the edge of the field, onto an earthen path and into cedar and grasses. Shortly the path veers back into the woods. At 0.8 mile keep left at a fork, under some cottonwoods. Come out into the open again, and you'll notice a large gash of a ravine to the left. As the guide notes, this area at the meeting of the open prairie and the thick woods is an excellent place for observing wildlife, as the animals have access to both food and shelter. The trail follows a chain-link fence around the overgrown end of a sports complex to a parking lot, and though you can follow deer tracks across the creek bed to your left, they lead only to a fence, so at this point you must turn around and head back through this thriving strip of woodland to the dam.

## Nearby Activities

Canyon Lake is popular with boaters, and there are several small parks on its shoreline that offer picnicking and camping as well as boat ramps. Several of these were closed after the 2015 floods. Check that they have reopened before visiting.

---

**GPS TRAILHEAD COORDINATES**

**N29° 52' 10.1"  W98° 11' 39.4"**

From I-35 north of New Braunfels, take Farm to Market Road 306 west 14.2 miles to South Access Road. Turn left on South Access Road, and continue 0.5 mile. Turn left into the second parking lot, south of the watercourse.

# 53 Hightower Trail

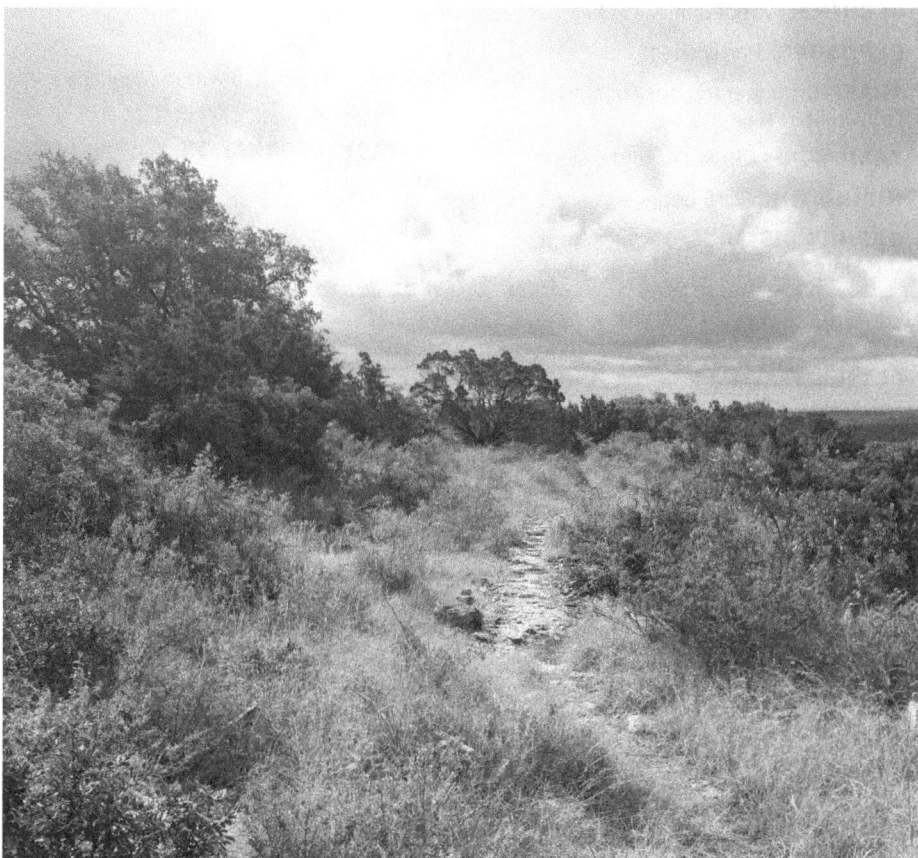

*The Hightower Trail leads you through typical Hill Country terrain.*

## In Brief

This fine loop around the southern tip of Hill Country State Natural Area has something for everybody—lonesome summit country, ranching history, views from Comanche Bluffs, and Chaquita Falls on West Verde Creek.

## Description

The views from Comanche Bluffs and the peaceful plashing of Chaquita Falls are the cherries on top of this satisfying hike through the Hill Country State Natural Area. The trail follows one old road up to high ground, then cuts across the brow to meet another.

**LENGTH:** 4.5 miles

**CONFIGURATION:** Loop

**DIFFICULTY:** Moderate

**SCENERY:** Wooded hills, creek

**EXPOSURE:** Partly shady

**TRAFFIC:** Moderate; busy on spring and fall weekends

**TRAIL SURFACE:** Rocks and dirt

**HIKING TIME:** 2.75 hours

**DRIVING DISTANCE:** 57 miles from the Alamo

**ACCESS:** Daily; office hours are 8 a.m.–5 p.m.; $6 day-use fee per person over age 13

**WHEELCHAIR ACCESS:** No

**MAPS:** tinyurl.com/hcsnamap

**FACILITIES:** Bottled water, privy at park headquarters

**CONTACT INFORMATION:** 830-796-4413; tpwd.texas.gov/state-parks/hill-country

This second track leads down to West Verde Creek and the way back. You walk through a slow unfolding of unspoiled Hill Country terrain, with juniper coppices predominating on the way up and at the top and denser, more varied woods covering the slopes on the way down. As you hike, you will encounter many reminders that, not that long ago, the area was a working ranch. Many things to contemplate and much beauty all around make this one of the best hikes in the state.

The Hightower Trail begins near the mailbox at the park headquarters. Trails at the park are marked with numbered plastic posts; this trail is number 8. Begin the hike with a climb away from the Bar-O Day Use Area. The limestone scrabble and the mix of grassland and juniper thickets are familiar Hill Country territory. Pass through the first ranch relic, a fence line, where you can take a look back at the Twin Peaks behind you. The path drops down into a little valley and crosses a wash. At 0.3 mile keep right at a fork to stay on Trail 8. To the left is Trail 8A, by which you will return.

Continue up the partly wooded hillside. The next 0.7 mile follows the doubletrack ranch road to a lonely tin barn set on a narrow spur, drifting through juniper groves and live oak mottes. Occasional open areas allow glimpses of the vistas to the west, but mostly the topography limits your horizon to the tops of the surrounding trees, allowing you to hike in a meditative frame of mind while observing the shifts in terrain and the plant life in this textbook Hill Country landscape.

At almost 1 mile, you come to the next set of ranch exhibits at the top of the hill. The path comes to another fence line, and then to a large tin barn. The breeze and the shorter cedar trees and scrubby bushes covering the rocky grassland are telltale signs of a summit, though even up here the vegetation blocks the view. Cut through a second gap in the fence, and descend into a grassy swale before climbing toward a small transmission line.

Turn left, and follow the poles to top a second hill, the hike's high point, a foot lower than Twin Peaks. The trail narrows and veers away from the line for a spell, then at 1.5 miles starts a very rocky downgrade. Boulders, pebbles, and stones of every size cover the trail. Ahead of you at the bottom of the hill is a water tower and other ranch remains.

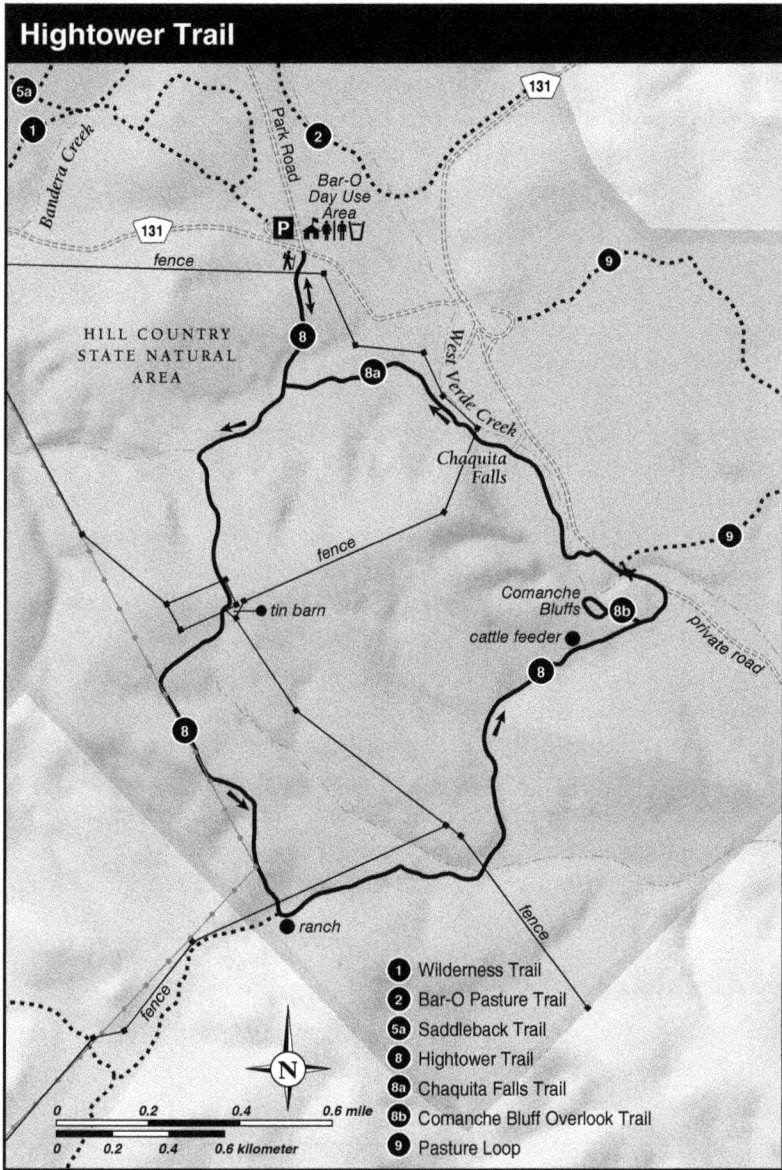

# Hightower Trail

HILL COUNTRY
STATE NATURAL
AREA

Bandera Creek

Park Road

Bar-O
Day Use
Area

West Verde Creek

Chaquita
Falls

fence

tin barn

Comanche
Bluffs

cattle feeder

private road

ranch

fence

N

1 Wilderness Trail
2 Bar-O Pasture Trail
5a Saddleback Trail
8 Hightower Trail
8a Chaquita Falls Trail
8b Comanche Bluff Overlook Trail
9 Pasture Loop

0   0.2   0.4   0.6 mile
0   0.2   0.4   0.6 kilometer

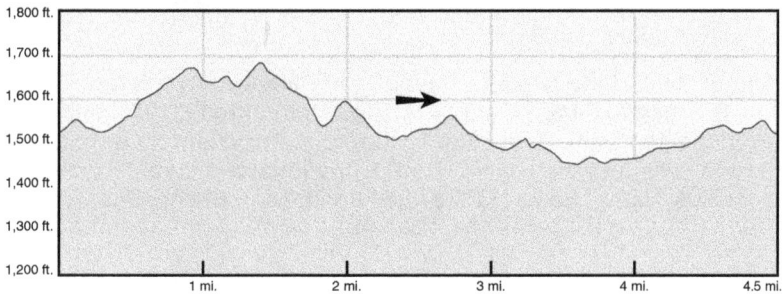

1,800 ft.
1,700 ft.
1,600 ft.
1,500 ft.
1,400 ft.
1,300 ft.
1,200 ft.

1 mi.   2 mi.   3 mi.   4 mi.   4.5 mi.

Descend and find a stock tank, a metal shed, and a corral close to the water well. This distant vale must once have been a center of activity. Now the only sounds are birds and the constant hum of insects. The trail turns left along a fence line and picks up the second ranch road, which undulates northeast past Comanche Bluffs to the road along West Verde Creek valley. Climb over a spur, and drop into a locale where two rocky washes converge; then shadow the second streambed up to a gap in a ridgeline. The hills to the right of the path are thickly wooded and lovely. Green treetops meet the blue sky.

Views over West Verde Creek valley open up as you descend from the second ridge. Pass a rock shelf and a pond to your right at 2.7 miles, and keep your eyes open for a side trail leading left. A sign points to the Comanche Bluffs. This path leads to these high cliffs that shade clear pools at a bend in the creek; there are views both up and down the valley. Huge oaks grow along the opposite bank. Behind them, more trees shade the Comanche Bluffs Camping Area. To the right is the low-water bridge that you will shortly cross.

Backtrack and descend to a road. To the right is the park boundary and beyond that the Davenport Ranch. Turn left and cross the bridge, the low point of the hike. An old barn and a ranch house, called the Chapa house, are to your right in the park's group camp area.

Continue along the road for a few yards, past the Comanche Bluffs parking area, and then turn left onto a path that is signed as Trail 9. Arrive at the creek. Trail 8A continues on the other side of the creek—you might get your feet wet at this crossing. (According to the park map, 8A starts at the path leading back past campsite 121. This does lead to a pleasant pool in the creek but ends there.)

Stroll along the creek in the shade of the riparian woods, and at 3.7 miles come to Chaquita Falls, where you may want to stop and cool off. Along the way, signs point to sites in the Chaquita Falls Camp Area. Look for high bluffs to your left, beyond the flat camping area. The trail starts to climb away from the creek, and at 4 miles it turns west and heads back to the junction with Trail 8. Turn right here, and backtrack a third of a mile to the trailhead.

## Nearby Activities

Hill Country State Natural Area offers walk-in tent camping, backpacking, bicycling, and horseback riding.

---

### GPS TRAILHEAD COORDINATES

**N29° 37' 37.5"  W99° 10' 51.8"**

From San Antonio, take TX 16 to Bandera. In Bandera, turn left on TX 173 S, following it 1 mile to Ranch Road 1077. Turn right onto FR 1077, and follow it 10 miles to the park, where the road turns to dirt. Turn right in the park, across West Verde Creek, and then again into the headquarters area. The trailhead is directly across County Road 131 (Tarpley Road) from the headquarters.

# 54 Hill Country Cougar Canyon Trek

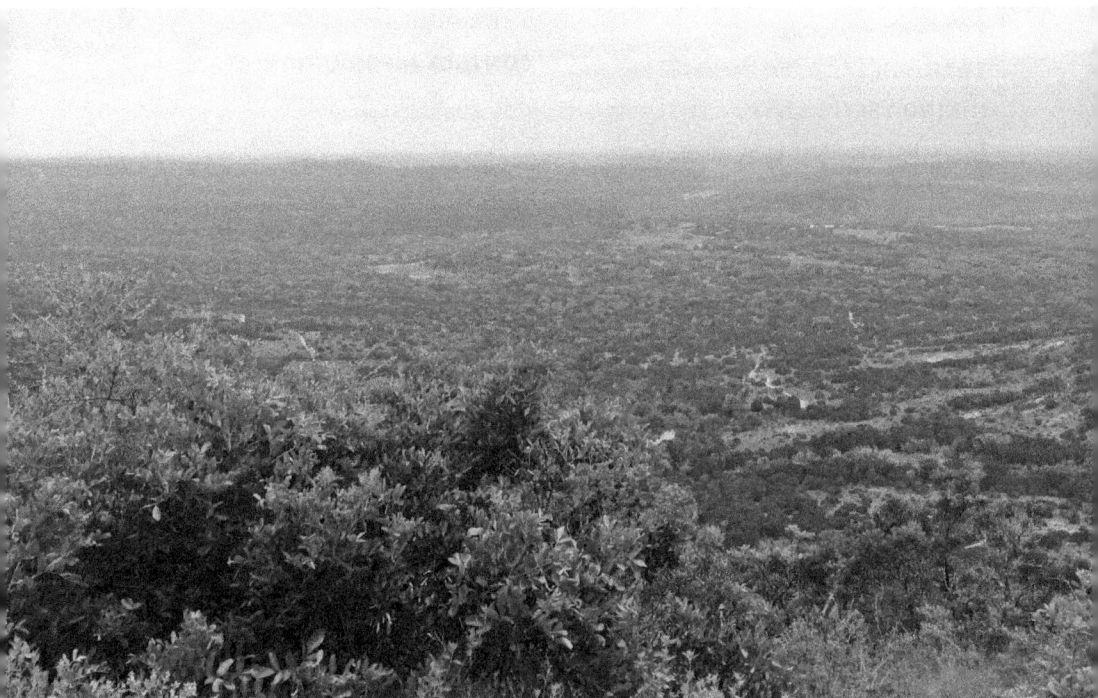

*A Hill Country vista from a high point in the Hill Country State Natural Area*

## In Brief

This demanding hike takes in the far elevations of the Hill Country State Natural Area, reaching three successively higher ridges. Start out in the West Verde Creek valley, and scout the park's more remote regions. You'll pass backcountry campsites and plunge into Cougar Canyon. A long downgrade takes you back to the trailhead.

## Description

This is one of the best—if by best you mean wild, scenic, and challenging—hikes in the entire Hill Country, taking you across terrain for which the word rugged was invented. From the wide West Verde Creek valley, you will climb up eroded hillsides onto limestone mesas with views across miles of rock and cedar. Advanced backpackers might

**LENGTH:** 10.3 miles

**CONFIGURATION:** Loop

**DIFFICULTY:** Difficult

**SCENERY:** Wooded and open hills, canyons, creek bottomland

**EXPOSURE:** Mostly open

**TRAFFIC:** Moderate

**TRAIL SURFACE:** Dirt, rocks

**HIKING TIME:** 5.5 hours

**DRIVING DISTANCE:** 57 miles from the Alamo

**ACCESS:** Daily; office hours are 8 a.m.–5 p.m.; $6 day-use fee per person over age 13

**WHEELCHAIR ACCESS:** No

**MAP:** tinyurl.com/hcsnamap

**FACILITIES:** Bottled water, privy at park headquarters

**CONTACT INFORMATION:** 830-796-4413; tpwd.texas.gov/state-parks/hill-country

consider making this an overnight hike, as the route passes two backcountry camping areas. Trails are open to hikers, bikers, and equestrians, with whom the park is extremely popular. Hikers and bikers must yield to horses.

Leave the parking area, and continue along the gravel access road up the West Verde Creek valley. At 0.2 mile turn right onto Trail 6 (Spring Branch). Though trails are named on the map, marker posts at trail junctions show only the numbers. Follow the hedge line across a broken pasture to meet Trail 2 (Bar-O Pasture). Turn left here. West Verde Creek is on your right, and the hills of Twin Peaks are to the left across the meadow. Birdsong fills the air. Trail 2B (Prairie Loop) leaves right; keep forward to meet Trail 2A (Creek Bottom) at 0.4 mile. Turn right here, immediately stepping over the creek bed, a deep channel gouged out by many floods. Begin to tunnel through the thick Ashe juniper forest growing in the sandy soil bordering the boundary fence.

At just over a mile, a gate leads out of the park to the private Hill Country Equestrian Lodge. Veer left here, and then find a quick right turn onto a singletrack path. Do not go forward on the wide roadbed, as you will find yourself back on the park road. The correct trail goes over a small berm and passes an old pond bed to the right.

Ahead, the woods open a bit. Songbirds accompany the deep green of the juniper and the brighter hues of the deciduous trees, and this array contrasts with the brownish grass and blue Texas sky. At about 1.4 miles the track starts to climb, and the woods thin out. At 1.6 miles, in a slight clearing, you'll meet Trail 3 (Hermit's Trace) coming in from the left. Continue forward on Trail 3, clambering over broken terrain as you go around the peaks to your right, which are outside the park boundary. At several points, brush piles block wrong turns. Climb over a couple of deep washes to reach a trail junction at 2.1 miles; turn right, picking up Trail 3A (Good Luck), where the the gloves come off. The steep ascent will remind you why it is called Hill Country. The junipers offer enough space between them to allow views all around, as well as the knowledge that you are heading into a bowl encircled by ridges. At 2.4 miles the trail levels off along the contour, and you get a view across the northern end of the park to the interlocking folds of spur and canyon you will soon be exploring.

## Hill Country Cougar Canyon Trek

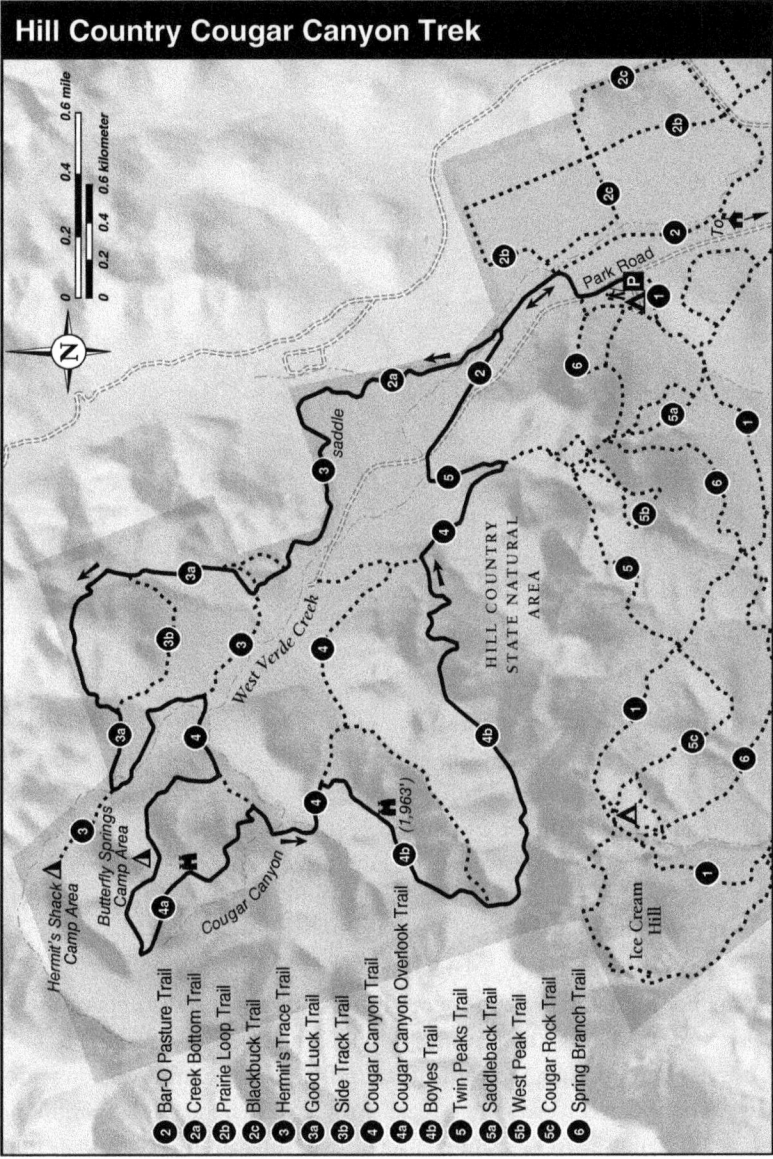

**2** Bar-O Pasture Trail
**2a** Creek Bottom Trail
**2b** Prairie Loop Trail
**2c** Blackbuck Trail
**3** Hermit's Trace Trail
**3a** Good Luck Trail
**3b** Side Track Trail
**4** Cougar Canyon Trail
**4a** Boyles Trail
**4b** Cougar Canyon Overlook Trail
**5** Twin Peaks Trail
**5a** Saddleback Trail
**5b** West Peak Trail
**5c** Cougar Rock Trail
**6** Spring Branch Trail

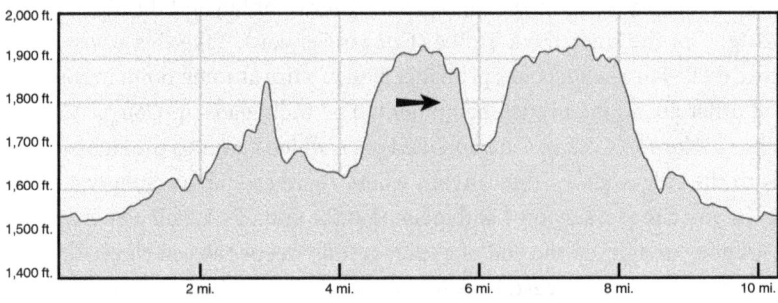

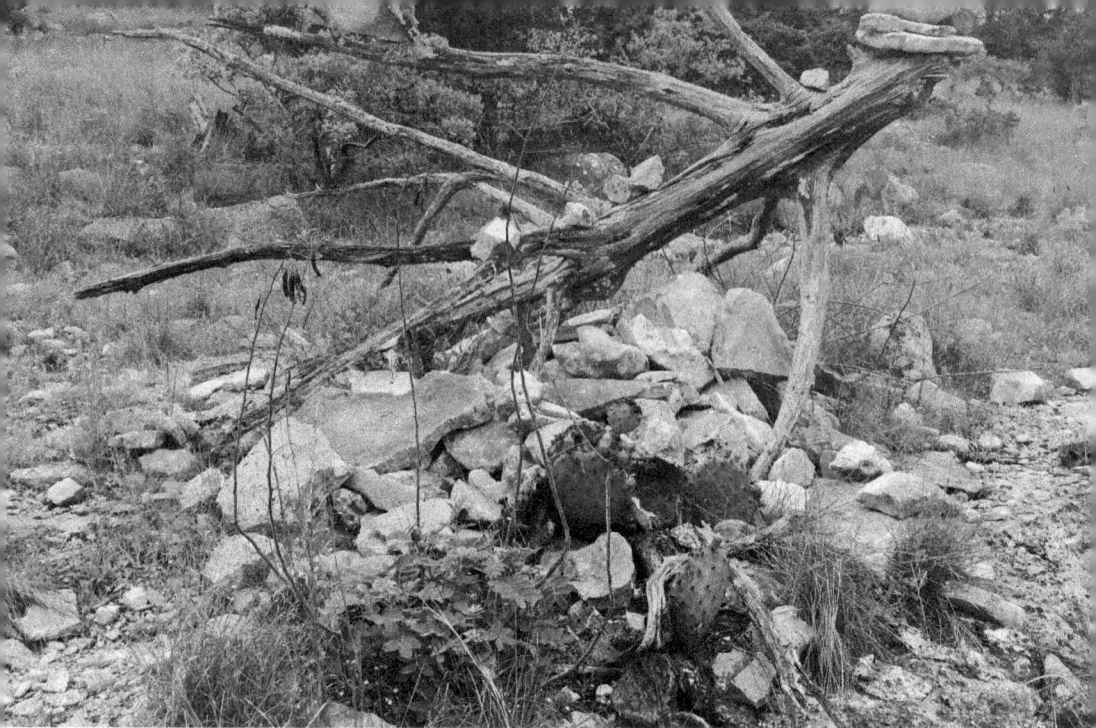

*Art—natural or man-made—along a high trail at the Hill Country State Natural Area*

The path starts to dip down into the bowl. At 2.6 miles Trail 3B (Side Track) leaves to the left. Continue on 3A, climbing up, and then dip into a densely wooded wash. Begin a lung-busting climb on a rocky trail to top out on a saddle. This is the first peak of the trek. Gather yourself, and then begin the treacherously steep descent into the next ravine. You will meet a rock wash at 3.2 miles, where you might catch a breath and enjoy the silence. Just ahead, Trail 3B comes in from the left. Stay right. You'll probably agree with the sign's rating of the trail as "most difficult." Keep going through the rocks and cedar to meet Trail 3, a doubletrack path, at 3.6 miles.

This is an important junction. To your right, 0.3 mile away, in the uppermost reaches of West Verde Creek valley, is the Hermit's Shack Camp Area for equestrians and back-packers. Turn left here, passing the verdant Butterfly Springs Camp Area on your right, for backpackers only. Cross West Verde Creek, and keep down the valley, working around a wide-open wash that used to be spanned by a bridge. You can still see the soil abutment of the bridge. Watch for an old wooden shack on your right beyond the abutment. At 4.1 miles look right for the singletrack Trail 4 (Cougar Canyon). Take this across the bed of West Verde Creek. The skeletal oaks probably died in a fire at some point in the past. Pass a fence and other abandoned ranch equipment. The trail heads up Cougar Canyon, but we are going to take 4A (Cougar Canyon Overlook), which leaves to the right at 4.4 miles. This leads to the ridges above the canyon, where there are far-reaching vistas and not much else. (If you choose, stay on 4 and meet us at the end of 4A, half a mile ahead.)

Trail 4A goes straight up the end of a spur, getting steeper as you climb, then leveling out as you reach the top. Look east, back to the saddle you climbed, and beyond that, over the ranches between you and Bandera. The rough trail continues, climbing up to a higher ridge—our second summit area—through grass, sotol, and low cedar and reaching an apex at 5.2 miles. A sharp left takes you south, following the contour along the back side of a ridge above a steep side canyon, its base invisible. Continue the stony descent into a vast green bowl, hidden from the world in remote Cougar Canyon. At 6 miles you meet Trail 4. Turn right, dipping to a small wash and ascending out of the canyon to the ridge dead ahead. At the top, at 6.3 miles, take in the view ahead down the long West Verde Creek valley, and then turn right onto Trail 4B (Boyles). This trail, a doubletrack balloon, takes us through the third and highest summit area, reaching 1,963 feet. It winds around the edges of a canyon on lonesome ridges far from the world, along which you will find several dramatic vistas. (If you prefer, stay on 4 to join the end of 4B a mile down the valley.)

The long descent into West Verde Creek valley and back to the trailhead starts at the 8-mile point, with half a mile of steep grade marked on the map as especially challenging. Small, loose rocks underfoot demand careful steps. There are now views to the east where ranch houses and other buildings break up the endless cedar. At 8 miles you come to an old barn and then sandy, easy Trail 4. Turn right, and pass a boarded-up house. Cross the dam of an old pond. Reach another trail junction in damp woods at 9 miles. Turn left onto Trail 5 (Twin Peaks). At 9.2 miles, the trail dips and turns right through a delightful oak glade, at a point where two feeder branches reach West Verde Creek. Sycamores line the banks of the stream bed. Soon you'll reach the park road. Look for Trail 2, veering left after a few yards. The grass and soil footing and the wide-open valley bottom contrast greatly with the rocky hills through which you've been traveling.

Keep in grassland through the heart of the valley. At 9.8 miles intersect Trail 2A. This completes the loop portion of the trek. Keep forward on Trail 2, backtracking to Trail 6, and return to the trailhead.

## Nearby Activities

Hill Country State Natural Area offers walk-in tent camping, backpacking, bicycling, horseback riding, and fishing. Many ranches around the park offer horse-riding experiences within its boundaries. Bandera has several decent restaurants and a coffee shop.

---

### GPS TRAILHEAD COORDINATES
#### N29° 38' 4.2"  W99° 11' 3.7"

From San Antonio, take TX 16 to Bandera. In Bandera turn left on TX 173 South, following it for 1 mile to Farm Route 1077. Turn right onto FR 1077, and follow it 10 miles to the park, where the road turns to dirt. Turn right in the park across West Verde Creek, and then turn right again, passing the Bar-O Day Use Area and park headquarters. Once you have your permit, continue to the trailhead, 0.5 mile farther up Park Road.

# 55 Kerrville-Schreiner Park Loop

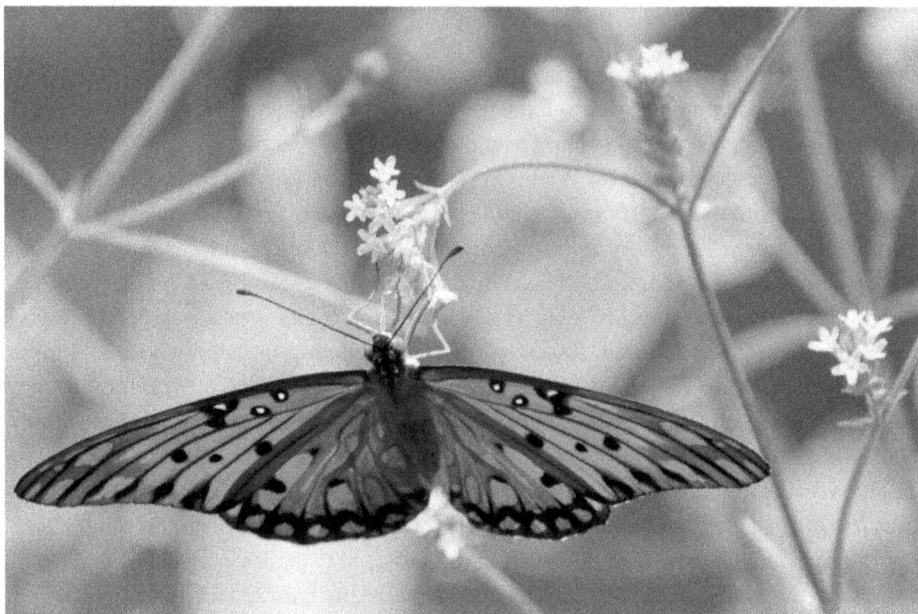

*Kerrville-Schreiner Park's Butterfly Garden is a certified Monarch Way Station.*

## In Brief

This loop of loops covers all the trails at Kerrville-Schreiner, a well-maintained Kerrville city park. Wander through juniper woods, topping out at a point where you can overlook the Guadalupe River Valley below. Hikers and mountain bikers can combine the trails in many different ways for a multitude of possible routes.

## Description

Be sure to pick up or download a map before starting your hike at Kerrville-Schreiner Park, or risk getting turned around in this labyrinth of interconnected paths that has been organized into five color-coded trails and then further subdivided alphabetically. Signs and posts on the trails clearly announce each trail's color and letter, making it simple to stay on track—if you have the map. The trails make the kind of winding loops that suggest as much attention to the needs of bikers as those of hikers, and given the uniformity of the scenery they pass through, you might have more fun exploring them by bike.

| | |
|---|---|
| **LENGTH:** 5.8 miles | **ACCESS:** Daily, 8 a.m.–10 p.m.; $4 day-use fee per person ages 13 and older; $2 day-use fee per senior ages 65 and older; $1 day-use fee per child |
| **CONFIGURATION:** Loop | |
| **DIFFICULTY:** Moderate | |
| **SCENERY:** Juniper woods | |
| **EXPOSURE:** Mixed | **WHEELCHAIR ACCESS:** No |
| **TRAFFIC:** Moderate | **MAPS:** tinyurl.com/kerrvilletxparkmap |
| **TRAIL SURFACE:** Gravel, rock, dirt | **FACILITIES:** Water, restrooms at nearby campground |
| **HIKING TIME:** 2–3 hours | |
| **DRIVING DISTANCE:** 64 miles from the Alamo | **CONTACT INFORMATION:** 830-257-7300; tinyurl.com/kerrvilletxpark |

That scenery is an unbroken tract of juniper forest corralled by a country club and a subdivision. No other species of tree seems to have managed to get more than a foothold on these slopes; I saw one or two live oaks, and that was it. Overall the understory is sparse, with occasional grassy areas. The route goes from Yellow to Orange to Green to Red to Blue and back to Yellow, the colorful names making up for any marked difference in the scenery. Some are rated as more difficult than others, but the Orange Trail, with its steep ascent to an overlook, is the only one that demands a concerted effort.

Leave Trailhead 3, and immediately enter the shady forest on the Yellow Trail, a wide swath of pea gravel. At 0.1 mile keep right at a fork; the surface changes to cedar shavings and then to dirt and rocks. At half a mile you arrive suddenly to the fence at the edge of the park and therefore the forest; across the fence are some rough fields, and beyond them the Comanche Trace subdivision.

The woods open up a bit as the Yellow Trail winds around the head of a valley, passing the end of the crossover to the Blue Trail, the return path. Some rocky ups and downs account for the "moderately difficult" rating. Look for narrow deer paths crisscrossing the trail, which then turns north and climbs around the shoulder of a little hill to meet the Orange and Blue Trails at 1.8 miles. Go left onto the Orange Trail and left again at the 2-mile mark, where the Orange Trail forks. This junction, where there is an information board, is also the end of the Green Trail. You will already have begun a steep climb on a rooty track, and that climb continues, eventually reaching an altitude of 1,830 feet above sea level by a water tower that is just the other side of the fence line and has been visible from the trail for a while. A few feet farther, at a rock lip, a view over the Guadalupe Valley opens up, the vista extending out beyond the park's green woods over the city of Kerrville to a distant line of hills.

Descend alongside the fence marking the park boundary until you come to a gate, where the trail doubles back on itself. In this shady section, I noticed a couple of live oaks standing out against the ranks of cedar. Turn left onto the Green Trail, rated moderately difficult like the Yellow, which heads northwest, shadowing the two Orange tracks and crossing a wash before turning south and making its way across a wider valley, crossing a

# Kerrville-Schreiner Park Loop

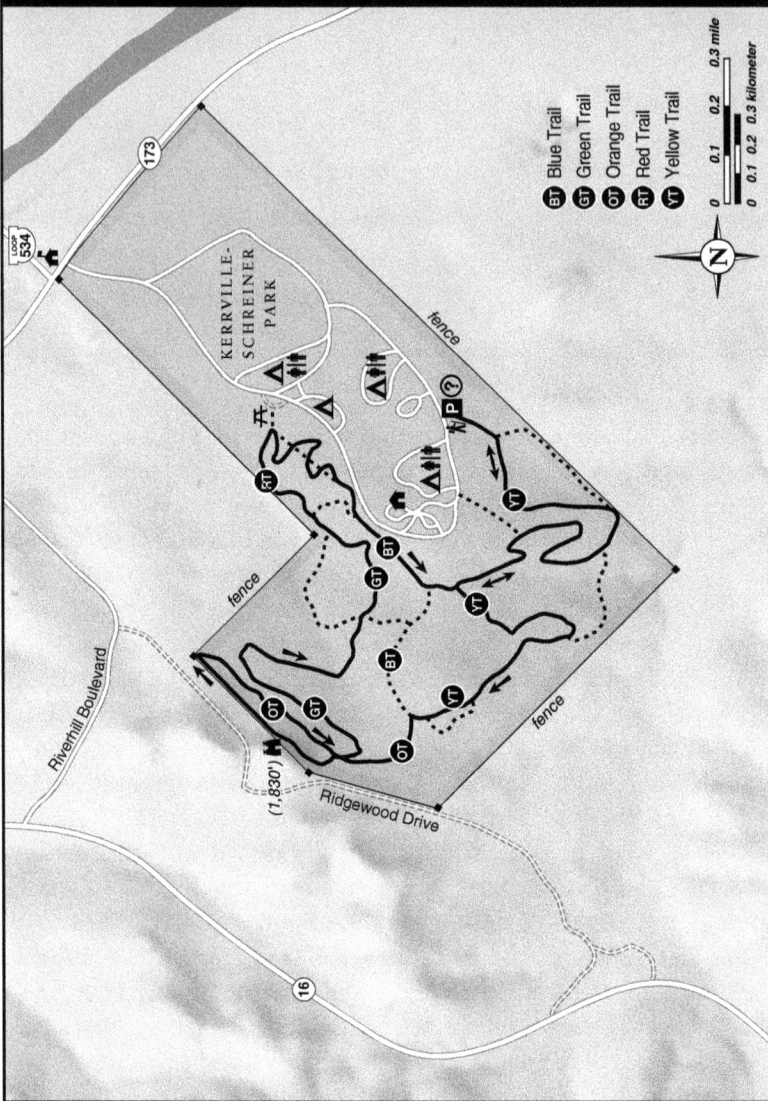

**Map legend:**

- **BT** Blue Trail
- **GT** Green Trail
- **OT** Orange Trail
- **RT** Red Trail
- **YT** Yellow Trail

0.1  0.2  0.3 mile

0  0.1  0.2  0.3 kilometer

KERRVILLE-SCHREINER PARK

Riverhill Boulevard

Ridgewood Drive

(1,830')

fence

173

LOOP 534

16

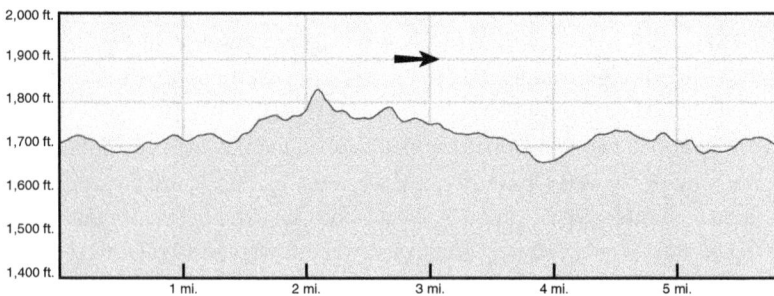

few more drainages as it does. The last of these is at 3.3 miles, when the path begins to climb out of the valley bottom. Pass a crossover trail leading to the Blue Trail, and then a dramatic lone live oak, defiant amid a sea of juniper.

The trail makes another dip, then at 3.6 miles comes to a junction with a branch of the Red Trail, which you will take, turning left. Keep an eye out for this junction, as the sign is not easily visible from your direction of approach. In just over another 0.1 mile, the Red Trail forks. I did not see any signage at this junction. Go left here, too, over a little rock drop-off, stepping into a grassier part of the forest. This path will make the full loop of the Red Trail. You'll know you are on the right track when you see the "A" section marker.

At 4 miles, make a sharp right to keep on the Red Trail loop, or end up at Trailhead 1. A sign warns of possible encounters with snakes, fox, coyotes, and even mountain lions. No doubt you will be too concerned with all these trail junctions to notice them.

At 4.3 miles you will arrive at a triangular junction. Go left here, and climb up to come to Trailhead 2 at the road. Find the Blue Trail, which is the last trail to the right; it's a wide jeep track and very soon goes through a metal gate. At 4.6 miles come to the crossover trail that links the Blue Trail to the Yellow. Turn left here, and soon come to the Yellow Trail. Turn left, and retrace your steps 1.2 miles to come back to Trailhead 3, where you started.

## Nearby Activities

Kerrville-Schreiner Park has fishing and kayaking on the Guadalupe River, along with tent and RV camping. You can rent kayaks, canoes, paddleboards, and bicycles at the park.

### GPS TRAILHEAD COORDINATES
**N30° 0' 3.6"  W99° 7' 40.3"**

From San Antonio, head north on I-10 to Exit 508, TX 16. Take TX 16 south and travel 0.5 mile to Loop Road 534. Turn left on Loop Road 534. Keep forward on Loop 534, crossing the Guadalupe River, and reach TX 173 at 4.3 miles. Turn left on TX 173, and immediately turn left to enter Kerrville-Schreiner Park. The park headquarters and registration are by the entrance. The trailhead is in the section of the park on the other side of TX 173. Leaving the headquarters, turn right, and the entrance is on the left before Loop 534. Turn in, turn left on Park Road 19, and travel 0.4 mile to an intersection. Turn left again toward the camping area. Trailhead 3 will be on your left after 0.4 mile, just beyond the right turn into the park group shelter.

# 56 Panther Canyon Nature Trail

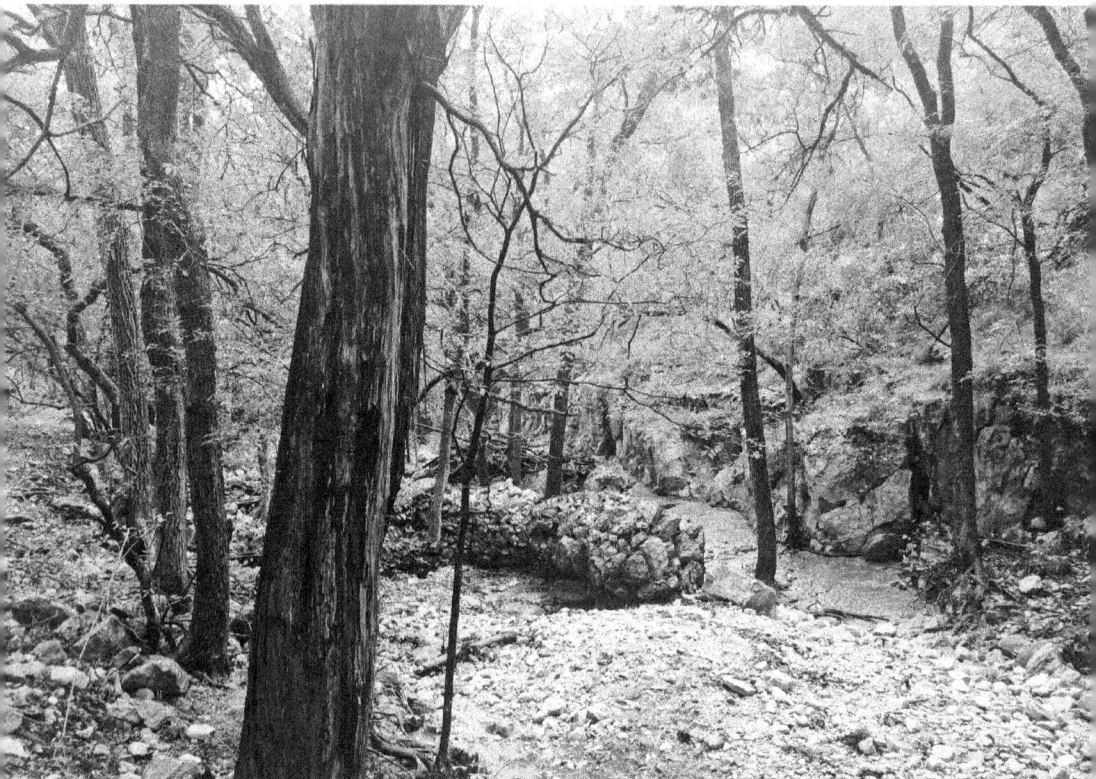

*Panther Canyon*

## In Brief

This is a pretty hike up a surprisingly lush canyon in Landa Park, a popular New Braunfels city park by the Comal River with paddleboats and picnic tables. Give yourself time to enjoy not only the trail but the rest of the park as well.

## Description

The trail begins at Comal Springs, the headwaters of the Comal River, around which Landa Park is centered. However, Panther Canyon is dry, unless there have been heavy rains. Along the way you will crisscross the wet-weather streambed beneath rich woodland

| | |
|---|---|
| **LENGTH:** 1.6 miles | **ACCESS:** Daily, 6 a.m.–midnight; no fees or permits required (except a $10 picnic-table fee) |
| **CONFIGURATION:** Out-and-back | |
| **DIFFICULTY:** Moderate | |
| **SCENERY:** Wooded canyon | **WHEELCHAIR ACCESS:** No |
| **EXPOSURE:** Shady | **MAPS:** USGS *New Braunfels West* |
| **TRAFFIC:** Moderate; busy on warm weekends | **FACILITIES:** Restrooms, water fountains at park |
| **TRAIL SURFACE:** Rocks, dirt | **CONTACT INFORMATION:** 830-221-4350; nbtexas.org/1429/panther-canyon-nature-trail |
| **HIKING TIME:** 1 hour | |
| **DRIVING DISTANCE:** 33 miles from the Alamo | |

covering the canyon floor and hills. Sheer rock bluffs add more scenery to the walk. Landa Park also has a paved walking and jogging trail that winds through the park.

Landa Park and Comal Springs have an interesting history. Located along the Balcones Fault, the springs, heralded as the biggest in Texas and the Southwest, flow from the Edwards Aquifer. The level land of the park area was a popular camping spot for Texas's American Indians. Many artifacts and burial sites have been found around the springs. A Spanish mission was built here in 1756. Later, German settlers came to the area, naming the community New Braunfels. William H. Merriweather bought the Comal Springs tract in 1847, building a cotton gin and gristmill. Joseph Landa purchased it in 1860. In the late 1800s, the area known as Landa's Pasture became a popular picnicking place. Comal Springs' reputation as a tourist destination grew, attracting a railroad line and hotel. An excursion train ran from San Antonio and Austin, carrying passengers to visit and bathe in the springs.

The property was sold, and the tract suffered during the Great Depression and was eventually closed. The city of New Braunfels moved to purchased the land in 1936. Since then, the park has been expanded through further acquisitions to become the destination it is today. Panther Canyon was one of these later purchases.

At the parking area, stop for a moment to admire the majestic oaks that shelter the picnic tables. Then walk toward the trailhead along a sidewalk, past Comal Springs, where the water is clear, cool, and clean as it busts directly out of a limestone wall. The spring is home to the fountain darter, a small, endangered fish.

Pass the springs, and enter the natural surroundings of narrow, deep Panther Canyon. This gash of green extends northwest out of the river basin toward TX Loop 337, contrasting greatly with the rest of the park, with its pagodas and golf courses. Currently the difference is exacerbated by work on the Landa Park River Front Rehabilitation Project, though that is slated to be completed by the summer of 2015.

Immediately cross the first wash. Overhead is a dense tree canopy that will shelter the entire route. Look for live oak, elm, buckeye, and mountain laurel, as well as juniper.

# Panther Canyon Nature Trail

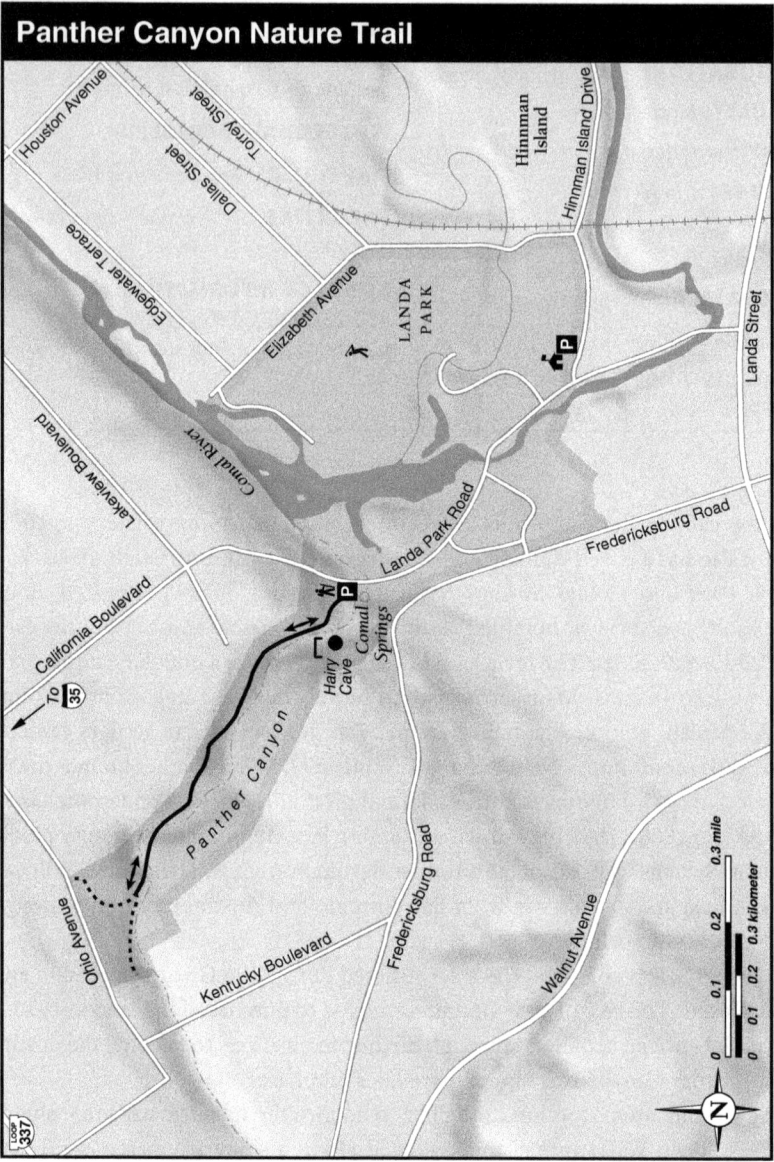

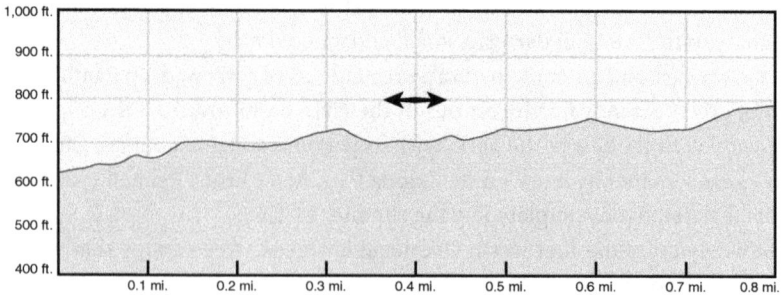

Turn back and admire the arches of the stone road bridge that crosses the canyon. The liquid calls of many birds abrogate any noise from Landa Park. If you keep quiet as you ascend the canyon, you may see deer, especially in the morning and evening.

At 0.1 mile find a bench, and scan the bottom of the bluff along the rocky streambed for a small cave, really more of a narrow, tunnel-like opening. This is an old spring mouth, now dry, known as Hairy Cave. During the summer, the cave is so thick with granddaddy longlegs that the inside appears to be hairy.

Keep making your way up the canyon, crisscrossing back and forth over the streambed. The sides of the valley are sometimes sheer walls, sometimes softer grass- and tree-covered banks. The canyon opens up and widens in places. Here and there, the hardwood trunks make elegant patterns over a grassy understory. Look for limestone shelves at some of the crossings. The trail curves with the canyon, continuing to ascend. Side washes come in occasionally. At the half-mile mark, you'll notice a rock outcrop and a large oak, after which the canyon makes a turn to the left. At the next crossing, an iron trestle in the creek bed is all that remains of what must have been a bridge.

You'll notice that the path is getting closer to the ridgetops on either side as you proceed, and quite soon you will see a pink house on a tall bluff to your left. This is a sign that you are close to the park boundary. You'll end up in a little valley, by what would be an island in the stream if water were flowing. Look for a wooden post just across the creek. This is a good turnaround spot, though you may wish to explore farther along the unofficial paths that lead out to Ohio Avenue.

## Nearby Activities

Landa Park is a fun family destination. Swim in a spring-fed pool or an Olympic-size conventional pool, picnic, ride a mini-train, and fish. Other pastimes include golf, miniature golf, and tennis. The park also has a concrete walking and jogging trail. Don't forget to tour the William & Dolores Schumann Arboretum, with more than 50 species of trees.

---

**GPS TRAILHEAD COORDINATES**

**N29° 42' 47.2" W98° 8' 15"**

From Exit 184 on I-35 in New Braunfels, take TX Loop 337 North 4.1 miles. Turn right on California Boulevard. Continue 0.8 mile to the park. The Panther Canyon trailhead is just on the right at the bottom of the hill that descends into the Comal valley. The parking area is a few yards on, over a bridge.

# 57 Purgatory Creek Natural Area: Dante's and Beatrice Trails

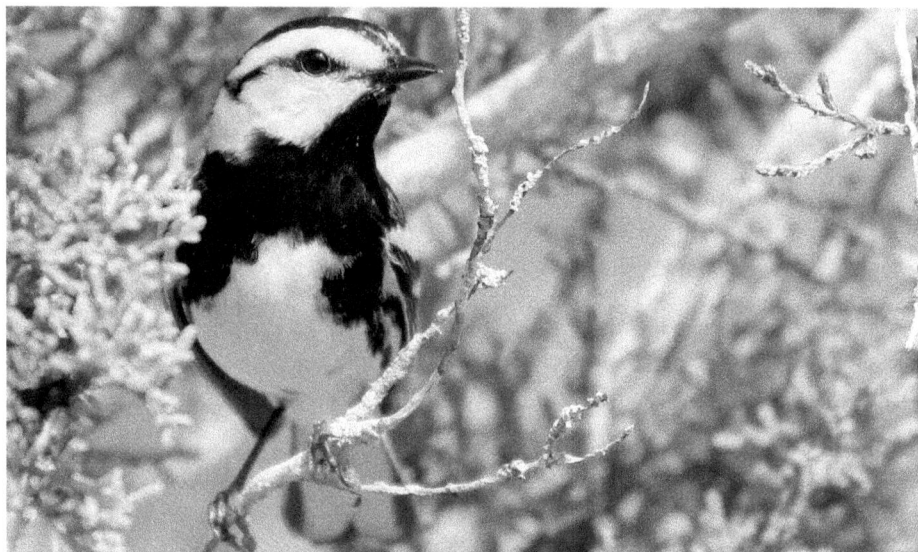

*Golden-cheeked warbler*

## In Brief

Kudos to the San Marcos Greenbelt Alliance for working to ensure that America's fastest-growing city of 2014 has several new parks for hikers and bikers to enjoy, of which the 570-acre Purgatory Creek Natural Area is the largest. Wander through open meadows and dense woodland, and enjoy views over the high cliffs along Purgatory Creek.

## Description

Getting to the trailhead requires driving along a few hundred yards of dirt road alongside the gleaming divided highway—Wonder World Drive (Ranch to Market Road 12)—that now bypasses San Marcos on its way to I-35. Apartments have sprung up along Craddock Avenue, and the park itself encloses three sides of a large construction site that will surely be a new neighborhood by the time you read this. But even though its vistas often include neighboring subdivisions, the park is large enough that within its boundaries you can

| | |
|---|---|
| **LENGTH:** 6.9 miles | **ACCESS:** Daily, 6 a.m.–11 p.m.; free |
| **CONFIGURATION:** Balloon loop | **WHEELCHAIR ACCESS:** This route is not; however, there is a short section of accessible trail beginning at the Lower Purgatory Creek parking lot. |
| **DIFFICULTY:** Moderate | |
| **SCENERY:** Juniper and oak woodland, with some open areas | |
| **EXPOSURE:** Mostly shady | **MAPS:** tinyurl.com/purgcreekmap |
| **TRAFFIC:** Moderate–busy | **FACILITIES:** None |
| **TRAIL SURFACE:** Natural surfaces | **CONTACT INFORMATION:** 512-754-9321; smgreenbelt.org |
| **HIKING TIME:** 3 hours | |
| **DRIVING DISTANCE:** 35 miles from the capitol | |

forget the neighbors and lose yourself in nature. By the way, "lose yourself" is not just a metaphor, particularly in the many trails and tracks of the Lower Purgatory, so take a picture of the map at the trailhead when you get there, or print one out from the website beforehand.

Our route follows Dante's Trail from the Upper Purgatory area, a maze of rock mounds and ravines, all the way to the Lower Purgatory, where we will loop around the Beatrice Trail (and a portion of the Ripheus Trail) and return the way we came. It's a good long hike—nearly 7 miles—so make sure that, as always, you are prepared with water and sunscreen. There are many options to shorten the hike, should you choose.

From the Upper Purgatory parking lot, we immediately enter familiar Hill Country oak-and-juniper woodland. At less than 0.1 mile a large sign points right along Dante's Trail, and the crunch of gravel underfoot soon gives way to a rockier surface. To the left is the Paraiso Trail. You meet it again in 0.4 mile, at the corner of an open upland meadow area, and you can add another mile to the hike by taking this loop to the north. It is closed March 1–May 31, when the golden-cheeked warblers are nesting. Otherwise continue along Dante's Trail, passing the large tree known as Grandma's Oak. Here, the trail takes a slight left to head south through the dense cedar. In another 0.1 mile you emerge briefly from under the branches and get the first look across Purgatory Creek canyon to the trees (and houses) along Summit Ridge.

Immediately after this viewpoint, the track veers left and then makes a dogleg to the right, heading east along the northern edge of the smaller canyon formed by Pandemonium Creek, the stream that bisects the Upper Purgatory. Sunlight filtering through the tall trees growing on the bank spreads mottled shadows on the rocks and fallen leaves underfoot. This sloping terrain makes for one of the prettiest parts of the hike, in which you drop around 50 feet to come to the creek crossing. Larger limestone outcrops are a feature of the boulder-strewn creek bed (usually dry), and to your right is a throne that someone has built out of boulders. This delightful spot is a popular hangout for casual visitors, including, naturally, many Texas State University students.

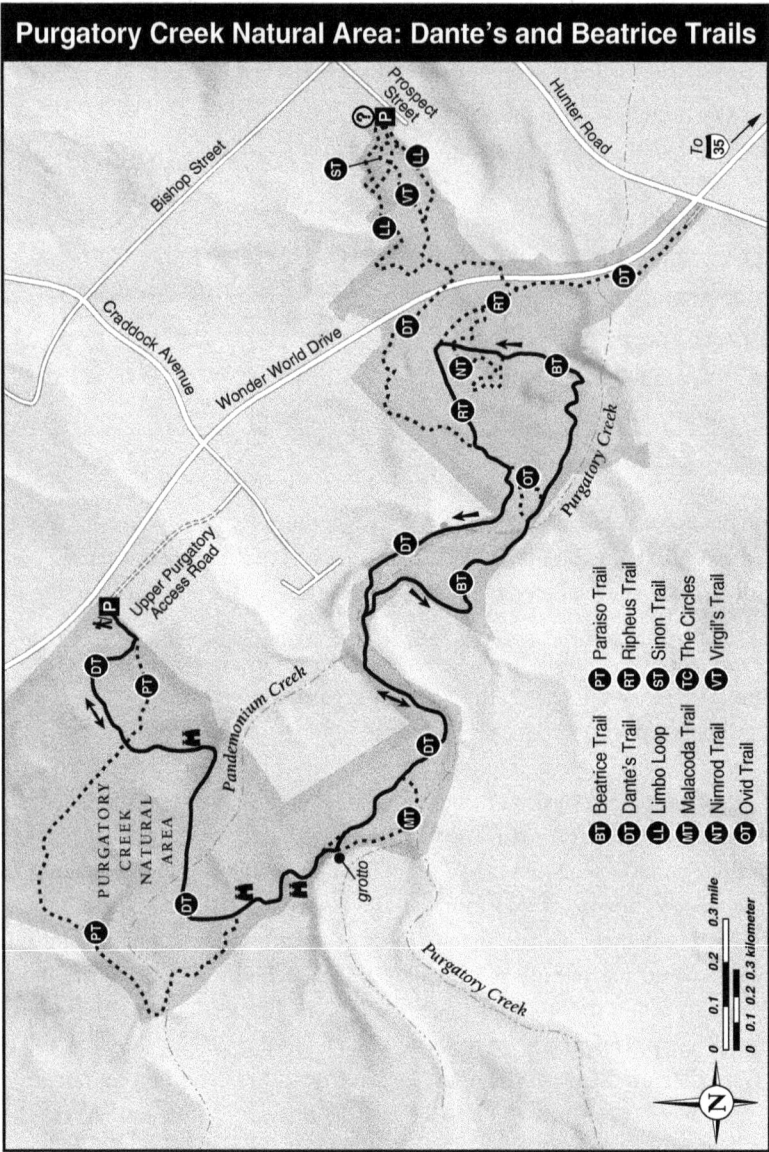

## Purgatory Creek Natural Area: Dante's and Beatrice Trails

**PT** Paraiso Trail
**RT** Ripheus Trail
**ST** Sinon Trail
**TC** The Circles
**VT** Virgil's Trail

**BT** Beatrice Trail
**DT** Dante's Trail
**LL** Limbo Loop
**MT** Malacoda Trail
**NT** Nimrod Trail
**OT** Ovid Trail

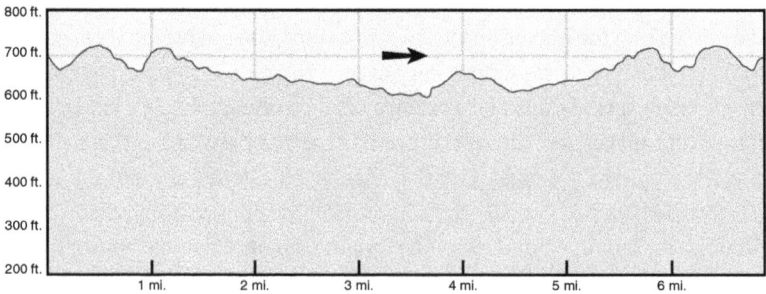

Rocks and roots under your feet make for a somewhat hazardous climb away from the creek bed through thick, scrubby woods and around a long curve to the south. At 1.1 miles you arrive at the junction with the end of the Paraiso, having regained all the altitude you lost to cross Pandemonium Creek. This is the highest point on the hike, close to the park's long southeastern boundary, which you will follow for a while. After 0.1 mile cross a jeep track where there's a glimpse into the central open grassland that our route skirts. At 1.4 miles you cross a little side canyon, and the path comes to the threshold of a vertiginous drop, the top of the high cliffs carved from the rock by Purgatory Creek as it makes a wide right turn southwest. The view down across this hidden valley is an unexpected and lovely surprise. You can also take the short detour 150 yards farther on that takes you to the edge of the flat shelf of red rock at the top of the bluff.

From here, the route descends slowly for most of a mile to where the Beatrice Trail crosses Purgatory Creek, but this route adds a half mile there-and-back detour along the Malacoda Trail. This path goes back up the canyon to a large cave cut out of the cliffs, known as the grotto, the park's semisecret attraction. (The trail continues past the grotto—if you find yourself doubling back to the left, you've gone too far.) It's about a third of a mile from the detour I mentioned to the junction with the Malacoda, and along that stretch you'll see at least three unsanctioned tracks to your right where people have scrambled down the rock face to join that trail.

At 2.4 miles take another sharp turn northwest, following the narrow dogleg of land along Purgatory Creek that links the upper and lower portions of the park. Gradually the path emerges from the trees, and you cross a jeep track (the same one you saw earlier) and turn east to walk to the other side of the flat, grassy valley and around the end of Summit Drive. After you cross the stream, you arrive at the junction with the Beatrice Trail. Turn right on the Beatrice, and begin the loop around the Lower Purgatory area.

The first section of this trail is somewhat drab: the ground is flat, the woods sparse, and the fences along the back of the houses quite visible. Soldier on, though, and the trail starts to descend through thick forest. After a sharp left turn, you will find an alternative Purgatory Creek watercourse and then, a few steps farther, a couple of oaks that have taken advantage of a little side stream to grow to an impressive size. Here begins the prettiest part of the hike, a half mile or so where your path takes you through enchanting deciduous bottomlands. The deep river channel is just to your right, and beyond it imposing bluffs interspersed with steep, tree-covered, grassy banks. Dappled shadows dance across the bright green leaves and thick grass. At 3.2 miles you pass the first of three mystery tracks going off to your left, any one of which will take you back to Dante's Trail, should you wish to cut the hike short. The officially signed junction with the Ovid Trail, which is marked on the map and joins with Dante's Trail, is at 3.5 miles. Quite soon after that, there is a junction with another unmarked singletrack. Turn right, and emerge from the woods right in front of the vast stone flood-control dam, guarded here by a graffiti-covered concrete pylon, a sudden slap of the urban at the lowest point of the hike.

The trail turns left, north, climbing up along the curve of the dam. At the top of the first sharp rise, pause to look to your left, where a deep hollow has become an impromptu rock art gallery. A tenth of a mile farther, at a fork, you could choose to add a half mile to the hike by turning left into a small coppice, following the Nimrod Trail, or continue straight up the steady incline between the trees and the dam. If the sun is out, the woods might be the better choice, as the Lower Purgatory trails are quite open to the elements. A few yards after the Nimrod Trail rejoins the Beatrice, you turn left along the jeep track that is the Ripheus Trail, walking along the edge of a large boomerang-shaped dry lake, possibly an abandoned quarry. At 4.2 miles the end of the Ripheus Trail, there's a slightly tricky junction. Turn right, back into the woods, then immediately left to pick up Dante's Trail. You stay under cover on the flat, winding path 0.3 mile before turning sharply northwest at the junction of the Ovid Trail. (Bonus points to the San Marcos Greenbelt Alliance for inventive trail names reflecting the literary theme.)

Walk through a wide valley to come to another Purgatory Creek crossing at 4.7 miles. The path stays on the north side a few yards, crossing back over just before a spot where some lovely bluffs loom over a pond. From here, it is less than 0.3 mile to the Beatrice Trail junction, where you left Dante's Trail on your way out. From this point out, you retrace your steps 2.1 miles through the woods back to the trailhead.

## Nearby Activities

San Marcos has several other greenbelt areas. The caves of Wonder World Park are close by on Prospect Street.

---

### GPS TRAILHEAD COORDINATES

**N29° 53' 1.3"  W97° 58' 39.8"**

From I-35 in San Marcos, take the exit for RM 12, and head north. After 1.2 miles turn left at Craddock Avenue; then after 100 yards, turn right at the T-junction. A dirt road leads to the parking lot and trailhead.

# 58 Spring Lake Natural Area

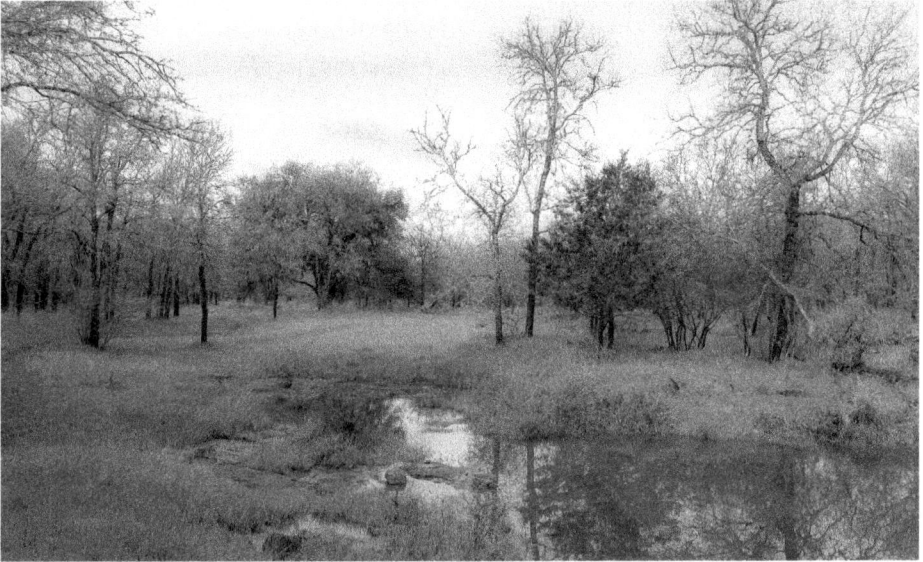

*A hotel and conference center were almost built on land that is now the Spring Lake Natural Area.*

## In Brief

This jigsaw piece of parkland at the northern edge of San Marcos is named for a lake that is outside its boundaries, but no matter; these 251 acres compose one of the best-preserved tracts of the typical Edwards Plateau woods and meadows in the Hill Country, with plenty of trails for hikers and bikers.

## Description

Since there were people, they have been drawn to the beautiful San Marcos Springs—and more recently, up until the 1990s, Aquarena Springs (as it was known) and its famous mermaid show, a popular Texas tourist attraction. When Texas State University bought the property, they planned to sell the area that is now the preserve for development, but a chorus of objections forced a change of plans, and this practically perfect example of Hill Country ecology is now a lovely public park. The route takes you almost to the end of the area, with a loop up to a thickly wooded hill along singletrack that is also great for cyclists. Be aware that the latest map (from January 2012) doesn't accurately reflect the current state of the park, listing a Grey Fox Trail that doesn't exist.

From the trailhead in the golf maintenance area, walk up a gravel road 0.1 mile before crossing the park's official boundary, and then swing right to stay on this road another 0.1

**LENGTH:** 4.3 miles

**CONFIGURATION:** Loop

**DIFFICULTY:** Moderate

**SCENERY:** Juniper and oak woodland, with some open areas

**EXPOSURE:** Mostly shady

**TRAFFIC:** Moderate

**TRAIL SURFACE:** Natural surfaces

**HIKING TIME:** 2 hours

**DRIVING DISTANCE:** 30 miles from the capitol

**ACCESS:** Daily; free; some trails closed March 1–May 31

**WHEELCHAIR ACCESS:** The Tonkawa Trail (0.9 mile) is accessible.

**MAPS:** tinyurl.com/springlakemap

**FACILITIES:** Restrooms at the Meadows Center and at the Lime Kiln Road access; parking at the Meadows Center ($3 on weekdays)

**CONTACT INFORMATION:** 512-754-9321; smgreenbelt.org

mile to reach the actual entrance to the trail system, with its welcoming pagoda. Here you turn left, stepping briefly onto the Tonkawa Trail, where you are in the familiar juniper woodland of the Edwards Plateau. Immediately turn right onto Blind Salamander Way. This shorter but more energetic route might soon have you sweating as you climb over roots and rocks to a ridge covered with juniper and mountain laurel. At 0.3 mile you come to a slight clearing where you can take in a view over the trees. A few yards farther, you turn right on the crunchy, wide, gravel-topped Tonkawa Trail. After another couple of yards, on your left you see the rather grand entrance to the Blue Stem Trail, our return path. For now, keep forward past clusters of cactus and a sundial made of limestone blocks to the end of the Tonkawa. Step into the woods onto the rocky natural surface of the Exogyra Trail. You have now covered 0.6 mile.

At 0.8 mile turn right onto the Blue Heron Trail, and shortly you will descend steeply through cedar thickets down the side of the hill at the northern end of the ridge. At 1.1 miles, you will see one end of a fair-sized pond, but the trail veers away and does a loop to the east before coming back to the other end of the pond, where there is a dock. Pause for a few moments, and you might see a blue heron. The loop around the pond connects with the alternative access to the trail system from Lime Kiln Road, where there is a restroom.

When you leave the dock, keep right at the fork (the sign says Red Oak) to stay on the Buckeye Trail. After 20 yards you pass the end of Skink Link Trail to the left. The track turns left, and on your right is a large, dead tree after which the trail makes a steep descent into the Sink Creek valley, a very different locale. After rainfall, this can be a lush, grassy meadow. A large oak stands out among many smaller trees. After 200 yards or so, the track turns left out of the valley and up an incline toward the junction with the Blue Stem Trail. This trail leads all the way to the northern end of the preserve. Between March 1 and May 31, this point is as far as you can go, as the area is closed to protect golden-cheeked warblers during their nesting season.

Keep right to follow the Blue Stem Trail 0.6 mile along an old jeep track through a more open, grassy plain. Ignore the singletrack that bisects the trail, pass the junction

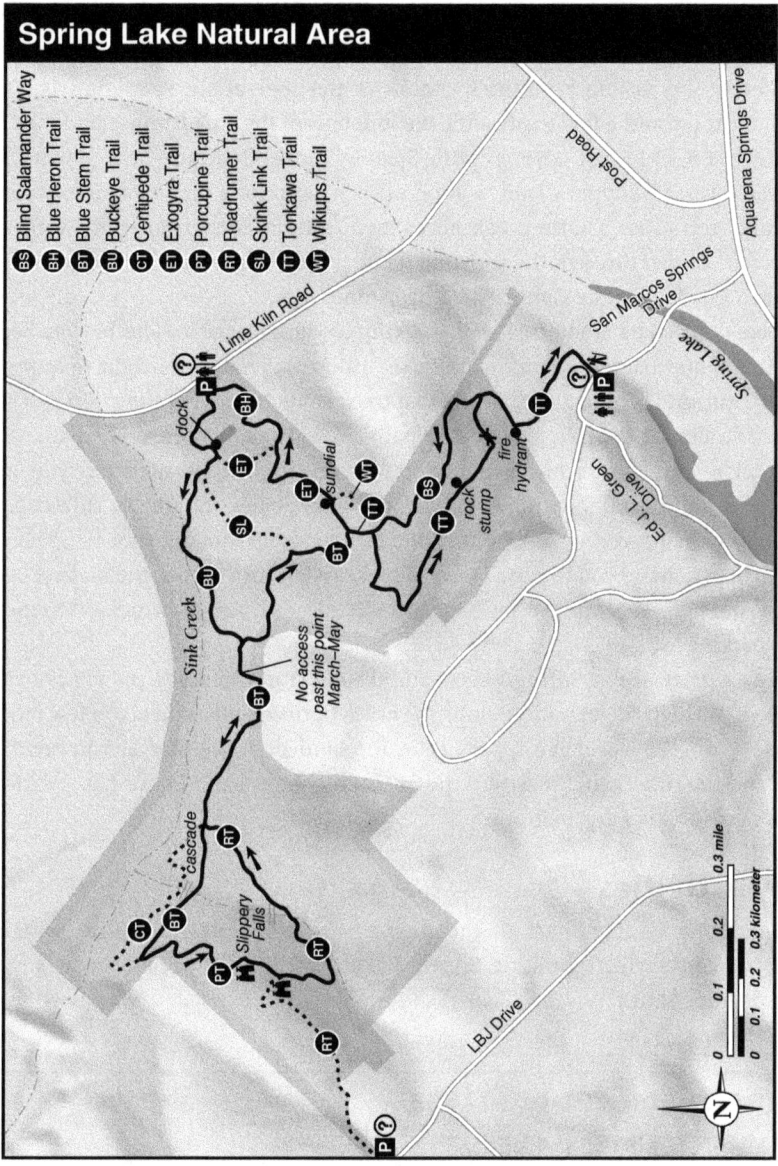

## Spring Lake Natural Area

- **BS** Blind Salamander Way
- **BH** Blue Heron Trail
- **BT** Blue Stem Trail
- **BU** Buckeye Trail
- **CT** Centipede Trail
- **ET** Exogyra Trail
- **PT** Porcupine Trail
- **RT** Roadrunner Trail
- **SL** Skink Link Trail
- **TT** Tonkawa Trail
- **WT** Wikiups Trail

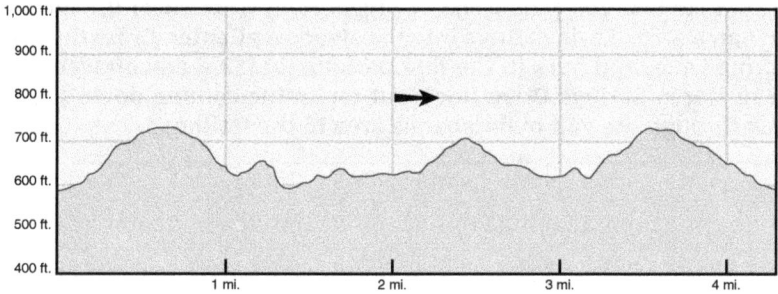

with the Centipede, and step over a narrow stream that goes down to Sink Creek. At the second signpost, turn left, and head into the woods up the Porcupine Trail, scrambling up the hill that was visible from the meadow. At the apex of our route, nearly 100 feet above the meadow and a few yards after the junction of the Roadrunner and Porcupine tracks, there is a large oak covered with Spanish moss. Continue back down the hill through the forest to Slippery Falls, a good place to stop for a picnic or simply contemplate nature. You cross a little creek here; then, a little farther, keep forward across another track. Zigzag through the thinning woods at the edge of the open area to return to the Blue Stem Trail at the Centipede/Roadrunner sign.

Retrace your steps along this trail, walking along a clearing. The bushes begin to close in as you approach the junction with the Buckeye Trail. Turn right to stay on the Blue Stem Trail, and for the next 0.3 mile that track gains 100 feet of elevation as it strides up the hillside along a wide, boulevard-like path flanked by taller trees. The path narrows and gets rockier as it approaches the junction with the Tonkawa Trail, where you emerge through the grand portal mentioned earlier into a small clearing on the ridgetop. Turn right to follow the gravel surface for 0.1 mile to a peaceful-looking spot where a picnic table and a bench invite you to rest. The trail makes a left turn at this, the highest point of the hike. From here, a gentle 0.8-mile-long descent leads through woodland to the trailhead and parking lot.

There's a lot to see at Spring Lake Natural Area. You can enjoy the views over San Marcos from the high ridge; ramble along the creek bottomlands; and take a few moments to step back from the world at Slippery Falls, the sundial, or the Blue Heron pond. With this park and the others that make up the city's greenbelt, San Marcos has transformed itself into a great hiking destination.

## Nearby Activities

At the Aquarena Center (part of the Texas State University complex, where you parked), you can navigate pristine Spring Lake on a glass-bottomed boat, kayak, or stand-up paddleboard.

### GPS TRAILHEAD COORDINATES

**N29° 53' 44.4"  W97° 55' 43.5"**

From I-35, take Exit 206 (Aquarena Springs Drive) west. After 0.7 mile turn right on San Marcos Springs Drive into the Meadows Center. Cross the bridge over Spring Lake, and park in the first parking lot ($3 a day on weekdays). Cross San Marco Springs Drive (look out for traffic coming down the hill), and walk through the golf maintenance area to the trailhead.

# 59 Twin Peaks Trek

## In Brief

Energetic types who want the best of the Hill Country without preamble should tackle this short, strenuous loop that climbs to the top of the Twin Peaks in the Hill Country State Natural Area. Here, you and the soaring vultures can enjoy the sight of green peaks and valleys stretching to the horizon in every direction.

## Description

Hill Country State Natural Area is probably as rugged as a park can get and still accommodate visitors. This marvelous preserve is heaven for horse lovers, mountain bikers, and hikers alike and was designed solely for their use. As it was deeded to the Texas Parks & Wildlife Department under the condition that it be kept as wild and natural as possible, little has been done in the way of improvements. There is no water or electricity available at the campgrounds, most of which have only primitive walk-in sites. Nonetheless, you could make it to the top of Twin Peaks in the morning and be back in San Antonio for lunch.

These peaks are a pair of connected hills that stand guard over the intersection of the West Verde Creek and Bandera Creek valleys. From the Equestrian Camp Area, the closer peak is a long, shallow bowl under a green ridge. This route will climb into the bowl and around the ridge to the pass between the mountains, where it will turn left to scramble up to the summit area of the western peak. Before you start, remind yourself of trail etiquette. Bikers should yield to hikers, and both must yield to horses. This preserve is intended to be as natural and wild as possible, so please stay on the trails— a ranger will give you a ticket if you do not. Pets are allowed, but on leash only. Bring a bird book and binoculars.

A short connecting spur leads away from the trailhead between sites 214 and 215 to the junction with Trail 6 (Spring Branch). Although the park map gives the trails names, the signs use the numbers, so that's how I will refer to them. A couple of vague paths lead into the grass from a point just after the trailhead, but keep straight on the more distinct track, and in 0.1 mile see the marker at the junction. Turn left onto Trail 6, and immediately begin a steep ascent up a wide, rocky path, heading straight for the deepest part of the bowl. It's rugged hiking, with rocks liable to slip underfoot. The trail climbs about 150 feet and then turns left, staying at about 1,700 feet above sea level as it comes around the mountain to the pass. A mixture of sotol and juniper covers the rocky limestone. There are already views across the West Verde Creek and Bandera Creek valleys, as you are already high above the campground. You will see hikers and horses making their way along the lattice of trails in the distance. From this vantage point, you will notice how trail creep has turned many of the paths into a random weave of dirt tracks.

| | |
|---|---|
| **LENGTH:** 2.3 miles | **DRIVING DISTANCE:** 57 miles from the Alamo |
| **CONFIGURATION:** Loop | |
| **DIFFICULTY:** Moderate | **ACCESS:** Daily, 8 a.m.–10 p.m.; $6 day-use fee per person ages 13 and older |
| **SCENERY:** Typical Hill Country vegetation, rocky hills | **WHEELCHAIR ACCESS:** No |
| | **MAPS:** tinyurl.com/hcsnamap |
| **EXPOSURE:** Open | **FACILITIES:** Bottled water, restroom at park headquarters and trailhead |
| **TRAFFIC:** Moderate | |
| **TRAIL SURFACE:** Loose rocks, dirt | **CONTACT INFORMATION:** 830-796-4413; tpwd.texas.gov/state-parks/hill-country |
| **HIKING TIME:** 1.5 hours | |

At 0.7 mile Trail 5A comes in from the right. Keep straight at this complex junction. Trail 6 leaves to the left; follow 5A up some rocky steps onto the saddle, a little climb that surely helps the trail earn its "most difficult" rating. Shortly you come to the junction with Trail 5B. Turn left to keep climbing up the saddle on a path that's been washed away in many places. Don't let your guard down—watch your step on all these trails. The climb eases off as you approach the summit area, and you start to have stunningly good views over the Bandera Creek valley. Feel the breeze blow the cobwebs away, filling your lungs as you make the final part of the ascent.

Remarkably, the beginning of the loop around the cap is less than a mile from the trailhead. There are benches just off the trail, where you can rest and enjoy the views, but don't leave without completing the circuit, as the views west from the bench at the far end are better, even comparable to those from the South Rim at Big Bend. Flowering plants bloom in profusion among the rocks and cedar. Vultures cruise so close by you can hear their wings flap. It's noticeable that most of the cedar has survived the long drought, in contrast to some other parks, and that dark shade is the deepest note in the palette of greens around you. As clouds pass over, the light shifts and plays across the hills and valleys around you. It feels like another world. At 1.1 miles (if you turned right at the start of the summit loop), a signpost announces the elevation: 1,868 feet above sea level.

At 1.3 miles you have completed the loop and are back at the first benches. Take some time here. When you are ready, descend back down the hill to the junction with Trail 5A. The return path goes via Trails 5A and 1, crossing the wide valley to come to dry Bandera Creek and then roughly following that creek before a spur trail leads back to the campsites.

Trail 5A is quite steep to begin with, tracking a deep ravine cut by a stream coming off the mountain to join Bandera Creek. Look for an old shelter and corral to your right. The path turns away from the feeder creek, and by 1.8 miles you find yourself on a single-track that makes a gentle decline across more or less open meadows to the line of trees along the creek. There are birds everywhere, flitting from tall grass to bush and back again. At 2 miles, at the dry creek bed, you come to Trail 1. Turn left to head back to the

## Twin Peaks Trek

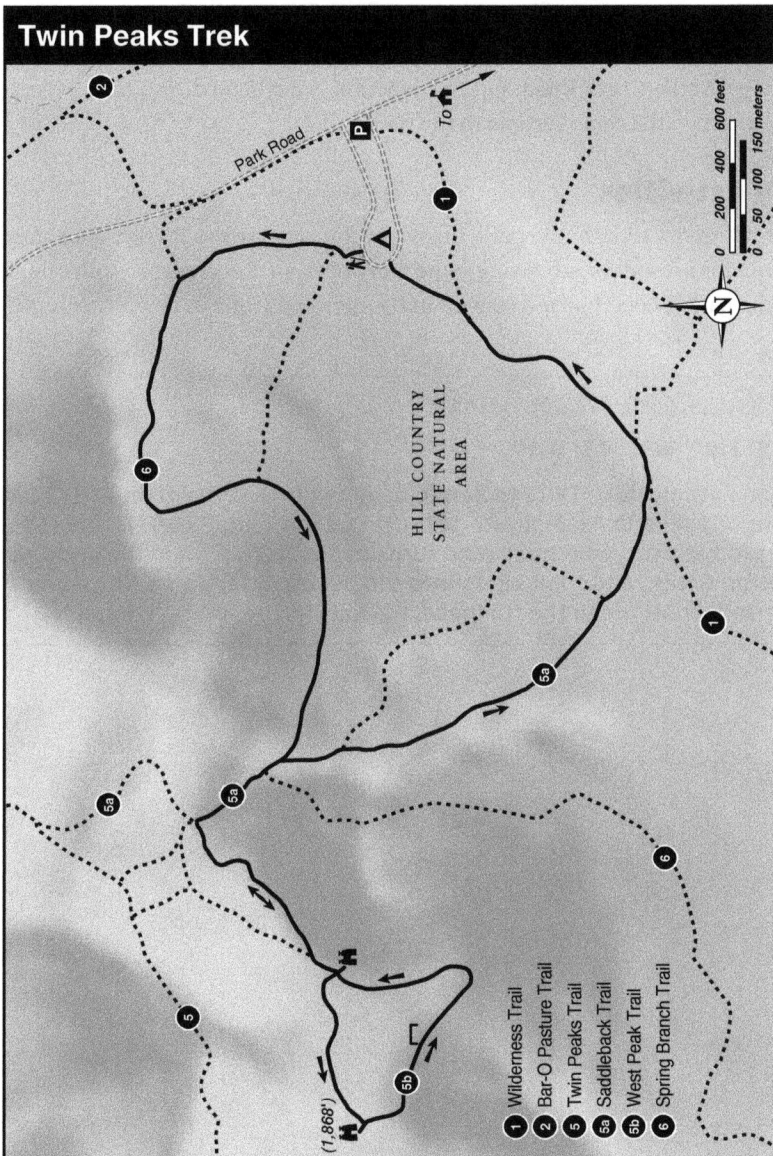

Park Road

To

600 feet
400
200
0

150 meters
100
50
0

HILL COUNTRY STATE NATURAL AREA

(1,868')

1 Wilderness Trail
2 Bar-O Pasture Trail
5 Twin Peaks Trail
5a Saddleback Trail
5b West Peak Trail
6 Spring Branch Trail

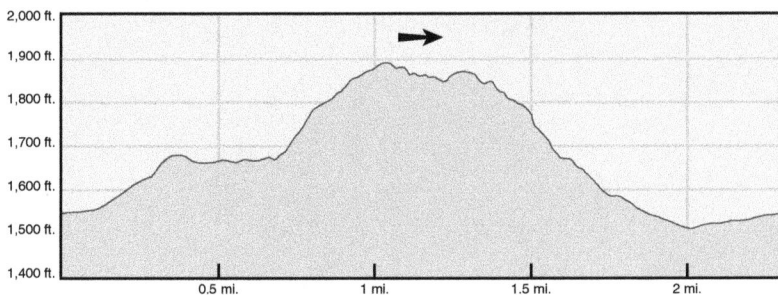

trailhead along this wide, easy path. Soon 5A goes off to the right, over a hill and back to the Bar-O Day Use Area. Trail 1 also leaves to the right shortly before the campsites, joining with West Verde Creek Road, but this junction is not signed, and the obvious route leads back through the camping area to the trailhead.

## Nearby Activities

There are numerous trails in the park, many of which are covered in this book. Consider camping out for a few days and trying some more of them. Local ranches offer horseback riding in the park. Make sure you stop off in Bandera and enjoy its cowboy culture.

---

### GPS TRAILHEAD COORDINATES

**N29° 38' 3.9"  W99° 11' 8.3"**

From San Antonio, take TX 16 to Bandera. In Bandera, turn left on TX 173 South, following it 1 mile to Farm Route 1077. Turn right onto FR 1077, and follow it 10 miles to the park, where the road turns to dirt. Turn right in the park, across West Verde Creek, and then again into the headquarters area. Once you have your permit, continue to the trailhead, 0.5 mile farther up Park Road.

---

# 60 Wilderness Trail at Hill Country State Natural Area

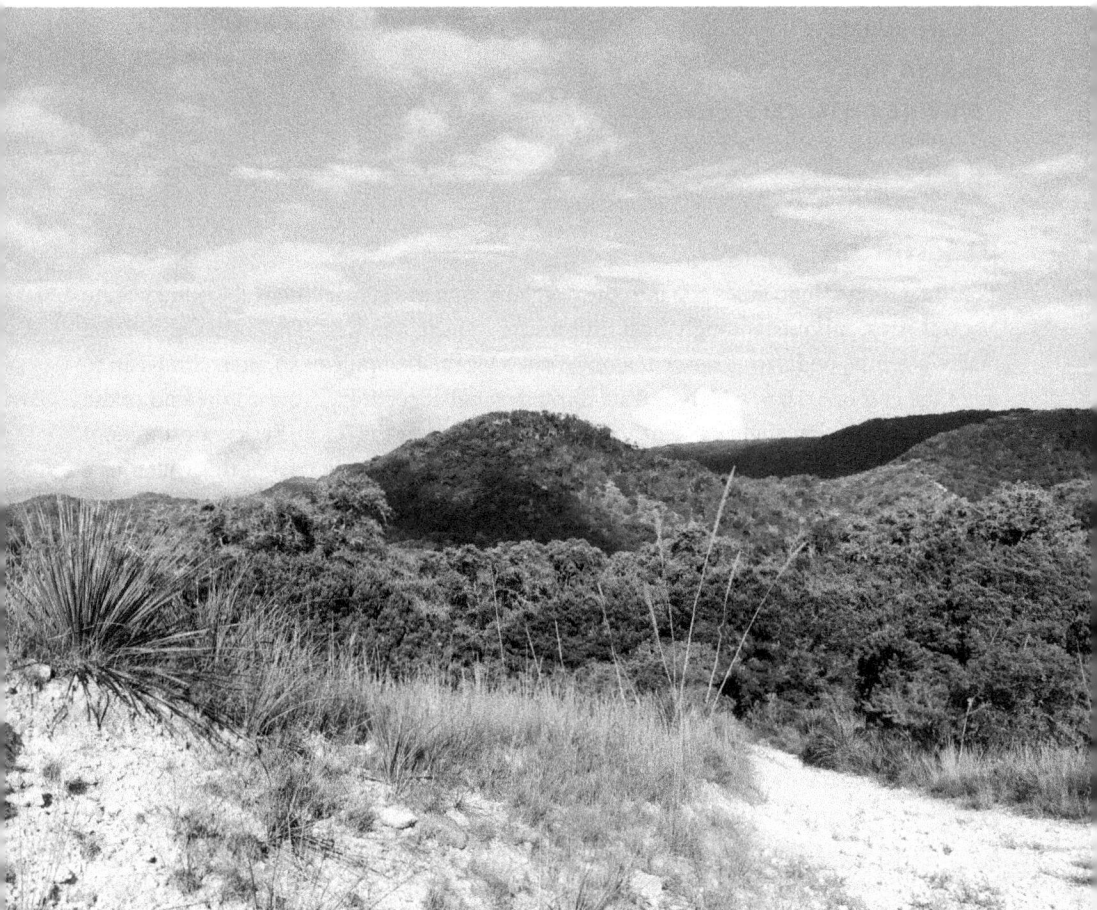

*The backcountry at Hill Country State Natural Area*

## In Brief

A good introduction to the Hill Country State Area, this figure eight can be tailored to your limits. The first half is easy, and the second, more challenging. You'll see wildlife and explore a corner of the park's more remote regions, returning via the foothills of Twin Peaks.

**LENGTH:** 5.1 miles

**CONFIGURATION:** Figure eight

**DIFFICULTY:** Moderately challenging

**SCENERY:** Cedar scrub, rocky hillsides, creeks, and woodland

**EXPOSURE:** Mostly exposed

**TRAFFIC:** Light–moderate

**TRAIL SURFACE:** Rocks, dirt

**HIKING TIME:** 2–3 hours

**DRIVING DISTANCE:** 57 miles from the Alamo

**ACCESS:** Daily; office hours are 8 a.m.–5 p.m.; $6 day-use fee per person ages 13 and older

**WHEELCHAIR ACCESS:** No

**MAPS:** tinyurl.com/hcsnamap

**FACILITIES:** Bottled water, restroom at park headquarters and trailhead

**CONTACT INFORMATION:** 830-796-4413; tpwd.texas.gov/state-parks/hill-country

## Description

This figure-eight loop eases you into the rugged hiking available at the Hill Country State Natural Area, an outstandingly beautiful preserve near Bandera. The outward portion makes a gentle, undulating descent along Trail 1 for the first mile or so, then climbs up to meet the end of Trail 6, which returns through rougher territory. Toward the end of the hike, there is a challenging ascent to the saddle between the Twin Peaks, a prominent feature of the park. Casual hikers can comfortably tackle the first part of this route for a taste of unspoiled Hill Country terrain.

Trail 1 leaves from the southern edge of the parking area at the Equestrian Campground. Step onto the path, and keep right at the junction with Trail 7. Cross a little rise, and come to a wide, grassy path. Trail 1 follows this double-wide path, an old ranch road, all the way to the Wilderness Camp Area, 2 miles away. The first mile of the hike gently descends to the middle point of the figure eight, passing through the lightly wooded meadow along Bandera Creek. Birds love this habitat, and your walk will be serenaded by an array of different calls.

At 0.4 mile the trail forks; keep left. Trail 5A leaves to the right, heading toward Twin Peaks. If you complete the full hike, you will cross the other end of it on your return. Trail 1 continues along the peaceful valley, the surface alternating between grass, sand, and rock. A line of low hills marks the southern boundary of this verdant vale. To the right, you can see the sloping ridges of the Twin Peaks. Trail 1A, a shortcut to Tarpley Road and Trail 7, leaves to your left at 0.9 mile. At 1.1 miles you arrive at the center of the figure eight, where Trail 1 crosses Trail 6.

You might decide to turn back here, having sufficiently experienced the delights of this green valley. After this point, Trail 1 gets rockier and rougher, and the ascents and descents are sharper. The Bandera Creek valley narrows, blocked by the hills ahead of you. Trail 1 follows a side canyon to the right of those hills, which this route will circumnavigate. At 1.4 miles you cross an earth bank. Immediately Trail 5 leaves to the right, and 5C goes to the left. Trail 5C heads past a pond and over the hills you will go around. It

## Wilderness Trail at Hill Country State Natural Area

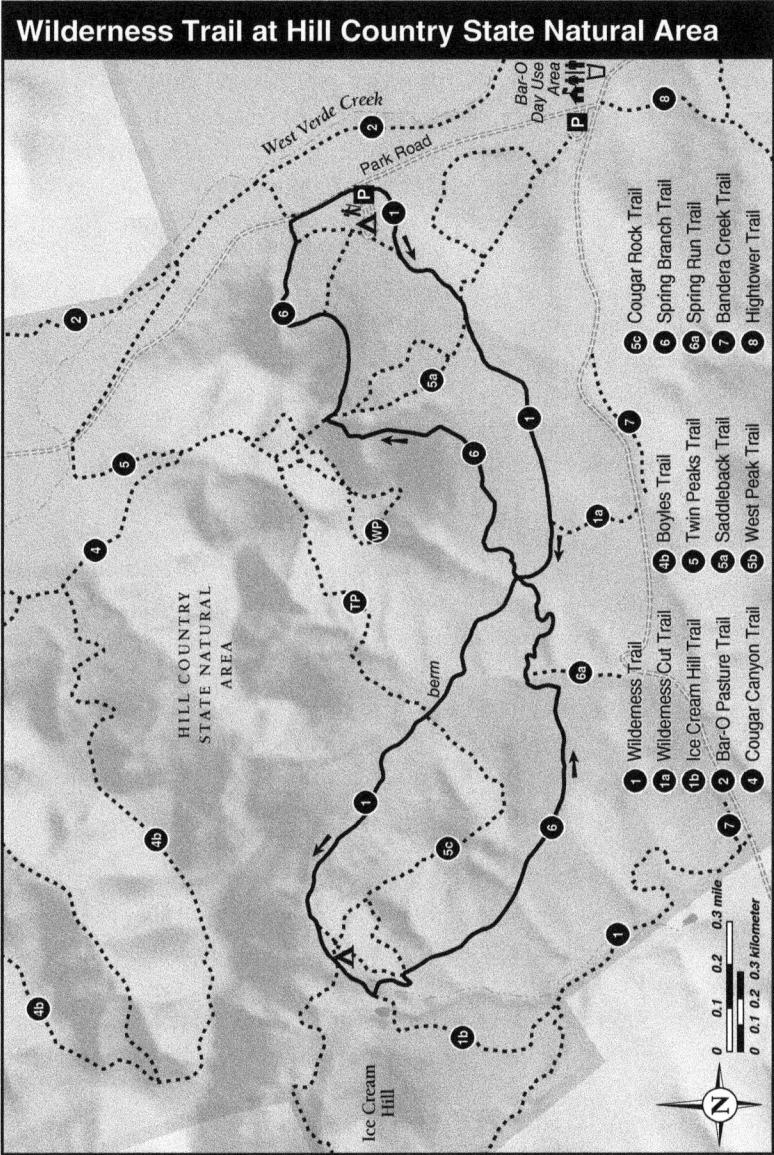

| | | | | |
|---|---|---|---|---|
| 5c Cougar Rock Trail | 6 Spring Branch Trail | 6a Spring Run Trail | 7 Bandera Creek Trail | 8 Hightower Trail |
| 4b Boyles Trail | 5 Twin Peaks Trail | 5a Saddleback Trail | 5b West Peak Trail | |
| 1 Wilderness Trail | 1a Wilderness Cut Trail | 1b Ice Cream Hill Trail | 2 Bar-O Pasture Trail | 4 Cougar Canyon Trail |

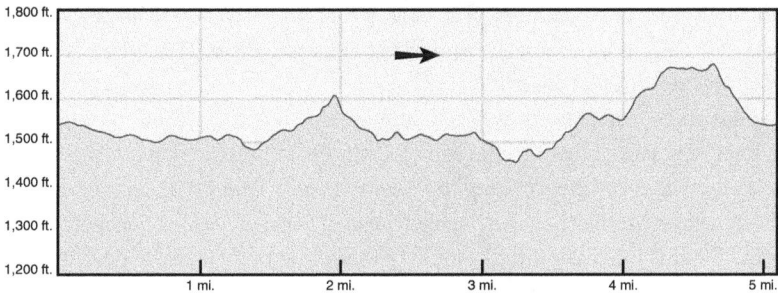

rejoins this route at the Wilderness Camp Area and is an option if you want to add more elevation to your hike.

Crest a rise in the open, and cross a drainage—the path might be muddy—and then another as you begin the 0.3-mile ascent to the spur that links the hills on your left to the peaks on your right. Trees and vegetation crowd the trail but afford little shade. Once you've arrived at the top of the pass, stop and take a moment to take in the wild canyon between you and the cedar-covered summit of Ice Cream Hill, more than 1,800 feet above sea level.

Continue the descent, and come to a fork. The left path leads to the grassy Wilderness Camp Area. Continue around the edge of the campground, passing an attractive site under some spreading oaks. If you had put a sleeping bag and some jerky into your pack, you could be spending the night here. The campground is just over 2 miles from the trailhead, and perhaps this is the place you decide to turn back, after a satisfying 4-mile hike and with a taste of the wilderness that you can take home. From here on, the path gets decidedly more rugged.

Past the campground, Trail 1B leaves to the right to go around Ice Cream Hill. Trail 1, quite eroded at this point, arrives at the farthest point of the hike, the junction with the end of Trail 6, at an open area. Turn left onto a rough and narrow path, leaving the ranch road behind. Cross a creek bed, and then climb up onto an exposed spur to the junction with Trail 5C, which you may remember was an option earlier. If you took it, you'll meet us here. Turn right (left if you came down 5C), staying on Trail 6, which now works its way around the other side of the hills to complete the far loop of the figure eight. For a while, the scenery is not much more than the bare Hill Country essentials—rocks, cedar, and, very likely, sun—the very essence of rugged and remote.

Eventually you will come to a T-junction, just after a fence line. At this point, you have hiked 3.1 miles. To the right, Trail 6A leads to Trail 7. Turn left, staying on 6, and cross a little wash. You have returned to the wide Bandera Creek Valley at an area where two drainages come together. These thicker woods afford some welcome shade. The path shadows a pretty ravine, then makes a stiff climb to meet Trail 1 at the center point of the figure eight. You've hiked 3.6 miles and must make another choice: turn right to return on the easy trail, or keep forward on Trail 6 to attempt the most challenging portion of this hike.

The first 0.1 mile on this last quarter of the hike is a stiff, rocky climb up the southern flank of the Twin Peaks. The path levels off at 1,500 feet above sea level and follows the contour through thicker vegetation. Next comes the most strenuous ascent of the hike, the 0.3 mile to the 5A junction on the saddle between the Twin Peaks. The grade on this section hovers around 20%.

Pause and catch your breath while taking in the view from the junction, 4.3 miles into the hike. If you've not been to the top of Twin Peaks and you have some breath left, consider turning left at this point along the 5A and taking Trail 5B up to the summit.

Trail 6 continues to the right. Stay left at the next fork, where the 5A heads across the valley back to Trail 1. Walk around the southern shoulder of the eastern peak and into the bowl area under the lee of the ridge, staying with the contour. The terrain of limestone, cedar, grass, and cactus will be familiar by now. At 4.6 miles turn right and descend sharply to Park Road, a few yards beyond the parking area at the Equestrian Campground. When you are almost at the end, a spur leaves to the right, heading for the campground. The last few yards of the trail from here to the road are ill-defined, but the end is clearly visible ahead.

## Nearby Activities

Some of the local ranches offer horse rides in the park, an iconic way to explore the old frontier territory.

---

**GPS TRAILHEAD COORDINATES**

**N29° 38' 3.2"  W99° 11' 2.8"**

From San Antonio, take TX 16 to Bandera. In Bandera, turn left on TX 173 south, following it 1 mile to Farm Route 1077. Turn right onto FR 1077, and follow it 10 miles to the park, where the road turns to dirt. Turn right in the park, across West Verde Creek, and then again into the headquarters area. Once you have your permit, continue to the trailhead, 0.5 mile farther up Park Road.

---

# Appendix A
## HIKING STORES

## Austin

**Backwoods**
12821 Hill Country Blvd.,
Ste. C2-110, Bee Cave, TX 78738
512-263-3610
backwoods.com/austin
Quality outdoor gear and apparel

**Cabela's**
15570 IH-35, Buda, TX 78610
512-295-1100
cabelas.com
A huge inventory of hunting and
outdoor gear

**Gossamer Gear**
3512-B Montopolis Drive,
Austin, TX 78744
512-374-0133
gossamergear.com
This company, headquartered
in Austin, makes ultralight
backpacking and hiking gear.

**Patagonia Austin**
316 Congress Ave.,
Austin, TX 78701
512-320-8383
patagonia.com
Boutique, high-quality outdoor gear

**REI**
9901 N. Capitol of Texas Highway,
Ste. 200, Austin, TX 78759
512-343-5550

601 N. Lamar Blvd.,
Austin, TX 78703
512-482-3357
rei.com
Popular chain carries gear for
most outdoor activities

**Whole Earth Provision Co.**
1014 N. Lamar Blvd., Austin, TX 78703
512-476-1414

2410 San Antonio St.,
Austin, TX 78705
512-478-1577
wholeearthprovision.com
Austin-grown outdoor and fashion
retailer

## San Antonio

**Bass Pro Shops**
17907 IH-10 W, San Antonio, TX 78257
210-253-8800
basspro.com
Popular chain with everything you
might need for the outdoors, including
hunting and fishing gear

**Gander Mountain**
8203 TX 151, Ste. 104,
San Antonio, TX 78245
210-202-2822
gandermountain.com
Chain with a range of outdoor
and hunting equipment

**Good Sports Outlet**

5039 Beckwith Blvd., Ste. 102,
San Antonio, TX 78249
210-694-0881
goodsports.com
Sporting goods outlet store

**MoonTrail**

722 W. Craig Place,
San Antonio, TX 78212
210-682-9881
A full range of backpacking
and hiking gear

**National Outdoors & Army Surplus**

5600 Bandera Road,
San Antonio, TX 78238
210-680-3322
Mostly military surplus

**REI**

11745 IH-10 W, Ste. 110,
San Antonio, TX 78230
210-877-2329
rei.com
Popular chain with gear for
most outdoor activities

**Whole Earth Provision Co.**

255 E. Basse Road,
San Antonio, TX 78209
210-829-8888
wholeearthprovision.com
Toys and knickknacks as well as
outdoor gear

# Appendix B
## HIKING CLUBS

## Austin

**Meetup (meetup.com) has many hiking groups in Austin.**

> meetup.com/topics/hiking/us/tx/austin
> Below are a few of the most active.

**Austin "Crack Of Dawn" Hiking Meetup Group**

> meetup.com/hiking-586

**Austin Hiking Group**

> meetup.com/austin-hikers

**Austin Sierra Club Outings**

> meetup.com/austin-sierra-club-outings

**Outside in Texas**

> meetup.com/outsideintexas

**Also try:**
**Hill Country Outdoors**

> hillcountryoutdoors.com

## San Antonio

**Meetup (meetup.com) has many hiking groups in San Antonio.**

> meetup.com/topics/hiking/us/tx/san+antonio
> Below are a few of the most active.

**Alamo Sierra Club Outings & Events**

> meetup.com/alamo-sierra-club-outings

**The San Antonio Hiking & Outdoors Meetup Group**

> meetup.com/saoutdoors

**San Antonio Hill Country Hikers**

> meetup.com/sanantoniohillcountryhikers

**San Antonio Outdoor Adventurers**

> meetup.com/sa-outdoor-adventurers

**Also try:**
**Adventure Club San Antonio**

> adventureclubsa.com or meetup.com/adventureclubsa

# Appendix C
## WHERE TO FIND MAPS AND MORE

### Overview

National Geographic sells a map of the Texas Hill Country, available at Amazon.
amazon.com/texas-country-national-geographic-destination/dp/1597755168

### State Parks

Find Texas state park maps at the parks and online at tpwd.texas.gov.
It's a good idea to download maps and plan your route before you go.

### GPS Devices

Garmin device owners can buy very detailed maps online.
garmin.com/en-US/maps/outdoor

### Apps

MotionX-GPS is great for GPS navigation. (iOS)
AllTrails has over 50,000 trails. (iOS and Android)
MapMyHike gives detailed feedback on hike duration, distance, pace, speed, elevation, calories burned, route traveled, and more. (iOS and Android)
iBird is a comprehensive guide to birds of North America. (iOS and Android)

# Index

# About the Authors

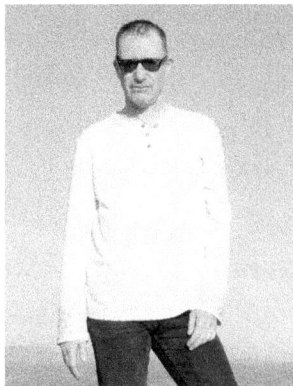

CHARLIE LLEWELLIN moved to Austin in 1991 and soon started exploring the state's varied landscapes, from woods to desert and from the prairies to the coast. A writer and photographer, he now lives in Blanco and continues to wander the Hill Country and beyond.

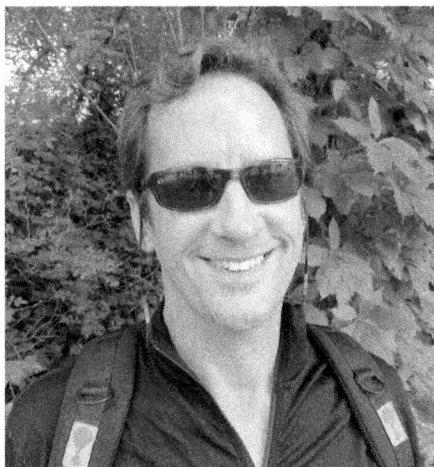

JOHNNY MOLLOY is an outdoor writer based in Johnson City, Tennessee. Born in Memphis, he moved to Knoxville in 1980 to attend the University of Tennessee (UT). During his college years, he developed a love of the natural world that has since become the primary focus of his life. After graduating from UT with a degree in economics, Johnny spent an ever-increasing amount of time in the wild, becoming more skilled in a variety of environments. Friends enjoyed his adventure stories; one even suggested that he write a book. He pursued that idea and soon parlayed his love of the outdoors into an occupation. The results of his efforts are more than 30 books. These include hiking, camping, paddling, and other comprehensive guidebooks, as well as books on true outdoor adventures. Johnny has also written for numerous publications and websites. He continues to write and travel extensively to all four corners of the United States, exploring a variety of outdoor activities. For the latest on Johnny, please visit johnnymolloy.com.

**DEAR CUSTOMERS AND FRIENDS,**

**SUPPORTING YOUR INTEREST IN OUTDOOR ADVENTURE,** travel, and an active lifestyle is central to our operations, from the authors we choose to the locations we detail to the way we design our books. Menasha Ridge Press was incorporated in 1982 by a group of veteran outdoorsmen and professional outfitters. For many years now, we've specialized in creating books that benefit the outdoors enthusiast.

Almost immediately, Menasha Ridge Press earned a reputation for revolutionizing outdoors- and travel-guidebook publishing. For such activities as canoeing, kayaking, hiking, backpacking, and mountain biking, we established new standards of quality that transformed the whole genre, resulting in outdoor-recreation guides of great sophistication and solid content. Menasha Ridge Press continues to be outdoor publishing's greatest innovator.

The folks at Menasha Ridge Press are as at home on a whitewater river or mountain trail as they are editing a manuscript. The books we build for you are the best they can be, because we're responding to your needs. Plus, we use and depend on them ourselves.

We look forward to seeing you on the river or the trail. If you'd like to contact us directly, visit us at menasharidge.com. We thank you for your interest in our books and the natural world around us all.

**SAFE TRAVELS,**

*Bob Sehlinger*

**BOB SEHLINGER
PUBLISHER**

www.ingramcontent.com/pod-product-compliance
Lightning Source LLC
Chambersburg PA
CBHW051905090426
42811CB00003B/472